Health for Pilots

Health for Pilots

A Complete Guide to FAA Medical Certification and Self-Care

PAUL M. GAHLINGER, M.D., PH.D.

sagebrush PRESS

Distributed by the Independent Publishers Group

Health for Pilots is directed to the 650,000 pilots and air traffic controllers in the United States, and those overseas under American licenses, who need to stay healthy to fly safely. This book will benefit everyone interested in aviation—from the flying student and weekend pilot to the airline captain, flight manager and air traffic controller.

How is it possible to refer to all these individuals? The FAA uses the term airman, but that seems a bit old-fashioned and ignores the increasing number of aviators who are women. For convenience, I use the term *pilot* for everyone—even though this book is useful to many who have other roles in aviation.

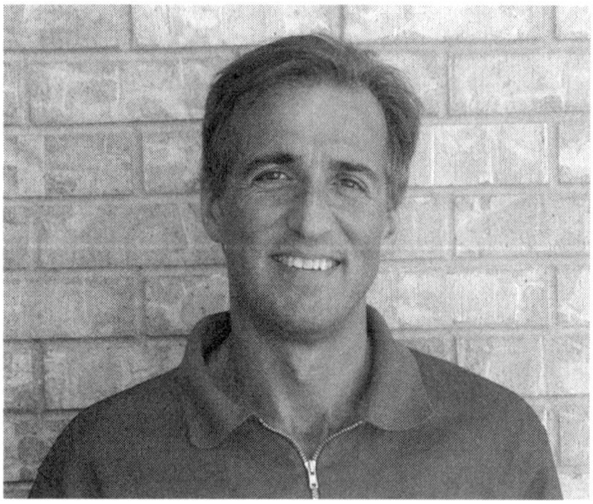

ABOUT THE AUTHOR:

Paul M. Gahlinger, M.D., Ph.D., M.P.H., FACOEM, is Adjunct Professor in the Department of Family and Preventive Medicine, University of Utah, Salt Lake City, and a Senior Aviation Medical Examiner at the Kaysville Clinic. His research interests have taken him from Antarctica to NASA at the Kennedy Space Center, where he studied motion sickness and continues to serve as a consultant on space science research. He is the author of *The Cockpit: A Flight of Escape and Discovery*, *Northern Manitoba from Forest to Tundra*, *Computer Programs for Epidemiologists*, and *Illegal Drugs: A Complete Guide to Their History, Chemistry, Use and Abuse*. He is a commercial and multi-engine instrument-rated pilot.

to my teachers

the flight instructors
who taught responsibility
and
the medical professors
who taught compassion

Printed in the U.S.

Library of Congress Cataloging-in-Publication Data

Gahlinger, Paul M.
Health for pilots : a complete guide to FAA medical certification and self-care / Paul M. Gahlinger.
p. cm.
Includes bibliographical references and index.
ISBN 0-9703130-3-9
1. Air pilots—Health and hygiene. 2. Air pilots—Medical examinations. I. Title.
RC1062 .G345 2002
616'.0088'6291—dc21
2002000547

The purpose of this book is to provide health information for pilots. This information is descriptive only and is not intended to be, and nor should it be considered, a substitute for competent medical care, counseling, flight training, or legal advice. While every attempt has been made to ensure accuracy, some errors may persist. The author and publisher assume no responsibility whatsoever for any use the reader may make of the information provided herein.

Sagebrush Press
Salt Lake City, Utah
www.sagebrushpress.com

Distributed by the Independent Publishers Group
www.ipgbook.com

CONTENTS

Introduction Fit for Flight **1**
Why is there a special aviation medical exam? 1
Aviation safety yesterday and today 3
Is flying dangerous? 6
Why do accidents occur? 7

Chapter 1 How Can I Pass the FAA Medical Exam? **11**
The aviation medical examination 11
Family doctor vs AME 11
Appropriate medical certificate 13
Combination medical certificate and student pilot certificate 14
Three classes of medical certification 15
Medical certificate duration 16
Physical requirements 16
Age 16
Height and weight 18
Visual acuity 18
Color vision 19
Hearing 19
Ear, nose, throat 19
Blood pressure 19
Electrocardiogram (ECG) 20
Mental status 20
Disqualifying conditions 20
If you don't meet the requirements 21
Special Issuance Authorization 22
Statement of Demonstrated Ability (SODA) 23
Appealing a denial 23
Disabled pilots 24
Preparing for the medical exam 24
Finding an Aviation Medical Examiner 24
Choosing an AME: what to look for 25
Preparing for the exam 26
If you have a health problem 27
What to bring for the exam 28
Application for Airman Medical Certificate (FAA form 8500-8) 29
Allowable medications 37
FAA-accepted medications 40
Medical status changes after certificate is issued 47
Getting caught flying without a medical certificate 47
Medical certificate replacement 47

Chapter 2 Conditions That *May* Disqualify You **49**
A. Frequent or severe headaches 49
Migraine headaches 49
Cluster headaches 50
B. Dizziness or fainting spell 50
Fainting 51

C. Unconsciousness for any reason 51
Head injury 53
D. Eye or vision trouble 53
Visual acuity requirements 55
Eyeglasses and contacts 57
Sunglasses 58
Glare 59
Night vision 59
Color vision 60
Macular degeneration 63
Eye surgery 63
Glaucoma 67
One-eyed pilots 68
E. Hay fever or allergy 68
Decongestants 69
Antihistamines 69
Hives 70
Earwax 70
F. Asthma or lung disease 71
Asthma 71
Chronic bronchitis and emphysema 72
Pneumothorax 73
G. Heart or vascular trouble 73
High cholesterol 73
Heart disease 75
Irregular heart beat (arrhythmias) 78
Bundle Branch Block 80
Cardiomyopathy 80
Pacemaker 81
Heart valve replacement 82
Deep vein thrombosis 83
Raynaud's disease 85
Automatic external defibrillators 86
H. High or low blood pressure 87
Hypertension 87
Blood pressure medications 90
Low blood pressure 91
I. Stomach, liver, or intestinal trouble 91
Ulcers 92
Intestinal disease 93
Medications 94
Passengers 94
J. Kidney stone or blood in urine 94
Kidney stones 94
Kidney transplant 96
K. Diabetes 96
Oral medication only 98
Insulin 99
L. Neurological disorders 102
Loss of consciousness 103
Migraine and other headaches 103

Epilepsy 103
Stroke 104
M. Mental disorders 105
Depression 106
Bipolar disorder 109
Anxiety 109
Attention Deficit Hyperactivity Disorder 110
Personality disorder 112
Psychosis 113
Psychiatric and psychological evaluation 113
N. Substance dependence or abuse 114
Drug conviction 116
Transporting intoxicated passengers or drugs 116
O. Alcohol dependence or abuse 116
Alcoholism 118
Alcohol and pilots 119
How to get a medical certificate after recovery 121
P. Suicide attempt 123
Q. Motion sickness requiring medication 123
Simulator sickness 125
Motion sickness medications 125
How to prevent airsickness without medication 127
Flicker vertigo 129
R. Military medical discharge 129
S. Medical rejection for military service 130
T. Rejection for life or health insurance 130
U. Admission to hospital 130
V. History of traffic conviction 131
W. History of non-traffic conviction 134
X. Other illness, disability, or surgery 134
How sick do you need to be? 135
Surgery 135
Arthritis, muscle, or skeletal problems 135
Sleep disorders 136
Cancer 137
HIV 139
Amputations or paralysis 140

Chapter 3 Getting a SODA 141

What does it mean to be disqualified? 141
Special issuance authorization 142
Status reports 145
Withdrawal of special issuance 145
Denials and appeals 146
Statement of demonstrated ability 147
Functional limitations 147
Old SODAs 147
Impairments and disabilities 148
Disabled pilots (Capt. Sheri Coin Marshall) 149

Chapter 4	**Flying High: Drug-Testing Programs**	**153**
	The long, strange history of drug abuse	153
	Drug use and aircraft accidents	154
	Federal regulations: the NIDA 5	156
	Americans with Disabilities Act	157
	Drug surveillance programs	158
	How are people tested for drugs?	159
	Chain of custody	161
	Tampered specimens	161
	The "shy bladder" excuse	162
	Laboratory analysis	162
	Screening tests	163
	Confirmation tests	163
	Can drug tests be fooled?	163
	Adulteration products	164
	Diluted urine	165
	Legal medications that can cause positive drug tests	167
	What happens when a drug test is positive?	169
Chapter 5	**Cleared for Flight**	**171**
	Taking care of yourself	171
	Back pain	171
	Dehydration	173
	Skin care	174
	Stress	175
	How to reduce stress if you are a member of a crew	176
	How to reduce stress if you are the leader of a crew	176
	Vaccines	177
	Weight and balance	178
	Diets	179
	Exercise	181
	Cholesterol	182
	Vitamins and supplements	183
	Hearing loss	184
	Hearing requirements	187
	Hearing protection	189
	Hearing aids	190
	Ear block	190
	Sinus block	191
	Teeth pressure (barodontalgia)	192
	Vibration exposure	192
	Smoking	192
	The real poison—carbon monoxide	193
	How to quit	194
	Using oxygen	194
	From sea level to outer space	194
	Altitude and hypoxia	196
	Stages of hypoxia	198
	Rapid decompression	200
	Altitude chamber	201

Sickle cell anemia 203
Hyperventilation 204
Using oxygen 204
SCUBA diving 206
Depressurization and the bends 206
Flying after diving 207
Undersea and Hyperbaric Medical Society recommendations 208
High altitude and Nitrox diving 208
Recompression chambers 209
Women's health 209
Oral contraceptives 210
Menstrual discomfort 210
Pregnancy 211
Sleep and fatigue 211
Stages of sleep 212
Snoring 213
Sleep apnea 214
Fatigue 215
FAA regulations for flight time and rest schedules 216
Jet lag 217
Sleep hygiene 218
Sleeping pills 219

Chapter 6 Military Pilots (Col. Christopher Kleinsmith, USAF) 221
Military medical requirements 221
Air force 222
Army 222
Mental health 223
Critical Incident Stress Management (CISM) 224
Substance abuse 225
Allowable medications 226

Appendix I Further Information 231
FAA addresses 231
Pilot resources 232
Regional flight surgeons 233

Appendix II FAR: Medical Standards and Certification 235

Notes and References 250

Acknowledgments 256

Index 257

INTRODUCTION

Fit for Flight

Why is there a special aviation medical exam?

For just about everyone who begins the long road to becoming a pilot, one of the first questions is: "Can I pass the medical test?" They ask, "Is my eyesight good enough?" "What about my medications?" "My doctor said I had a heart murmur—is that allowed?" "I had epilepsy as a child, and just assumed I'd never be allowed to fly." And so on. There is no question that the health requirements for pilots *are* strict, but the intention of this book is to make it clear that almost everyone can pass the medical examination. Certain additional tests may be required, and perhaps there will be restrictions on flight, but if you follow the directions detailed here, there is every chance you will get your certificate.

The aviation medical examination is seen not only as a barrier to learning how to fly, but often as a threat to existing pilots, whether they fly for personal or professional reasons. It can be unnerving to know that your hobby, or even your career, is on the line with every visit to the doctor. A look at the advertisements in *Trade-A-Plane* tells a sadly common story: 1980 BONANZA A36TC, BEAUTIFULLY KEPT, LOW PRICE ... OWNER LOST MEDICAL. Who knows what could have been done if this pilot had had the help of a good aviation medical examiner?

The requirement for such a rigorous aviation medical has often been questioned. Certainly, there are medical examinations for operators of other types of heavy equipment—trucks and ships and nuclear reactors, for example. Even for a basic driver's license there are visual requirements, and it is technically illegal to drive or operate a boat while "impaired" (by illness, medications or drugs). But these exams are far less detailed than the flight physical. They also occur less often, and any physician can do them.

Flying is different. It is the only general activity that requires a specific, stringent, and recurrent medical examination, which must be carried out by an FAA-certified physician. Once you get a driver's license, it is pretty much up to you to make sure you are fit to drive. To drive an airplane, on the other hand, you need a special medical examination at least every three years, and as often as every six months if you fly professionally.

The reason for the exam is simple: Safety. Air travel has become much less hazardous over the years. Nowadays, the most dangerous part of a flight is the drive to or from the airport. But although almost a century has passed since the first powered aircraft, there is still something a little unnerving about flying. People who feel completely relaxed in an express train going 130 miles per hour feel a twinge of anxiety every time they get on an airplane and the wheels leave the ground. One of the ways to minimize this anxiety is to make sure that whoever is operating the aircraft is fit to do so.

Over 70 percent of aviation accidents are at least partly due to "human factors"—in other words, there was something wrong with the pilot or crew.

Pilots tend to be somewhat healthier than the average person, but not much. Most pilots would never consider treating their aircraft as badly as they treat their own bodies. Any aircraft owner will tell you that an airplane must be inspected routinely (at least annually or every 100 hours of flight), all problems corrected immediately, and the airplane should be flown frequently, at least once per week. Now ask that airplane owner how often he or she has a routine medical exam, whether all problems are corrected immediately, and if he or she exercises at least once a week—and you might get a different answer!

The purpose of the aviation medical exam is to help screen out any obvious deficiencies and, hopefully, to encourage the pilot to maintain good health. Would you go to a mechanic who just glances at your airplane and signs off on your annual inspection? Probably not. Would you prefer a mechanic who not only checked the required maintenance, but also advised you on how to prevent future problems and get the very best performance out of your aircraft? Definitely. Even so, many pilots pay little attention to their own health and try to get through their aviation physical as quickly as possible.

I learned about medicals from that...
Fresh out of medical school, I worked for a while as a rural physician in the Hawaiian Islands, and bought a part-ownership in a Piper Warrior. In fact, I still own the airplane. I would like to fly it, except that it is 8 miles off Diamond Head, about 2,000 feet below sea level, resting on the bottom of the Pacific Ocean. The last flight was by the other owner, who did not survive the accident. I learned later that he had falsified his medical. Therefore, insurance payment was denied.

Good health plays a vital role in a safe and legal flight. It is the purpose of this book not only to help you pass your medical examination, but to take good care of yourself.

Aviation safety yesterday and today

The effects of flying on health have been known for a long time, and were suspected even before the first flight took place. By the time of the Wright brothers, a number of adventurous individuals were already familiar with motion sickness and the problems of high altitude: low temperatures, lack of oxygen, and pressure changes. With the beginning of powered flight in 1903, it did not take long for accidents to follow. The first fatal aviation accident victim was First Lieutenant Thomas Selfridge of the United States Army Signal Corps. While flying with Orville Wright on September 17, 1908, at Fort Myer, Virginia, a crack developed in the starboard propeller and the Wright Flyer crashed. Orville survived, but Selfridge died from a skull fracture. The following investigation recommended that aviators wear some sort of head protection.

The high risks associated with flying prompted concern about pilots' fitness. Germany was the first to develop minimum medical standards for aviators, in 1910. In 1912, the United States War Department published its first instructions on the physical examination of candidates for aviation duty. It included requirements such as good visual and hearing acuity. There was also an instruction for the examiner to: "Have the candidate hop around the room … first with the eyes open and then closed, on both feet and then on one foot, and hopping forward and backward." The need for this ability is not clear, given the tight open cockpits of those days, but a similar activity can be observed on today's airliners among people waiting for the restroom.

During the First World War, Great Britain reviewed aviation casualties and discovered that 60 percent of deaths were due not to

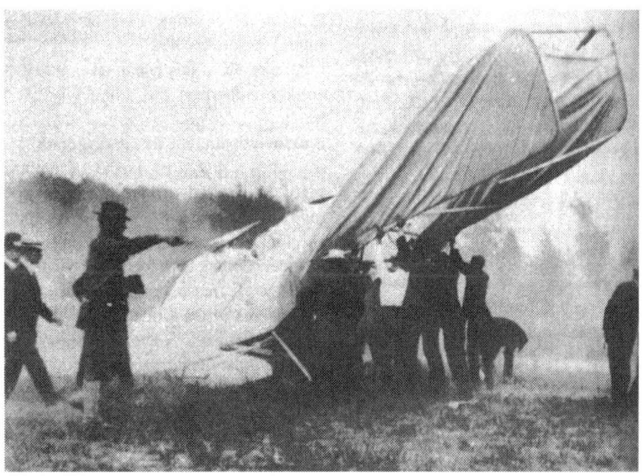

Wright Flyer crash

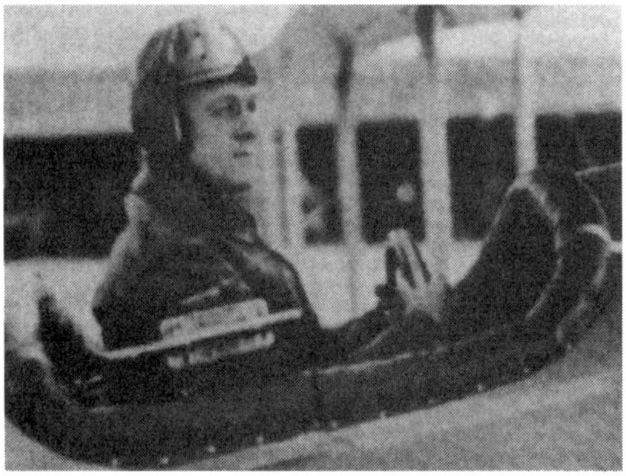

Army pilot Benjamin Foulois wearing his own football helmet for head protection

the enemy or defects in the airplane, but to physical defects of the aviators. The military developed tests to screen out deficient pilots, such as a "needle test:" the blind-folded candidate was told to hold the pointy ends of a needle between his thumb and forefinger, and then a pistol was fired unexpectedly behind him. If he punctured his finger with the sudden noise, he was disqualified because of "excessive excitability." Hearing impairment, evidently, was not as great a concern.

It was not long before the Royal Air Force learned that judgment was more important than physical qualities. The RAF medical officer reported:

> "Every now and then one meets the type with splendid physique and apparently unshakeable courage and finds that he learns to fly indifferently or is unable to learn at all, and again one meets the weedy, pale type learning quickly to fly and turning out to be a first-rate pilot."

Indeed, some of the greatest pilots were those who would have failed a modern medical test. One of Britain's air aces, Edward Mannock, had severe astigmatism and was essentially blind in one eye. The French pilot Guynemer had pulmonary tuberculosis. Oswald Boelcke of Germany had severe asthma. Frank Luke, the American ace, would have failed a psychiatric examination due to his moodiness and antisocial behavior.

By the 1920s, aircraft were becoming commonplace and accidents continued to increase. Crashes in the United States were occurring at the rate of one for every 241 flying hours, and a death every 721 hours.

In 1926, President Calvin Coolidge signed the Air Commerce Act, giving responsibility for civil aviation to the Department of Commerce, and recommending a physical examination as part of the requirement for the pilot license. The first medical standard for pilots was published on December 31, 1926. It specified three classes of physical requirements: private pilot, industrial pilot, and transport pilot. This framework still exists today.

Was the Red Baron medically fit to fly?

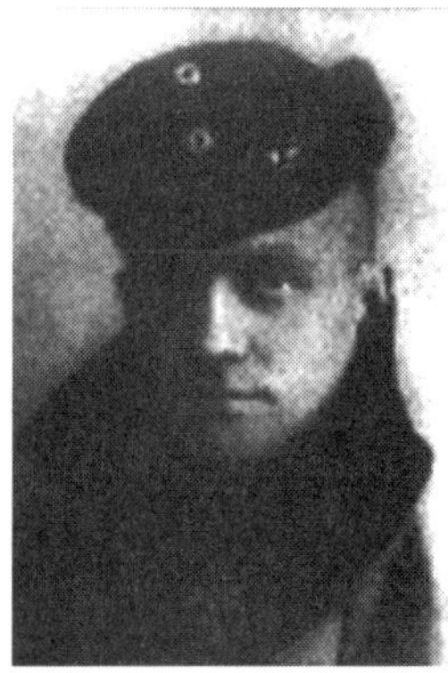

Manfred Freiherr von Richthofen entered the military cadet corps in 1903, at age ten. By 1911 he was serving in the trenches and then as a cavalry officer, rising to the rank of Captain. Four years later he was accepted into the newly established flying force. His success was almost immediate and he thrilled in combat, taunting the enemy by painting his triplane a scarlet red. Among the French, he was known as the "Red Devil." The British, in humor and in grudging respect, called him the "Red Baron." By July 6, 1917, he was credited with bringing down 57 enemy planes. That day, he was shot in the head during aerial combat and left totally blind and paralyzed, regaining just enough sight and strength to make a rough landing, after which he staggered from the aircraft and collapsed. He spent the next 20 days in a hospital, with a large open head wound that exposed sections of his skull. Meanwhile, the tide of war turned and his men suffered increasing losses. He was determined to go back to help them. With his head bandaged to hide the still-open wound, he snuck out of the hospital and took to the skies again on August 18, 1917, achieving his 58th aerial victory. Back on the ground, he felt sick and the surgeons removed another piece of bone from his skull. Each subsequent flight left him feeling worse. He became depressed, staying in his room between flights and refusing to see or speak to anyone. By the end of January 1918, his mother worried that her son had become distant, moody, and almost unapproachable. The Kaiser offered him a high-level desk job, but he refused to leave his squadron and continued to 80 victories. On April 21, 1918, his luck ran out. He was shot dead, probably from the ground, on a routine patrol flight. He was 25 years old.

"Success flourishes only in perseverance — ceaseless, restless perseverance." —*Manfred von Richthofen*

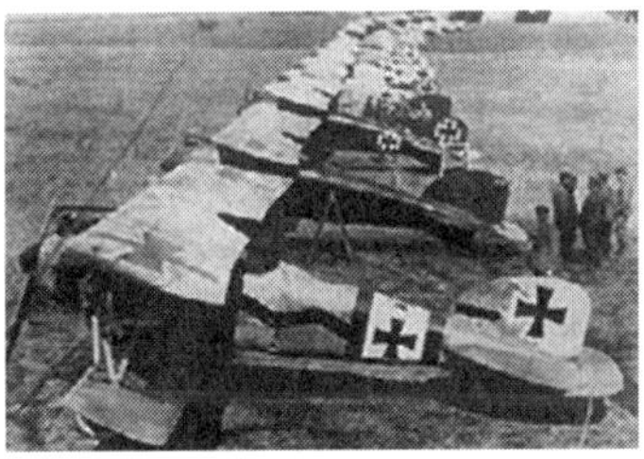

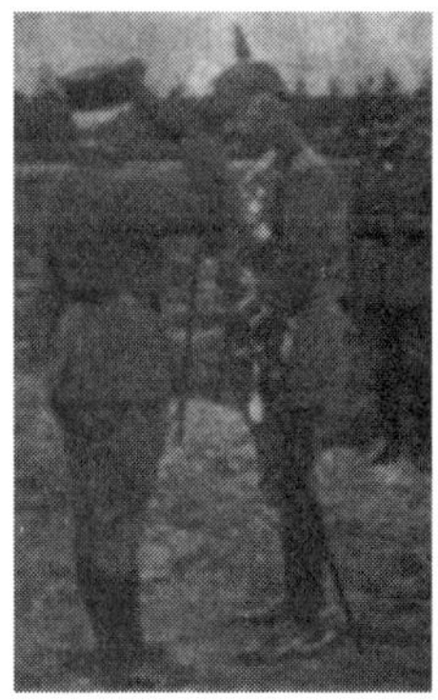

In headwound dressing, saluting the Kaiser

"If I should come out of this war alive, I will have more luck than brains."

The number of pilots grew rapidly, as did the number of aviation physicians and the study of aerospace medicine. In 1958 the FAA Act created the Office of Aviation Medicine to keep up with medical technology. The foremost concern was safety—specifically, the risk of pilot incapacitation. The regulations were not designed to evaluate overall health, although advice might be offered, but simply to reduce the risk of sudden incapacitation of the pilot.

In the 1920s, the French Breguet mail planes used in the Western Sahara were equipped with carrier pigeons to be released in the event of a crash.

The current airman medical standards are minimum requirements. There is no practical way for all possible medical conditions to be addressed in a regulation. The standards are necessarily quite general, and they are subject to interpretation by the FAA doctors who make the decisions. Although there are basic requirements for an applicant to hold a medical certificate, each case is ultimately evaluated on an individual basis.

Is flying dangerous?

In a 1972 decision, the U.S. Supreme Court said that "safe is not the equivalent of risk free." The only way to eliminate risk from any particular activity is to completely avoid it. Therefore, some risk must be considered acceptable. Over one billion passengers are carried on scheduled air services each year and therefore even a tiny risk can translate into a frighteningly large number of fatalities.

Aviation is a vast enterprise in the United States: there are about 650,000 active pilots, 170,000 active general aviation aircraft, and 18,700 air carrier aircraft. The country has 18,200 airports, and the FAA operates 476 control towers. It is by far the greatest, most efficient, and most user-friendly air travel system in the world. Pilots from every country like to train in the United States.

According to the National Transport Safety Board (NTSB) year 2000 statistics, there were 5.96 accidents and 1.11 fatalities for every 100,000 hours flown. This was an all-time low. The numbers showed 1,835 general aviation accidents (with 341 fatalities), the fewest since record keeping began in 1938, even though the number of flights and flight hours has dramatically increased.

Despite the statistically low number of aircraft accidents, compared with other types of travel, the risks associated with flying engender disproportionately high fear among the public. In fact, most accidents are relatively minor and do not involve serious injury. A study of 1,086 accidents with 34,369 occupants found that:

- There were no serious injuries in 82 percent of the accidents.

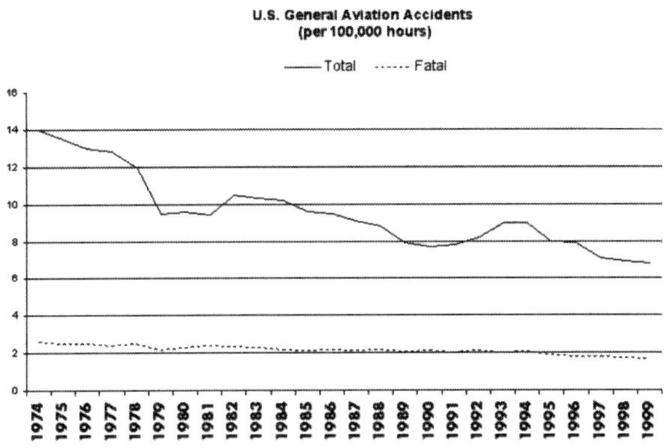

Your odds of dying from...

Heart disease	1 in 388
Cancer	1 in 499
Stroke	1 in 1,658
Diabetes	1 in 4,009
Flu or pneumonia	1 in 4,107
Motor vehicle accident	1 in 6,585
Gun shot	1 in 8,802
Bad medical care	1 in 83,720
Railway accident	1 in 524,753
Airplane crash	1 in 659,779

- More than 50 percent of serious injuries occurred in less than 1 percent of crashes.
- In 95 percent of crashes, less than 25 percent of the occupants were seriously injured.

Aviation therefore seems to be one of the safest modes of transport, and each year brings a further reduction in the accident rate.

Why do accidents occur?

An "accident" is defined as an unforeseen or unplanned event. (The U.S. Armed Forces prefer the term "mishap.") A study by Boeing found that most accidents result from a sequence of events rather than a single, catastrophic event. Their research team identified as many as 20 events in a flight that led to the eventual accident. The chain of events often begins with a fatigued or distracted crew, or poor crew communications, which is followed by a combination of other factors—weather, mechanical issues, etc.—to result in the accident. Each factor decreases tolerance for the others. In 76 percent of all accidents, and 82 percent of fatal accidents, the primary cause was considered to be the pilot. Operating an aircraft involves six basic kinds of activity. In rough order of importance, these are:

1. Flight path control
2. Vigilance to avoid other aircraft or obstacles
3. Communication
4. Navigation
5. Aircraft systems operation
6. Ancillary housekeeping tasks

Each of these requires pilot alertness and judgment, which are impaired by illness or medications. Accidents are more common, and much more likely to be fatal, during instrument conditions and at night. This is because the margin of error is much lower, and the pilot is more likely to be fatigued.

Suicides and aviation terrorism

As this book was being written, I did an FAA medical examination on one of the flight instructors of the 9/11 terrorists. His feelings of guilt were only partly relieved by the fact that he was in no way responsible for the disaster. In retrospect, yes, there were a few clues and even some warnings, but it is impossible to anticipate every outcome.

A founding principle of the United States is the freedom to pursue individual goals. This freedom has led to unparalleled opportunities, and attracts people from around the world to achieve their dreams. In other countries, flight training is a privilege restricted to the rich and the favored few. In the U.S., it is open to everyone, including foreign visitors. All freedoms come at a cost. It is our choice to keep open the privilege to fly, even though some might abuse it.

Strictly speaking, a suicidal aircraft crash is not an accident and is not used in accident rate calculations by the National Transportation Safety Board. Pilot suicides have been rare in the past. Because of new requirements stemming from the events on Sept 11, 2001, they are likely to become even more rare in the future.

About 90 percent of all fatal accidents are now followed by some sort of medical investigation of the pilot. These investigations have discovered the following major causes:

40%	Flying into weather beyond the pilot's abilities
30%	Inappropriate low-level maneuvers
15%	Pilot using alcohol or drugs
15%	Other causes, such as carbon monoxide poisoning, heart attacks, kidney stones, etc.

It is clear from these statistics that the great majority (85%) are due to deficient pilot judgment. Most of the others are due to medical problems that might have been avoided. However, these two conditions—judgment and illness—are usually given much less attention than mechanical concerns.

"Alas, many training programs teach only aircraft systems. Yet a systems failure is statistically rare as the cause of an aircraft accident."—*Professional Pilot*

Despite good health and adequate rest, it is possible for pilots to encounter health-related problems during flight. Even relatively brief or minor conditions can result in temporary loss of control of the aircraft.

Surveys of professional pilots found that they were sometimes affected by the following symptoms to the point of incapacitation:

Headache	Coughing attack
Faintness	Nausea
Eye injury	Vomiting
Earache	Severe indigestion
Toothache	Uncontrolled bowel action
Nosebleed	Leg or foot cramps
Sneezing attack	

It is impossible to avoid all such incidents, but it is important to prepare for them by keeping as fit as possible. One such method is the "I'M SAFE" checklist:

Illness:	Do I have any symptoms?
Medication:	Have I been taking anything that might affect my alertness?
Safe:	Am I stressed about anything? Can I focus on the flight?
Alcohol:	Have I had anything to drink in the last 24 hours?
Fatigue:	Am I tired? Did I get enough sleep?
Eating:	Have I eaten properly?

Safe flight depends on three factors: the equipment, the environment, and the operator. Of these three, the health of the pilot has repeatedly been shown to be the most frequent and most critical factor. The other two may be considered out of the control of the pilot, but this is an illusion. The proper maintenance and inspection of the aircraft are the responsibility of the pilot, as is the decision whether to fly given the weather conditions. Ultimately, it all comes down to the person sitting in the cockpit. A healthy, well-rested, and comfortable pilot is the key to a safe flight.

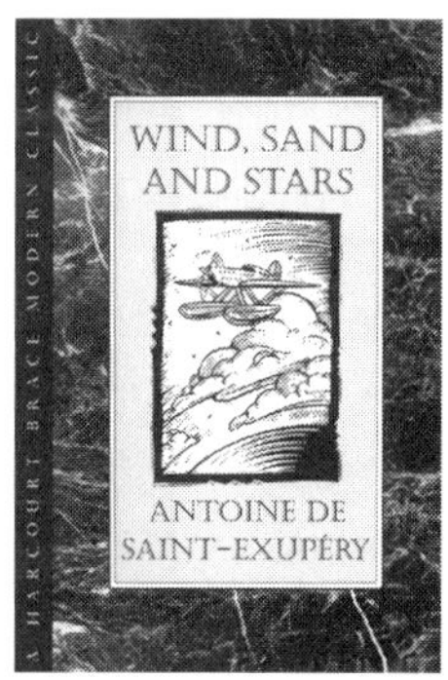

Antoine de Saint-Exupery was a courageous pilot and perhaps the greatest aviation writer of all time. He was also a notorious hypochondriac who treated his body like an untrustworthy machine, or even an enemy.

Some useful aviation terms for student pilots

Alternate airport	The area directly beyond the active runway when the engine quits on take-off.
Altimeter setting	The place where the altimeter sets. Usually hidden by the control column during a near-minimums instrument approach.
Bank	The folks who hold the mortgage on your aircraft.
Bi-plane	What you'll say to your bird if flying costs keep going up.
Carburetor ice	Phrase used by pilots when explaining accident caused by fuel exhaustion.
"Clear"	Warning shouted two seconds after hitting the starter button.
Control tower	A small shack on stilts inhabited by government pensioners who can't hear. When they become blind, they are sent to centers.
Critical altitude	Minus six feet.
Critical engine	The part of your airplane that used to be under the cowl, but is now in intensive care at the maintenance shop.
De-icer	A device designed to operate under all weather conditions, except icing.
Gliding distance	One-half of the distance from your present position to the nearest decent landing area at the time of complete power failure.
Gross weight	Maximum permissible take-off weight, plus an extra suitcase, a case of bourbon, rifle, ammo, golf bag, bowling ball, and diving weights.
Range	Five miles beyond the point where all fuel tanks have become filled with air.

1

How Can I Pass the FAA Medical Exam?

The aviation medical examination

The FAA is responsible for the licensing and medical certification of approximately 650,000 pilots in the United States, and in 93 other countries that have pilots with American licenses. Almost all FAA medical examinations are conducted by specially certified physicians in private practice. There are about 5,700 Aviation Medical Examiners (AME) in the U.S., and a few who practice in other countries.

Each year, the FAA processes almost a half-million applications for airman medical certification—an average of 10,000 per week.

FAMILY DOCTOR VS AME

Your personal physician may be an AME. However, the roles of a treating physician and an AME are very different. The job of your doctor is take care of you (or, more correctly, to help you take care of yourself). In order to get the best treatment, you should confide in your doctor and mention concerns about any aspect of your health. Your AME, on the other hand, is acting as a representative of the FAA. The AME's job is to screen out applicants with medical conditions that might impair performance as a pilot—not to treat you. Your personal doctor should optimize your health, while the AME is there only to detect any significant illness or handicap. For example, while an AME will issue you a certificate if your blood pressure is up to 155/95, your personal physician should be very concerned if your blood pressure is that high and should take urgent steps to reduce it.

Naturally, many pilots view the AME as a threat to their license, and they may be less than forthcoming about their health problems. If their personal doctor is the AME, this puts them at a conflict between wanting to share their personal health concerns while trying to look as healthy as possible.

An AME who is also your personal physician may feel he or she is in an awkward position. The doctor knows how important it is to you to fly, but is obligated to disqualify you if any information is discovered that is a safety hazard.

Pilot to family doctor: "Doc, I don't know what's the matter. I've just been feeling tired all the time. Run down. Can you help me?"

Pilot to AME: "No problems, sir. A bit tired now and then, understandable given my job and family. But really, I feel great!"

On the other hand, having a personal physician who is your AME can be quite efficient, and may be better for both your general health and aviation safety. The sort of medical concerns that someone might confide to a personal doctor, but hesitate to tell an AME, are generally things that will be approved anyway, although it might take an extra bit of paperwork. Doing so might be inconvenient but it can save a lot of trouble later on. For example, if you feel fine during your medical exam but know that you have attacks of hay fever at certain times of year, you should tell your AME. The AME will make a notation on your medical certificate limiting flight when you have symptoms or are using medication. Problem solved.

If you have a medical condition that your regular physician knows about and you did not confide this to your AME, you may be liable for falsifying your medical examination—which can cause a lot of problems besides safety. For this reason, the military not only prefers having your personal doctor be your AME, but insists on it: the military flight surgeon plays both these roles to military pilots, and is part of the team, ensuring pilots' health as well as certifying their medical condition (see *Chapter 6: Military Pilots*).

The job of the AME is to make the initial determination about whether an applicant meets the medical standards for acting as a pilot. AMEs have authority to do only one of three things:

1. Certify an apparently healthy applicant.

2. Deny certification to an applicant who does not meet the medical requirements, or has a disqualifying feature.

3. Defer the certification decision to the FAA physicians in Oklahoma City.

Again, it should be noted that the AME does not determine if a pilot is healthy, but tries only to rule out a future medical problem in flight. The AME exam is not a substitute for a regular medical examination.

Appropriate medical certificate

An FAA medical examination is required for all pilots. It is also required for other cockpit crew of larger aircraft, such as second officers and flight engineers, as well as air traffic controllers.

A pilot who is flying with an instructor (or someone else who can legally act as pilot-in-command) can do so without a valid medical certificate. For example, many students begin flying lessons before they get their medical certificate. However, the medical is required before the student will be allowed to fly solo. Therefore, new students should get their medical certificate as soon as possible. It is a nuisance to hold up the solo because you don't have the medical, and even more of a nuisance to discover that you have a disqualifying condition after you have already spent time and money on instruction.

Glider or free balloon pilots are not required to hold a medical certificate. To be eligible for the Glider or Free Balloon Airman Certificate, you must certify that you have no known physical defect that makes you unable to pilot a glider or free balloon. It is up to you to decide what is meant by "physical defect," as this is not specified but based on common sense.

A medical certificate is not necessary to pilot an ultralight aircraft (for that matter, you don't need a pilot's license either). Ultralights are an odd entity. Technically they are powered aircraft, but they are not certified as general aviation aircraft and have a great many restrictions on flight. Because of these restrictions, the safety standards are relaxed. Ultralight aircraft must weigh less than 70.3 kg and carry a maximum of 6.8 kg of fuel. There are an increasing number of such aircraft, and the relaxed standard exists partly to encourage continued experimentation and invention.

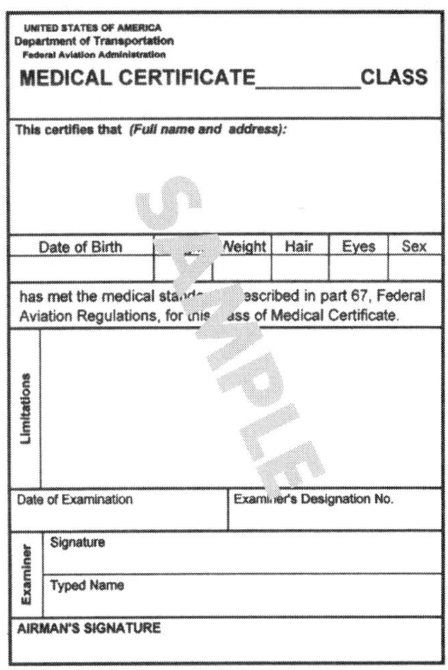
UNITED STATES OF AMERICA
Department of Transportation
Federal Aviation Administration

MEDICAL CERTIFICATE ________ CLASS

This certifies that *(Full name and address)*:

Date of Birth	Height	Weight	Hair	Eyes	Sex

has met the medical standards prescribed in part 67, Federal Aviation Regulations, for this class of Medical Certificate.

Limitations

Date of Examination | Examiner's Designation No.

Examiner: Signature / Typed Name

AIRMAN'S SIGNATURE

FAA Form 8500-9 (3-99) Supersedes Previous Edition

The recreational pilot certificate is another curiosity. In my opinion, it is the kind of proposal that seems to make sense to a government committee, but doesn't quite work in practice. The purpose of this certificate was to allow people to get a pilot license in about half the time and at half the cost of a private pilot certificate, in exchange for some restrictions on flight. Although well intended, this program appears to be more trouble than it's worth. With regard to the medical examination, the recreational pilot has the same requirements as the private pilot certificate. Some aviation experts believe that the time will come when licensed recreational pilots (not private pilots) may be able to medically certify themselves, but with the newly heightened public concern about aviation safety, I think this is unlikely.

Combination medical certificate and student pilot certificate

Anyone can apply for an FAA medical certificate. Interestingly, some people apply who have no plans to fly an airplane. For example, some professional automobile and speedboat drivers recognize the value of an FAA medical certificate and get one to show that they do not have medical deficiencies.

If you are planning to get instruction leading to a pilot's license, you will need the combination medical certificate and student pilot certificate. This combined certificate is required before your instructor can sign you off for solo flight. Once you have any type of pilot's license, you no longer need to get the combination certificate, even if you take instruction for a different type of pilot license.

The requirements for the combined medical certificate and student pilot certificate are:

1. You must be at least 16 years of age (see *Age*, below).

2. You must be able to read, write, speak and understand the English language.

3. You must qualify for at least a third-class medical certificate.

On the back of the combination certificate, you will notice a place for your instructor's endorsement to allow you to fly solo, once your instructor is satisfied that you have gained the necessary skills.

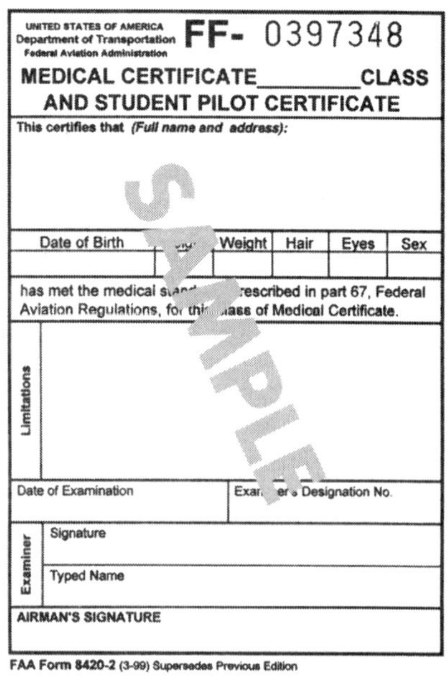
UNITED STATES OF AMERICA
Department of Transportation
Federal Aviation Administration
FF- 0397348
MEDICAL CERTIFICATE ________ CLASS
AND STUDENT PILOT CERTIFICATE
This certifies that *(Full name and address)*:

SAMPLE

Date of Birth	[illegible]	Weight	Hair	Eyes	Sex

has met the medical s[illegible] [illegible]rescribed in part 67, Federal Aviation Regulations, fo[illegible] [illegible]lass of Medical Certificate.

Limitations

Date of Examination | Exa[illegible]er's Designation No.

Examiner: Signature

Typed Name

AIRMAN'S SIGNATURE

FAA Form 8420-2 (3-99) Supersedes Previous Edition

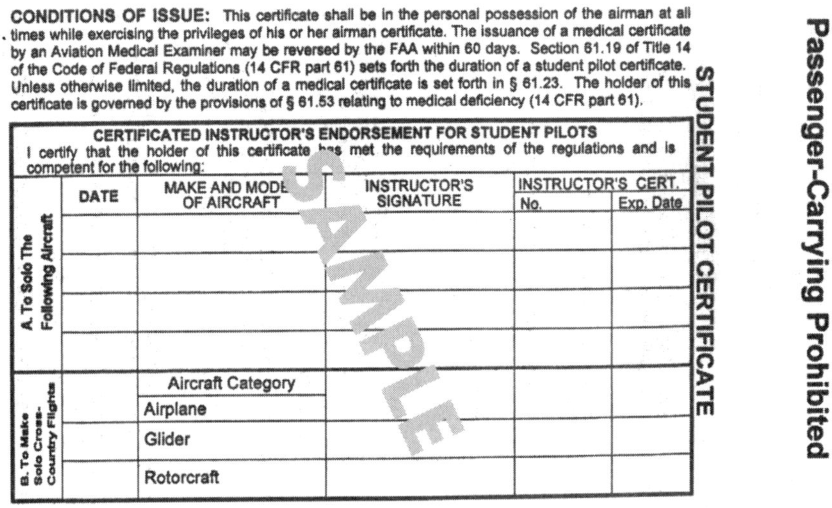

CONDITIONS OF ISSUE: This certificate shall be in the personal possession of the airman at all times while exercising the privileges of his or her airman certificate. The issuance of a medical certificate by an Aviation Medical Examiner may be reversed by the FAA within 60 days. Section 61.19 of Title 14 of the Code of Federal Regulations (14 CFR part 61) sets forth the duration of a student pilot certificate. Unless otherwise limited, the duration of a medical certificate is set forth in § 61.23. The holder of this certificate is governed by the provisions of § 61.53 relating to medical deficiency (14 CFR part 61).

CERTIFICATED INSTRUCTOR'S ENDORSEMENT FOR STUDENT PILOTS

I certify that the holder of this certificate has met the requirements of the regulations and is competent for the following:

	DATE	MAKE AND MODEL OF AIRCRAFT	INSTRUCTOR'S SIGNATURE	INSTRUCTOR'S CERT. No.	INSTRUCTOR'S CERT. Exp. Date
A. To Solo The Following Aircraft					
B. To Make Solo Cross-Country Flights		Aircraft Category			
		Airplane			
		Glider			
		Rotorcraft			

STUDENT PILOT CERTIFICATE

Passenger-Carrying Prohibited

SAMPLE

THREE CLASSES OF MEDICAL CERTIFICATION

The FAA issues three classes of medical certificate:

A third-class medical certificate is appropriate for student pilots, recreational pilots, and private pilots who fly for pleasure or personal business (but not for hire).

A second-class medical certificate is required for pilots who fly commercially—in operations such as crop dusting, delivering canceled checks, or carrying passengers or cargo for hire. A second-class certificate is required to act as a commercial pilot, flight engineer, or air traffic control specialist.

A first-class medical certificate is required for pilots who exercise Airline Transport Pilot (ATP) privileges; that is, those flying scheduled airliners and other pilots whose employers require this level of certification.

The difference between the classes of medical examination is minimal. There is a slight difference in the visual requirements, with first-class being more stringent than second, which is in turn more stringent than third. There is also a requirement for first-class pilots to get an ECG if they are over 35, which is not necessary for the others. Finally, it is likely (although not required) that the AME will take a more careful look at a first-class applicant. Any AME may conduct a third- or second-class physical, but only a Senior AME may conduct a first-class physical.

So, which one should you get? It depends on the type of flying you expect to do. If your ultimate goal is to fly for the airlines, you might as well go ahead and get a first-class physical, even though all you need is a student pilot/third-class. If all you plan to do is fly for pleasure, the third-class will suffice. It might also save you some money, since some AMEs charge more for a first- or second-class than for a third-class examination.

MEDICAL CERTIFICATE DURATION

A third-class medical certificate is valid for 24 months (36 months if the applicant has not reached his or her 40th birthday before or on the date of the examination). A third-class medical is valid for student, recreational, and private pilot privileges.

The second-class medical certificate is valid for commercial privileges for 12 months. After 12 months, it can serve as a third-class certificate for another 12 months (or 24 months if the applicant is younger than 40).

A first-class medical is valid for ATP privileges for six months. After six months, the first-class certificate can serve as the medical for another six months as a second-class, and another 18-30 months (to a total of 24-36 months) as a third-class, depending on the age of the applicant.

In each case, the certificate is valid for the remainder of the month of issue plus 6-36 calendar months thereafter, depending on class and age. Therefore, some thrifty pilots schedule their exam on the first days of the month, effectively extending the validity of their certificate by almost a month.

The medical certificate validity begins on the date stated on the certificate, which is the date of the examination, regardless of when the certificate is actually issued. It is entirely possible that the issuance of a certificate might be delayed if further information is required. The expiration date does not change.

Despite having a valid medical certificate, a pilot may be required to undergo a re-examination at any time if, in the opinion of the Federal Air Surgeon or a representative of the FAA, there is reason to question the pilot's ability to meet the medical standards. This is a decision of the FAA, however, and not the AME.

Physical requirements

AGE

It might seem odd, but the age requirements for a pilot license are not the same as those for an aviation medical certificate. A student pilot of a glider or balloon must be at least 14 years of age; for powered aircraft (not ultralights) he or she must be 16. For a private license, the requirement is 16 for glider or balloon, and 17 for powered aircraft. A commercial license cannot be obtained before age 18, and an airline transport pilot must be at least 23. (I once worked with a 17-year-old who had over 600 hours, including about 100 hours flying a cargo DC-6 for his father's airline, but he had to do so as a private pilot!)

For the combined medical certificate and student pilot certificate the applicant must have reached his or her 16th birthday. Other medical certificates are independent of the license and do not have specific age requirements.

I want to solo on my 16th birthday. How can I do that?

There are several ways to do this, assuming that the weather cooperates and your instructor signs you off for the solo:

1. Take the medical examination on your birthday, before the big flight.

2. Get the white medical certificate without the yellow student pilot certificate. Anyone, of any age, can apply for an aviation medical certificate. Then, on your birthday, get a student pilot certificate from the FSDO office or a designated Flight Examiner by presenting your medical certificate. You will then be given the yellow student certificate.

3. The best way is to find a sympathetic AME who may issue your combined certificate beforehand, with the following limitation: NOT VALID UNTIL SIXTEENTH BIRTHDAY (or NOT VALID UNTIL [date of your 16th birthday]). This may be done no more than 30 days before your birthday.

What about the rule that says you can't fly for an airline if you're over age 60?

On March 15, 1960 the FAA imposed an upper age limit of 60 for the pilot-in-command and copilot aboard airline transports. (There was no limit for flight engineers.) No scientific justification was given for this restriction, but it was felt that the risk of sudden incapacitation increased with age, and 60 seemed to be a suitable cut-off point. This rule was implemented as an operational restriction, under Part 121 of the regulations, and not as a medical restriction (Part 67), and therefore it cannot be waived.

In 1993 the FAA's Hilton Study demonstrated that there was really no decrease in flight performance as pilots reached the age of 60. A follow-up study in 1999 confirmed that there was no difference in the accident risk of pilots over age 60 compared with that of pilots aged 20-59. In fact, the highest risk was among the youngest pilots—something that might have been expected from automobile accident statistics.

However, until the law is changed, the age-60 rule stands for passenger airline operations. Many older pilots simply choose to work as a cargo airline pilot, or for foreign airlines that don't have this regulation.

As I write this, there are more than 2,600 pilots in their 80s, but just 30 pilots who are 90 years of age or older. John Miller, the founder of the United Flying Octogenarians, is still flying at 95 and looks up to Cole Kugel, an active pilot who is a sprightly 99.

Pilot age and accident rate

Age	*Accidents per 1,000 pilots*
16-19	15
20-24	5
25-29	4
30-34	4
35-39	4
40-44	4
45-49	3
50-54	3
55-59	4
60 or older	3

Height and weight

The FAA regulation disqualifies individuals who have "any congenital or acquired defect that would adversely affect flying safety or endanger the individual's well being." This regulation might be used for people who are extremely short or tall, underweight or overweight.

Although there are no specific medical standards for height, exceptionally short individuals may not be able to effectively reach all flight controls. However, they may be able to get a medical certificate under special issuance (see *Chapter 3: Getting a SODA*), and must fly specially modified aircraft. The AME will evaluate applicants of unusual height and may place operational limitations on the pilot certificate.

Obesity is a greater concern, not only for health reasons but also because the combined weight of a very heavy student pilot and instructor may easily exceed the operational limitations of a small training aircraft. Obesity in itself is not disqualifying, but the related conditions, such as diabetes or heart disease, may be. The same is true of an exceptionally thin person, who would provoke a closer examination to determine if there are underlying psychological or physical problems.

Visual acuity

There was a time when pilots were expected to have unusually good eyesight, but this is no longer a requirement, either in commercial flight or in the military, and certainly not for private or recreational pilots. The visual requirements, either with or without glasses or contact lenses, are:

Third class:	
distant vision	20/40 or better in each eye separately
near vision	20/40 or better in each eye separately
Second or first class:	
distant vision	20/20 or better in each eye separately
near vision	20/40 or better in each eye separately
intermediate vision (age 50 or over)	20/40 or better in each eye separately

Color vision

Since about 10 percent of American males are red-green color blind to some degree, this requirement has probably caused more anxiety and confusion than any other. The FAA specifies that the pilot be able "to perceive those colors necessary for safe performance of airman duties." In practice, this means being able to distinguish the red-green light gun signals from an airport tower. There are many ways to satisfy this requirement (see *Chapter 2: Eye or vision trouble*).

I knew a fellow who made his living transporting frozen fish in a Beechcraft B18. Once, after a particularly bad landing, he rode his airplane off the runway, spun it around twice, then wedged it into a muddy bog between taxiways. When asked about his landing he said, "I knew this was a bad landing but I didn't realize I was in trouble until I looked up and saw the face of cod."—*Rod Machado, AOPA Pilot*

Hearing

You must be able to show that you can hear an average conversational voice in a quiet room, using both ears at six feet, with your back turned to the examiner. If your hearing is worse than that, you can take an audiometric exam (see *Chapter 5: Ear problems*). Even if you are completely deaf, it is still possible to become medically certified.

Ear, nose, throat

You may not have any significant ear disease or condition manifested by vertigo or a disturbance of speech or equilibrium.

Blood pressure

The FAA does not specify a maximum blood pressure, but it should not be more than 155/95.

Electrocardiogram (ECG)

For a first-class certificate, you need an ECG once if you are over age 35, and every year after age 40.

Mental status

You may not have:

- A diagnosis of psychosis, bipolar disorder, or severe personality disorders.
- Alcohol or drug abuse in the past two years.
- Alcohol or drug dependence, unless there has been total abstinence for at least two years.

Disqualifying conditions

The FAA includes a list of 15 conditions that specifically disqualify an applicant, and the AME must either deny these applicants or defer them to the FAA for further evaluation. Some have called these the "fearful fifteen." In fact, it is possible (but not easy) to become certified even with these conditions if you can prove that you can fly safely, and many pilots have done so.

1. Diabetes mellitus requiring medication
2. Angina pectoris
3. Coronary heart disease
4. Myocardial infarction (heart attack)
5. Heart valve replacement
6. Permanent heart pacemaker
7. Heart transplant
8. Psychosis
9. Bipolar disorder (manic depressive)
10. Personality disorder with inappropriate behavior
11. Alcohol or drug dependence
12. Alcohol or drug abuse
13. Epilepsy
14. Loss of consciousness without a satisfactory explanation of the cause
15. Temporary loss of control of nervous system function(s) without a satisfactory explanation of the cause.

Chapter 2 describes each of these conditions in detail—and what to do about it to get your certification.

If you don't meet the requirements

Many times, a pilot's medical problems are not severe but increase the risk of sudden impairment or distraction. For example, high blood pressure can cause unexpected dizziness, headaches, or fainting; and kidney stones or ulcers can cause abrupt and overwhelming pain. If there is a medical condition of concern, the AME will require additional information to submit to the FAA to show that the pilot is safe to fly. There are no simple criteria for this: since the risk is a judgment call, each case is individually evaluated by the FAA. Once the FAA is satisfied that the medical condition is well controlled (for example, if blood pressure is lowered by approved medication), the pilot will be certified to fly.

"A denial, contrary to what many think, is never final."
—*Richard Reinhart, M.D., Flight Physiologist*

In some cases, the AME may not have enough experience, or be familiar enough with the regulations, to issue you the certificate and might choose to defer it to the FAA. If the problem is simply the need for some additional information, the AME can hold off issuing the certificate until this information arrives, without having to defer the application. Once the information is available and satisfactory, a medical certificate may be issued.

Although the aviation medical examination might seem daunting, the actual denial rate is very small—less than 0.7 percent. Of these, over 50 percent failed to provide the information needed by the FAA or did not pursue the recertification process. When these applicants provided the proper information, most of them were certified and the final denial rate was reduced to just 0.1 percent, or about one in 1,000 applicants.

"Persons who would have otherwise been summarily disqualified a few years ago are now given careful consideration and permitted to engage in aviation activities."—*Jon L. Jordan, M.D., Federal Air Surgeon*

The FAA has the authority to certify almost every medical problem, including all of the 15 disqualifying conditions. If you can show, with an examination and medical data, that you are safe to fly in the type of aircraft and position for which you are applying, there is a good chance that you will eventually achieve certification even with quite significant health problems.

In other words, *a denial is only final if you accept it as final.*

There are some deficiencies for which the AME may go ahead and issue you a certificate with certain limitations. The most common of these is poor vision, which requires corrective lenses such as glasses or contact lenses. In this case, the AME might issue your certificate with a printed notice on the front in the limitations block, "HOLDER SHALL WEAR CORRECTIVE LENSES."

If you need a hearing aid, it might read, "VALID ONLY WITH USE OF HEARING AMPLIFICATION." If you are completely deaf, your medical certificate will restrict you to areas in which radio communication is not required: "NOT VALID FOR CONTROL ZONES OR AREAS WHERE RADIO COMMUNICATION IS REQUIRED."

Any limitation is a part of the medical certificate, and its conditions must be met when flying.

I got my certificate from the AME—but the FAA denied it. How can they do that?

It rarely happens that the AME issues a certificate but the FAA then reverses the AME's decision and denies the certification.

A medical certificate is considered to be valid unless it is reversed by the:

- Federal Air Surgeon
- Regional Flight Surgeon
- Manager of the Aerospace Medical Certification Division

In this case, the FAA must inform the pilot within 60 days of the issuance by the AME. If the FAA requests additional information from the applicant (which they must do within 60 days after the certificate is issued), they have another 60 days after they get this additional information to decide whether to deny the certificate.

The FAA sent me a letter stating it is "unable to establish my eligibility to hold a medical certificate." The examiner had issued my medical, so may I still use it?

The FAA is questioning something about your medical history, medications, or visits to health professionals, and it is asking for further explanation. You need to provide this information. In the meantime, your medical certificate is valid as long as you have no other health problems.

Special Issuance Authorization

If you are medically disqualified, you may apply to the FAA for an Authorization for Special Issuance of a Medical Certificate. An Authorization states that the pilot does not meet the medical standard, but is considered to be safe to fly on the basis of further tests and an FAA review. Getting an Authorization is not easy, but it is being done increasingly for even quite extensive medical conditions. Between 1990 and 2000, the number of Authorizations more than doubled for medical conditions such as heart disease, pacemakers, and valve implants.

Authorizations are typically short-term solutions to allow you to fly, usually valid for only a few months and with very specific restrictions. They require close follow-up to re-evaluate the condition. Note that only the FAA, and not the AME, may grant an Authorization (see *Chapter 3: Getting a SODA*).

Statement of Demonstrated Ability

If you have a medical condition which is stable, non-progressive, and can be shown to present little risk for flight, you may apply for a Statement of Demonstrated Ability (SODA) rather than an Authorization. For example, a SODA may be issued when the pilot can demonstrate the ability to fly safely despite having a disability, such as an amputation or having only one eye.

Unlike an Authorization, a SODA does not expire and lasts until the condition is changed. After a SODA is granted, subsequent medical certification may be given by an AME without having to re-apply for the SODA. Getting a SODA may require a check flight in order for the pilot to demonstrate safe flying abilities. Like Authorizations, only the FAA, and not the AME, may grant a SODA (see *Chapter 3: Getting a SODA*).

There is no additional cost to getting an Authorization or a SODA, but you will benefit from the help of a supportive and interested AME.

Appealing a denial

If your AME finds that you are clearly not eligible for an aviation medical certificate, your application will be denied. You should be told the reason for the denial, your right to appeal this denial, and how to go about filing an appeal.

If your AME does deny your certification, you can appeal that decision within 30 days without the need to get more information. After 30 days, you will need to get another examination, and it is usually helpful to get further medical tests and reports to support your case.

If you do decide to appeal your denial, you will be given a fixed period in which to gather additional information or take further medical tests. This is usually 60 days, but depends on the severity of your medical condition and its effect on flying safely. Your file will be kept active during the appeal period. If you currently have a medical certificate, it will remain valid. After the deadline, you are no longer legally medically certified even if your previous certificate has not expired. If, for some reason, you can't get the additional medical information before the deadline, you should just submit what you have, and file for an extension. The FAA is generally quite considerate about this, and it is important to have a supportive AME who will work with them to help you get your certificate.

> Contrary to popular belief, the FAA really wants to certify as many pilots as possible. Very few applicants actually are finally denied medical certification.
> —*AOPA, Pilot's Guide to Medical Certification*

It is amazing how many pilots who fail their medicals simply don't provide the extra information that is required. For example, in 1994, with a total of 452,992 applications, there were 2,916 denials. Of these denials, 1,278 did not pursue reconsideration, and 1,116 failed to provide the FAA with the additional requested information. The result was that only 522 pilots were actually denied after the FAA reviewed their cases.

Can I still fly, even though my medical was denied?

You can always fly. You just can't legally act as pilot-in-command or as a required member of a flight crew. Many pilots who have lost their medical, either temporarily or permanently, continue to fly but do so with an instructor or other qualified pilot on board who is certified to act as pilot-in-command. Oddly enough, you can even log this time as pilot-in-command although you are not legally the PIC.

Disabled pilots

Following a flight test many pilots with disabilities—including deafness, amputations, and even paraplegia—have become certified. For more information (see *Chapter 3: Disabled pilots*).

Preparing for the medical exam

Finding an Aviation Medical Examiner

Unless you live in a remote area of the U.S., or in another country, it is likely that there is an AME in your community. The FAA has certified about 5,700 physicians to perform AME duties, and these physicians are selected in part by geographical need—ensuring very good coverage of the country. The methods by which pilots usually find an AME are:

- Ask other pilots whom they use, or call the local FBO. There will often be notices or advertisements posted at the FBO. If you are just starting to fly, the flight school will have recommendations.

- Check the yellow pages of the phone book under Physicians-Aviation.

- Check the online listings (see *Appendix: Further Information*). This is particularly useful if you are traveling and want to find someone in your area.

> I got my instrument rating in Lubbock, Texas, at a popular flight school for international students. One day, an Air India trainee took a Cessna 152 on a VFR cross-country to New Mexico. He lost radio contact after a couple of hours over the featureless desert, and became worried that he might have crossed the border into Mexico. He spotted a ranch airstrip and decided to put down to call the flight school. When the rancher pulled up in his pickup, the student politely inquired, in his heavy accent, "Excuse, Sir. I am from India. Please to tell me what country I am in." The rancher thought for a while. "Boy," he drawled, "that must have been one hell of a flight, because you are a LONG way from home."

The AME must personally conduct your exam (except for visual checks, blood pressure, collecting the urine sample, etc., which may be done by office staff), and the exam must be carried out in the AME's regular office. The AME is not allowed to conduct the exam at a temporary address or to permit another doctor to conduct the exam. If the particular AME you have chosen is not available, you must go to another one.

Choosing an AME: what to look for

In my opinion, it does not matter whom you choose if you have no medical concerns. All AMEs are certified by the FAA and the great majority are very competent physicians with a strong personal interest in flying. If you need a first-class medical certificate, make sure that the AME is a Senior AME, able to conduct first-class physicals. All AMEs can conduct second- and third-class physicals.

Although all AMEs are assumed to be competent, not all are willing to spend the time to help you if you run into trouble. If you think you might need extra attention, it is worth finding an AME who will assist you beyond the initial exam and not just defer or deny your application. A deferral may be necessary if you have a disqualifying condition, but a good AME can work with you and the FAA to get certification while a less aggressive AME might simply defer or deny it.

The best AMEs are those who do a *lot* of examinations and are very familiar with the FAA paperwork and procedures. They can really help expedite the process. On the other hand, an unsure or uninterested AME can tie things up waiting for the proper documentation or by filing the wrong paperwork. Ideally, the AME will identify and order all the necessary and appropriate tests and documentation and then prepare a neat and organized package for submission to the FAA. In some cases, the AME can get approval for immediate certification over the telephone while submitting the package.

If you have a special health concern, it may be useful to find an AME with skill in this area, to save time and frustration down the road as you prepare your paperwork for the FAA. Many of the AME listing services will recommend AMEs with particular specialties.

Should my AME be a pilot?

This is a recommendation that comes up often on web sites and in aviation advice columns. The reasons given are that physician pilots have a better understanding of flying and a greater appreciation of how much you want to fly.

My opinion is that this recommendation is over-rated. Although most AMEs are not pilots, all of them have an interest in aviation or they wouldn't be doing the job (the AME is the doctor driving the beat-up old Subaru, not the Mercedes). Of course, it is always fun to talk to someone about flying, turning the medical examination into a bit of a social visit, and Lord knows, if you get two pilots into a room, they'll happily talk for hours. But all AMEs take the same course at the Civil Aerospace Medical Institute in Oklahoma City, and non-pilot AMEs are very familiar with the physiological demands of flight. The only time I've found it helpful to be a physician pilot is when I examine student pilots and can help impress upon them the importance of their health in flying.

Preparing for the exam

If your regular doctor is also your AME, you don't need to do anything to prepare. Otherwise, the best way to prepare for an FAA exam is to see your regular doctor first and get a "pre-test" where you can check to see if you have any worrisome conditions. That way, you can take care of the problem before it results in a denial of your FAA medical certification and the subsequent piles of paperwork.

In addition to any particular concerns you might have, you should ensure that:

1. Your eyesight is satisfactory for near and distant vision.

2. You have adequate color vision.

3. Your blood pressure is within the normal range. Although the FAA allows a rather high blood pressure of up to 155/95, you should be treated if yours is over 140/90. Most blood pressure medications are approved for use by the FAA. (For more information, see *Chapter 2: High or low blood pressure*.)

4. Your hearing should be satisfactory. If you have any concerns, you should have an audiogram to see if there is a deficiency.

5. If you are going for a first-class medical examination, you should get an ECG beforehand. Make sure it is normal. If it is at all abnormal—even if your doctor tells you that the abnormality is not significant—you should get a further evaluation and a letter with an explanation of the finding and a statement that you do not have a heart condition that presents a safety hazard (see *Chapter 2: Heart or vascular trouble*).

If you have a health problem

This is where preparation really pays off. Contact the AME (or AOPA) before going for the test to see what, if any, special tests or documentation you might need. Bring a letter from your treating physician with a description of your condition and a statement that it is under good control and not likely to cause incapacitation. The letter should include:

1. Diagnosis
2. Dates of occurrence
3. Results of recent laboratory tests
4. List of medications, with a statement that these are well-tolerated and free of significant side-effects
5. Any functional limitations due to this condition, or risk of incapacitation.

AOPA's Medical Certification Department

If you know that you have a medical condition that will probably cause a problem with your certification, you can get help from AOPA's Medical Certification Department to prepare yourself before you see the medical examiner. Their specialists answer more than 20,000 calls a year from pilots with medical questions, and claim to be the best source of medical certification information outside the FAA. They will also help compile the necessary medical data into an organized file for submission to the FAA with an explanatory cover letter. This is one of the most popular and sought-after services available to AOPA members. (see *Appendix: Further Information*)

The Civil Aviation Medical Association (CAMA) is an organization that helps pilots with medical problems. Most CAMA members are highly experienced AMEs, and they are happy to advise your AME if he or she needs help with your certification. If your AME wants to defer your application, you might politely suggest contacting CAMA first.

The Flying Physicians Association (FPA) is another resource for pilots with medical problems. Not all of them are AMEs, but most are physician pilots with a special interest in aviation issues.

Airline pilots who belong to the Airline Pilots Association have the services of an aeromedical coordinator within their local union, and an aeromedical physician at the national level who specializes in directing grounded pilots to appropriate consultants. Since union dues pay for these specialists, airline pilots should take advantage of this service.

What to bring for the exam

I recommend that you arrive at the clinic at least 15 minutes early and bring:

1. Photo ID, such as your driver's license.

2. Your medical record and documentation, if you have had any illness, surgery, or hospitalization within the past three years. In general, you should bring a record of any medical visit other than routine physical exams.

3. If this is not your first exam, you should bring a copy of your previous examination form (FAA Form 8500-8). This is a legal document with controlled distribution. It used to be that pilots were not given a copy, and some old-fashioned AMEs may be hesitant to give it to you. The new form is in triplicate, and the third copy is for you. You should ask for it after the examination is completed. It will save some time in filling it out on the next examination, especially if explanations were added (this is explained later in this chapter).

4. Your glasses or contacts, if you use them.

5. A non-empty bladder, as you will be asked for a urine sample.

6. Cash, credit card, or checkbook to pay for the visit. The FAA does not set a standard fee for the examination. In general, AMEs charge $60 to

$90 for the exam; some charge the same for all exams, while others vary the fee with the class of the certificate.

7. A book or magazine—always be prepared for an unexpected wait.

The United States Office of Management and Budget (OMB) estimates that it will take two hours to fill out the form, provide the needed information, and undergo the physical exam. The reality is that most take only about 45 minutes, but be prepared and schedule accordingly.

Incidentally, if you have a tendency to high blood pressure, *don't* drink coffee, sodas, or anything with caffeine before your examination. It will also help if you arrive at the clinic early and take a little time to relax, chat with the staff, and calm yourself down before the examination.

Does the medical examination include drug testing?

No. Testing for illicit drugs is not part of the aviation physical. There is a urine test, but this is to test for diabetes or kidney disease.

If you are a professional pilot, you will probably be required to undergo drug testing, but this is separate from the aviation medical examination (see *Chapter 4: Flying High*).

Application for Airman Medical Certificate (FAA Form 8500-8)

Once you show up at the AME's clinic, you start a process that you cannot easily undo. If, for example, you refuse to show evidence of positive identification, this will be reported to the FAA. When you fill out the form, you must personally enter all the information. If you make a mistake, you must personally enter the correction on the form.

This form is a legal document, and each copy has a unique number and must be accounted for. If the form is only partially completed, torn up, or spoiled, it must still be submitted to the FAA.

The form must be completed in your own handwriting. If, for some unusual reason, you cannot complete the form yourself, someone else may complete it for you, but that person must put his or her initials beside each item and the AME should add a note explaining why you could not complete the form yourself.

All items (except for the Social Security Number, see below) must be completed. If you decide not to finish the form, it will still be sent to the FAA as an incomplete form.

The form is quite simple to fill out, and will probably only take you a

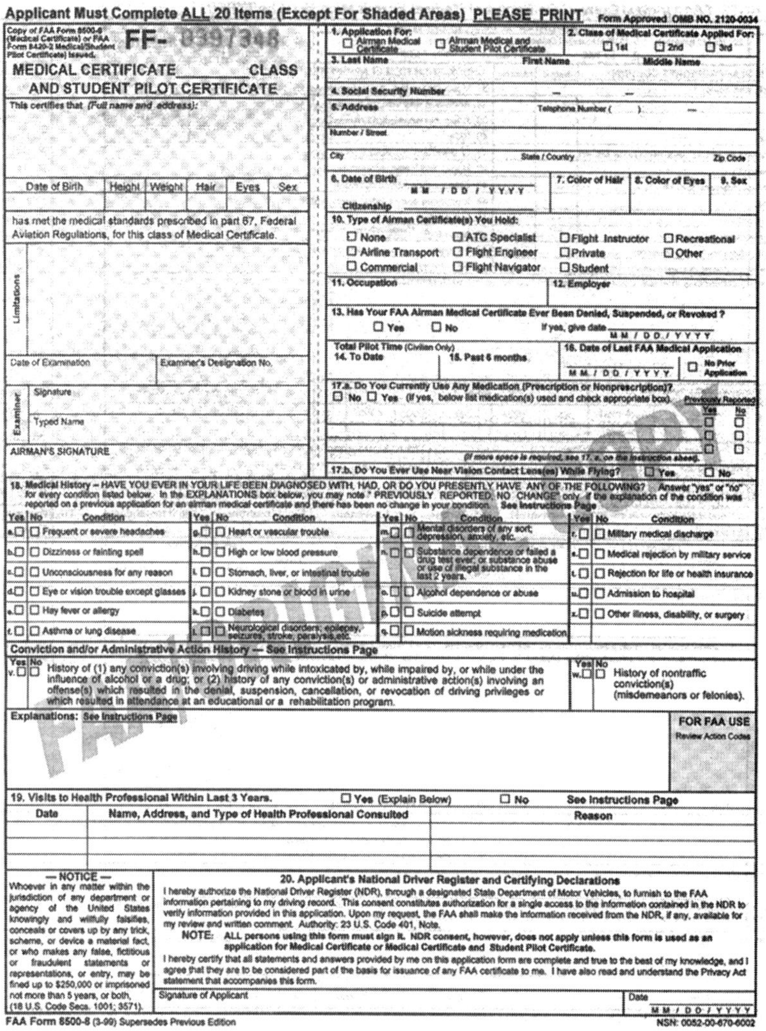

Applicant Must Complete ALL 20 Items (Except For Shaded Areas) PLEASE PRINT Form Approved OMB NO. 2120-0034

Copy of FAA Form 8500-9 (Medical Certificate) or FAA Form 8420-2 Medical/Student Pilot Certificate) Issued. FF-

MEDICAL CERTIFICATE ______ CLASS AND STUDENT PILOT CERTIFICATE

This certifies that (Full name and address):

Date of Birth	Height	Weight	Hair	Eyes	Sex

has met the medical standards prescribed in part 67, Federal Aviation Regulations, for this class of Medical Certificate.

Limitations

Date of Examination | Examiner's Designation No.

Examiner: Signature / Typed Name

AIRMAN'S SIGNATURE

1. Application For: ☐ Airman Medical Certificate ☐ Airman Medical and Student Pilot Certificate
2. Class of Medical Certificate Applied For: ☐ 1st ☐ 2nd ☐ 3rd
3. Last Name / First Name / Middle Name
4. Social Security Number
5. Address / Telephone Number ( ) — / Number / Street / City / State / Country / Zip Code
6. Date of Birth MM / DD / YYYY / Citizenship
7. Color of Hair
8. Color of Eyes
9. Sex
10. Type of Airman Certificate(s) You Hold: ☐ None ☐ ATC Specialist ☐ Flight Instructor ☐ Recreational ☐ Airline Transport ☐ Flight Engineer ☐ Private ☐ Other ☐ Commercial ☐ Flight Navigator ☐ Student
11. Occupation
12. Employer
13. Has Your FAA Airman Medical Certificate Ever Been Denied, Suspended, or Revoked? ☐ Yes ☐ No If yes, give date MM / DD / YYYY

Total Pilot Time (Civilian Only)

14. To Date
15. Past 6 months
16. Date of Last FAA Medical Application MM / DD / YYYY ☐ No Prior Application

17.a. Do You Currently Use Any Medication (Prescription or Nonprescription)? ☐ No ☐ Yes (If yes, below list medication(s) used and check appropriate box). Previously Reported: Yes / No

(If more space is required, see 17. a. on the instruction sheet).

17.b. Do You Ever Use Near Vision Contact Lens(es) While Flying? ☐ Yes ☐ No

18. Medical History – HAVE YOU EVER IN YOUR LIFE BEEN DIAGNOSED WITH, HAD, OR DO YOU PRESENTLY HAVE ANY OF THE FOLLOWING? Answer "yes" or "no" for every condition listed below. In the EXPLANATIONS box below, you may note "PREVIOUSLY REPORTED, NO CHANGE" only if the explanation of the condition was reported on a previous application for an airman medical certificate and there has been no change in your condition. See Instructions Page

Yes	No	Condition	Yes	No	Condition	Yes	No	Condition	Yes	No	Condition
a.☐	☐	Frequent or severe headaches	g.☐	☐	Heart or vascular trouble	m.☐	☐	Mental disorders of any sort; depression, anxiety, etc.	r.☐	☐	Military medical discharge
b.☐	☐	Dizziness or fainting spell	h.☐	☐	High or low blood pressure	n.☐	☐	Substance dependence or failed a drug test ever, or substance abuse or use of illegal substance in the last 2 years.	s.☐	☐	Medical rejection by military service
c.☐	☐	Unconsciousness for any reason	i.☐	☐	Stomach, liver, or intestinal trouble				t.☐	☐	Rejection for life or health insurance
d.☐	☐	Eye or vision trouble except glasses	j.☐	☐	Kidney stone or blood in urine	o.☐	☐	Alcohol dependence or abuse	u.☐	☐	Admission to hospital
e.☐	☐	Hay fever or allergy	k.☐	☐	Diabetes	p.☐	☐	Suicide attempt	x.☐	☐	Other illness, disability, or surgery
f.☐	☐	Asthma or lung disease	l.☐	☐	Neurological disorders; epilepsy, seizures, stroke, paralysis,etc.	q.☐	☐	Motion sickness requiring medication			

Conviction and/or Administrative Action History — See Instructions Page

v. Yes ☐ No ☐ History of (1) any conviction(s) involving driving while intoxicated by, while impaired by, or while under the influence of alcohol or a drug; or (2) history of any conviction(s) or administrative action(s) involving an offense(s) which resulted in the denial, suspension, cancellation, or revocation of driving privileges or which resulted in attendance at an educational or a rehabilitation program.

w. Yes ☐ No ☐ History of nontraffic conviction(s) (misdemeanors or felonies).

Explanations: See Instructions Page

FOR FAA USE Review Action Codes

19. Visits to Health Professional Within Last 3 Years. ☐ Yes (Explain Below) ☐ No See Instructions Page

Date	Name, Address, and Type of Health Professional Consulted	Reason

— NOTICE — Whoever in any matter within the jurisdiction of any department or agency of the United States knowingly and willfully falsifies, conceals or covers up by any trick, scheme, or device a material fact, or who makes any false, fictitious or fraudulent statements or representations, or entry, may be fined up to $250,000 or imprisoned not more than 5 years, or both, (18 U.S. Code Secs. 1001; 3571).

20. Applicant's National Driver Register and Certifying Declarations

I hereby authorize the National Driver Register (NDR), through a designated State Department of Motor Vehicles, to furnish to the FAA information pertaining to my driving record. This consent constitutes authorization for a single access to the information contained in the NDR to verify information provided in this application. Upon my request, the FAA shall make the information received from the NDR, if any, available for my review and written comment. Authority: 23 U.S. Code 401, Note.

NOTE: ALL persons using this form must sign it. NDR consent, however, does not apply unless this form is used as an application for Medical Certificate or Medical Certificate and Student Pilot Certificate.

I hereby certify that all statements and answers provided by me on this application form are complete and true to the best of my knowledge, and I agree that they are to be considered part of the basis for issuance of any FAA certificate to me. I have also read and understand the Privacy Act statement that accompanies this form.

Signature of Applicant | Date MM / DD / YYYY

FAA Form 8500-8 (3-99) Supersedes Previous Edition NSN: 0052-00-670-6002

few minutes, but I'm sometimes amazed at the questions that it can raise. Following is an item-by-item description that should answer most of these questions. The numbers correspond to the number of the box on the form:

1. If you are a student pilot, you will need the additional student pilot certificate, so you should check that box. All other pilots (as well as air traffic controllers and anyone else who wants to get an aviation physical) should check the box: Airman Medical Certificate.

2. Enter which class of medical certificate you want.

3. Enter your name, in the proper order. Nicknames and abbreviated names should not be used. If you don't have a middle name, you should enter NMN or NONE. If your name has changed, enter your current name and add any former names in the Explanations box of Item 18.

4. Your Social Security Number is not legally required here, but I recommend that you enter it to avoid mistakes in identification.

5. Enter your permanent address, with your 9-digit zip code, and your telephone number with area code. If your permanent address is not in the United States, include the country in the address. The idea of a "permanent address" is getting to sound a bit old-fashioned, if not absurd. Americans move, on average, once every three years and many—even high-status professionals—have no fixed place of residence. If you are one of these, just put down some proper address from which mail will be forwarded to you. Regardless of what address you use, it must be a real address; Post Office box numbers are not acceptable.

6. Enter your birth date as a two-digit number, in the following order: month, day, year. For example, March 7, 1964 is 03 07 1964. Also enter your citizenship, e.g., U.S.A.

   Enter the color of your hair. Do not abbreviate. You must enter one of:
   - Brown
   - Black
   - Blond
   - Red
   - Gray
   - Bald

If you are not sure which of these to enter, just put whatever is closest. If you're gray but you usually dye your hair black, you can enter Black. If you are balding and have a brown fringe of hair around the sides that you comb over the top, you can enter Brown. If you are bald and wear a hairpiece—well, it's up to you.

8. Enter your eye color. Do not abbreviate. Eye color is limited to:

Brown
Black
Blue
Hazel
Gray
Green

Once again, if you are not sure which of these to enter, just put whatever you think is closest.

9. Enter Male or Female. If you have had a sex-change operation, enter your new legal sex.

10. Check what type(s) of certificates you have. You may have more than one. If Other is checked, indicate the type.

11. Enter your occupation. This is for statistical reasons, so don't worry too much about what you put here, or if it is different from your previous medical certificate. Only enter Pilot if you actually make your living from flying.

12. Enter your employer. Again, you don't need to write a whole story here. Just a few words to identify your employer. "Self-employed" is okay, if that is the case.

13. If you had a previous medical certificate that was denied, suspended, or revoked, you must check YES here. The AME is not allowed to issue your certificate until you present a letter from the FAA stating that the problem has been resolved and you were subsequently medically certified. If you do not have this letter, your AME will have to get oral or written authorization from the FAA in order to issue you a certificate. It is very helpful to enter the date of your previous certificate; otherwise, expect a lengthy delay while all the details are established.

14. Total pilot time to date: enter your total number of civilian flight hours only. For example, if you are a military pilot with 3,000 hours and just started renting an airplane at the local FBO, with five hours so far in a civilian aircraft, you need to put down five hours. If you put down the

exact number of hours, add Log after the number. If you are estimating the number of hours, add Est after the number of hours.

15. Total pilot time last 6 months: enter the total number of civilian flight hours in the past six months. Again, add Log or Est after the number, as appropriate.

16. Date of last FAA medical application, if you have ever had one. Note that this is the date of the application, not the certificate. Even if you didn't get a certificate, but just started the application, you must put down that application date. Every application, including those that are incomplete or spoiled, gets sent to Oklahoma City and entered into the computer, so be sure you enter this date to avoid subsequent problems when the computer detects the discrepancy. If you don't remember, you can estimate the date (this is why it is useful to have your previous application or medical with you).

17a. If you take any medications (including prescription, non-prescription, or herbal remedies), check the box and list the medications. Check the box if you listed the medication on a previous FAA medical certificate.

17b. Check the box if you ever use near vision contact lenses while flying.

18a-u. For each of the conditions listed, check whether you have ever in your life been diagnosed with this condition. If you check YES for any of these conditions, you must put an explanation in the Explanations box below. The explanation should include the year or age when you had the condition, and whether the condition has resolved. The AME is likely to ask you more detailed questions about it. If you listed the condition on a previous FAA medical application, and there has been no change in the condition, you may state "PREVIOUSLY REPORTED, NO CHANGE." (If you are concerned that any of these conditions might disqualify you, see *Chapter 2*, where each of these conditions is discussed in detail—and advice given on how to qualify for the medical certificate despite having the condition.)

18v. Check here if you have ever had a conviction or administrative action for alcohol or drug use. This includes a fine, loss of driving privileges, loss or suspension of your license, or need to attend an educational or rehabilitation program. You need to enter a driving offense *only* if it involved alcohol or drugs. If your answer here is YES, enter the following in the Explanations box:

i. The alcohol or drug offense, and the administrative action (e.g., attendance at a treatment program, license denial or suspension, educational program, etc.).

ii. The name of the state or jurisdiction where the offense took place.

iii. The date of the conviction or administrative action.

18w. Check if you have ever had a criminal conviction. If your answer here is YES, enter the following in the Explanations box:

i. The charge for which you were convicted.

ii. The date of the conviction.

18x. Check here if you have had any other significant illness, disability, or surgery. You do not need to report minor problems such as colds or sore throats.

19. If you have had any visits to a health professional in the past three years—except routine physical examinations or minor illnesses and dental or eye exams—check YES, and enter the date of the visit and the name, address, type of health professional, and reason for the visit. Once the three years are up, NO can be checked.

Health professionals include physicians, physician assistants, nurse practitioners, psychologists, clinical social workers, and substance abuse specialists. If your visit was for counseling, list it only if it was for your own health condition.

Multiple visits to one health professional for the same condition may be grouped together on a single line.

20. Signing this form (and adding the date) gives your permission to the FAA to consult the National Driver Register for information about your driving record. Your signature is also your declaration that everything in the form is true and to the best of your knowledge. This form is a legal document, and you may be liable for knowingly entering false information.

If more space is needed for any of the answers in items 17, 18, or 19, use an extra sheet of plain paper, and sign and date it.

The other side of FAA Form 8500-8 is for the AME to fill out. It provides space for the results of the medical examination. Your AME may also record and submit additional information that is not on this form.

REPORT OF MEDICAL EXAMINATION

21. Height (inches)	22. Weight (pounds)	23. Statement of Demonstrated Ability (SODA) ☐ YES ☐ NO Defect Noted:	24. SODA Serial Number

CHECK EACH ITEM IN APPROPRIATE COLUMN	Normal	Abnormal	CHECK EACH ITEM IN APPROPRIATE COLUMN	Normal	Abnormal
25. Head, face, neck, and scalp			37. Vascular system (Pulse, amplitude and character; arms, legs, others)		
26. Nose			38. Abdomen and viscera (Including hernia)		
27. Sinuses			39. Anus (Not including digital examination)		
28. Mouth and throat			40. Skin		
29. Ears, general (Internal and external canals; Hearing under item 49)			41. G-U system (Not including pelvic examination)		
30. Ear Drums (Perforation)			42. Upper and lower extremities (Strength and range of motion)		
31. Eyes, general (Vision under items 50 to 54)			43. Spine, other musculoskeletal		
32. Ophthalmoscopic			44. Identifying body marks, scars, tattoos (Size & location)		
33. Pupils (Equality and reaction)			45. Lymphatics		
34. Ocular motility (Associated parallel movement, nystagmus)			46. Neurologic (Tendon reflexes, equilibrium, senses, cranial nerves, coordination, etc.)		
35. Lungs and chest (Not including breast examination)			47. Psychiatric (Appearance, behavior, mood, communication, and memory)		
36. Heart (Precordial activity, rhythm, sounds, and murmurs)			48. General systemic		

NOTES: Describe every abnormality in detail. Enter applicable item number before each comment. Use additional sheets if necessary and attach to this form.

49. Hearing	Record Audiometric Speech Discrimination Score Below		Right Ear					Left Ear				
Conversational Voice Test at 6 Feet ☐ Pass ☐ Fail		Audiometer Threshold in decibels	500	1000	2000	3000	4000	500	1000	2000	3000	4000

50. Distant Vision	51.a. Near Vision	51.b. Intermediate Vision – 32 Inches	52. Color Vision
Right 20/ Corrected to 20/	Right 20/ Corrected to 20/	Right 20/ Corrected to 20/	☐ Pass
Left 20/ Corrected to 20/	Left 20/ Corrected to 20/	Left 20/ Corrected to 20/	☐ Fail
Both 20/ Corrected to 20/	Both 20/ Corrected to 20/	Both 20/ Corrected to 20/	

53. Field of Vision ☐ Normal ☐ Abnormal	54. Heterophoria 20' (in prism diopters)	Esophoria	Exophoria	Right Hyperphoria	Left Hyperphoria

55. Blood Pressure (Sitting, mm of Mercury) Systolic / Diastolic	56. Pulse (Resting)	57. Urinalysis (if abnormal, give results) ☐ Normal ☐ Abnormal	Albumin	Sugar	58. ECG (Date) MM DD YYYY

59. Other Tests Given

60. Comments on History and Findings: AME shall comment on all "YES" answers in the medical history section and for abnormal findings of the examination. (Attach all consultation reports, ECGs, X-rays, etc. to this report before mailing.)

Significant Medical History ☐ YES ☐ NO Abnormal Physical Findings ☐ YES ☐ NO

FOR FAA USE
Pathology Codes:
Coded By:
Clerical Reject

61. Applicant's Name	62. Has Been Issued — ☐ Medical Certificate ☐ Medical & Student Pilot Certificate ☐ No Certificate Issued — Deferred for Further Evaluation ☐ Has Been Denied — Letter of Denial Issued (Copy Attached)

63. Disqualifying Defects (List by item number)

64. Medical Examiner's Declaration – I hereby certify that I have personally reviewed the medical history and personally examined the applicant named on this medical examination report. This report with any attachment embodies my findings completely and correctly.

Date of Examination MM DD YYYY	Aviation Medical Examiner's Name	Aviation Medical Examiner's Signature
	Street Address	AME Serial Number
	City State Zip Code	AME Telephone ( )

FAA Form 8500-8 (3-99) Supersedes Previous Edition NSN: 0052-00-670-6002

The form, and the regular medical examination, do *not* include:

1. Blood test.
2. Alcohol or drug test.
3. Strength or fitness test.
4. Lung function test.
5. Digital rectal examination (such as to check the prostate in men), or a pelvic examination for women. It is recommended that you have a regular physical examination that includes these, but this is not the purpose of the FAA medical examination. If you don't have a regular doctor, you may want to ask your AME to conduct a regular physical examination along with the FAA exam. Most AMEs will be happy to do so.

The AME will make comments on any abnormalities. There must also be a comment on any condition for which you checked YES on the front side of the form. If the condition is not related to flight safety, the AME may write "Reviewed with applicant. History is not significant or relevant to application."

If you have had a previous medical examination and were issued a SODA (see *Chapter 3*), you should tell your AME, who will want to see a copy of it.

All of the information on these forms is confidential. Access to this information is strictly on a "need to know" basis. By right of the Privacy Act of 1974, the FAA will not release this information unless it has your written permission or an order from an appropriate court of law. Great care is taken to protect your privacy during this process.

If, while acting as a pilot, you are involved in an accident or incident, the FAA will reveal the fact that you have a medical certificate, along with any pertinent information, to representatives of the National Transportation Safety Board (NTSB) for use in the subsequent investigation.

All applications (including incomplete ones) are immediately sent to the Aerospace Medical Certification Branch of the FAA in Oklahoma City. Applications are sent electronically, and the data are entered into the FAA computer. The application is compared with the previous application, if there is one. If anything is out of the ordinary, it is flagged and examined by a technician.

A copy of your application should be given to you. If it is not, you should ask for it.

What if I cheat on this form or the tests?

The law states that anyone who "falsifies, conceals, or covers up a material fact may be fined up to $250,000 or imprisoned not more than 5 years, or both." If you get caught taking the test on behalf of someone else, you will be ineligible for all aviation certificates or ratings for one year, and may lose one or all of the certificates you have.

Don't expect your AME to fudge facts or ignore findings—the AME is also legally bound to report the medical examination accurately. Failing to do so can bring the same penalties as for the applicant, and the loss of his or her license to practice medicine.

ALLOWABLE MEDICATIONS

Drugs affect people differently. For example, ibuprofen (Motrin, Advil, etc.) usually has no noticeable effect on people, but in some it can cause stomach pains or drowsiness. Those are the common side-effects, and there is an additional, long list of uncommon or rare reactions. Ultimately, any drug can have almost any side-effect—from simple discomfort to a life-threatening allergic reaction.

According to the FAA, "medication" includes any over-the-counter, prescription or herbal remedy.

Some drugs are well tolerated on the ground, but might cause serious problems at altitude, where pressure changes, dry air, lack of oxygen, and the stress of flying compound the effects of the drug.

Over-the-counter antihistamines or decongestants taken a half hour before a flight may seem innocuous until you're airborne. That's when altitude and pressure changes can cause uncomfortable side-effects that could render you "unable to safely perform airman duties." Drowsiness is common in many over-the-counter remedies that are frequently used by unsuspecting flight crew members.

Remember that the condition for which a drug is being taken may be disqualifying under FAR 61.53. A "medical deficiency" requires that you ground yourself, so a really bad cold and sore throat, combined with self-dispensed medications, may prompt you to have second thoughts about flying that day. If you decide to fly anyway, a good rule of thumb for any medication is to double the last dosage interval before flying. For example, if the prescription instructs you to take the medication every four hours, wait until eight hours after the last dose before leaving the ground. Your doctor or pharmacist should be able to answer any general questions about the proper usage of a medication, and possible adverse side-effects or drug interactions. Questions specifically about using medications while flying are best directed to an AME.

> The most important question is not "*What* medicine was taken?" but "*Why* was this medicine taken?"—The underlying health problem is the main concern.

While acting as a pilot, you should never take any medication for the first time, no matter how commonplace. Even the most ordinary and mild medications can have significant side-effects for some people. If you do know that you have adverse effects from a medication, you should wait at least two to three times the dosing interval before flying. For example, if you know that ibuprofen makes you drowsy, and you take it every eight hours, you should wait 16 to 24 hours after the last dose before flying.

> FAR 91.17(a)(3)
> No person may act as a crew member of a civil aircraft while using any drug that affects his faculties in any way contrary to safety.

There are two main concerns regarding the use of medication during flight:

1. *Why is the medication taken? Is there an underlying disease that affects pilot performance?*

   For example, the herbal medication St. John's Wort can be bought at most supermarkets and health food stores. It is not known to affect pilot performance. By why is the pilot taking it? Most people take it for depression. This condition has been shown to be a hazard to flight, and must be evaluated first. Depression should have been reported on the medical certificate application form, but many people think that if they are not taking a prescription medication, it is not really an illness. Let the AME be the judge of the significance of the health problem. If you are taking any medication, you should report it and appropriately assess the underlying reason for taking it.

2. *Does the medication have side-effects that might present a hazard to flight?*

   All medications have side-effects—there is no absolutely safe medication. The question then becomes whether the risk is low enough to allow its use. This is an individual as well as a regulatory matter. You should know your response to a medication before using it when flying.

Of the hundreds of thousands of medications available, there are very few that the FAA will not accept. However, this does not mean that the remaining medications are certified to be safe and free of complications.

In most cases, the medication is allowed if the prescribing physician presents a note with:

1. The reasons for the medication.

2. The dose.

3. A statement that no adverse effects are likely to occur or have been experienced, and there is no apparent risk to safety.

Flyin' the ointment
A fair-skinned pilot took the precaution of applying a sunscreen on his face just before take-off. (Apparently, he didn't know that you cannot get sunburned through a windshield.) As the cockpit became warm, he started to perspire. Then his eyes started burning and clouded up. Within a few minutes, he was completely blind. He just managed to set the automatic pilot on a heading away from the city. After about eight minutes, he regained partial sight and found that he had flown into a restricted area. He grabbed a can of soda he brought with him and poured it into one eye. This gave him enough sight to return to the airport and land.

With many medications, allowable use depends on the dose of the drug or how long it is used. For example, a short course of prednisone may be allowed to treat a flare-up of an inflammatory condition, but continuous use is not permitted. An antibiotic may be used, but only after having taken it for at least 48 hours to rule out side-effects.

Alcohol is often used as a solvent in liquid medicine, especially in cough and cold preparations. Up to 25% of the liquid may be pure alcohol—equal to a 50 proof drink.

If you take any medication, the best strategy is to check on the approval of the medication beforehand. If you wait until your medical examination, it may result in a deferred certificate and a lengthy delay, and possibly a denial. It is much better to make sure your medication is approved, or wait until you no longer use the disqualifying treatment. You will most likely have no problems with certification after the medication is discontinued and there is no recurrence of the condition that required it in the first place.

What about herbs and pills sold in health food stores? They are not really drugs, are they?

Herbal or other "natural" remedies are one of the fastest growing industries in the United States, with a multi-billion dollar market. It is ironic that they are sold in so-called "health food" stores—which look more like a regular pharmacy. The biggest difference between herbs and pharmaceuticals is that herbs are not recognized as medications by the Food and Drug Administration, and are therefore largely unregulated.

Pharmaceuticals, on the other hand, are highly regulated. The result is that you need a prescription to buy amphetamine, or estazolam (a strong sedative drug), but anyone can buy Ma Huang, which contains equally powerful amphetamine-like substances, or Sleeping Buddha, which actually contains estazolam!

In other words, many herbs *are* drugs and the FAA views them in the same way.

Can I fly after taking Viagra?

Sildenafil (Viagra) is used for erectile dysfunction. It works by causing the relaxation of smooth muscles, allowing blood to flow into the penis to help create and sustain an erection. This smooth muscle relaxation affects the entire body, including the heart and blood vessels, and may present a safety hazard in flight. Nitrate medications also cause smooth muscle relaxation, so users must be careful not to combine the two. Common side-effects include headache, flushing and upset stomach. About 3 percent of Viagra users experience light sensitivity and an inability to discriminate blue and green colors. It is recommended that you wait at least six hours after taking Viagra before flight duties.

I'm taking medication for weight loss. It does not affect me—in fact, I feel more alert!

Sorry. Almost all medications for weight loss, including herbal remedies, are similar to amphetamines. These are not allowed. There are better ways to lose weight (see *Chapter 5: Weight and balance*).

My doctor put me on Ritalin for Attention Deficit Disorder. Is it allowed for flight?

In general, the use of any psychoactive medication (anti-psychotic, antidepressant, anti-anxiety, etc.) is not allowed. But there are always exceptions. Ritalin for attention deficit disorder is specifically not allowed, yet it has been approved by the FAA in a small number of cases. Lithium carbonate, used to treat certain types of depressive disorders, may also be approved after very careful case evaluation. All antidepressants, including selective serotonin reuptake inhibiting (SSRI) medications, such as Paxil, Prozac, and Zoloft, are currently disqualifying, regardless of the reason for their usage.

FAA-ACCEPTED MEDICATIONS

There are over 13,000 prescription drugs currently approved by the United States Food and Drug Administration (FDA). This doesn't include over-the-counter drugs. However, approval by the FDA does not mean approval for flight.

When it comes to flying, the FAA organizes drugs in the following way:

- **Flight duties are normally permitted when taking the drug (e.g., aspirin taken as a blood thinner).**

- Flight duties are permitted if an AME or the FAA gives permission (e.g., an antibiotic taken for an infection).

- Flight duties may be approved by the FAA (e.g., thyroid medications).

- Flight duties are not permitted until the drug is cleared from the body (e.g., codeine taken for cough or pain).

- Flight duties are not permitted because of the condition for which the drug is taken (e.g., digitoxin taken for a heart condition).

- Flight duties are not permitted because of the side-effects of the drug (e.g., diazepam taken for anxiety).

- Flight duties are not permitted because the drug is prohibited (e.g., marijuana, taken for any reason).

Following is a list of medications that are generally approved by the FAA for flight duties, with their usual indications. Most of these are allowed if there is no problem, side-effect, or evident safety concern with their use. Some require additional evaluations for the underlying condition for which they are used.

Some medications are used "off label"—prescribed for a use other than the health condition for which the manufacturer obtained approval. If so, the drug may not be approved by the FAA for flight. For example, proprananol may be approved if it is used to manage high blood pressure, but not if it is used to control nervousness; Evista may be approved if it is used to control bone loss, but not if it is being used for severe depression, which is a disqualifying condition.

The medications listed here are just some of the more common drugs that the FAA has allowed (brand names are capitalized, generic names are not). It is by no means a complete list, and the restrictions change regularly. You should always check with the up-to-date list or ask an AME.

If you have any questions at all about the appropriateness of a drug, you can call the AOPA Medical Certification Department on the Pilot Hotline, 800-872-2672, or other information services listed in the *Appendix: Further Information.*

Medication	**Treatment for**	**May be approved if**
acarbose	diabetes	diabetes evaluation
Accupril	high blood pressure	heart evaluation
Accutane	acne	restriction: not valid for night flying
acebutelol	high blood pressure	heart evaluation
Aceon	high blood pressure	heart evaluation
acetaminophen	pain	no problems
Aciphex	stomach acid reflux	no problems
Actigall	gall stones	liver evaluation
Actos	diabetes	diabetes evaluation
acyclovir	viral infection	requires FAA approval
Adalat	high blood pressure	heart evaluation
Aerobid	asthma	lung evaluation
albuterol	asthma	lung evaluation
Aldactazide	high blood pressure	heart evaluation
Allegra	allergies	no problems
allopurinol	gout	no problems
Altace	high blood pressure	heart evaluation
amantadine	Parkinson's disease	neurologic evaluation
Amaryl	diabetes	diabetes evaluation
amiodarone	irregular heart beat	heart evaluation
amlodipine	high blood pressure	heart evaluation
amoxicillin	infection	no problems
Amoxil	infection	no problems
Arthrotec	inflammation, pain	no problems
Asacol	ulcerative colitis	gastrointestinal evaluation
aspirin	inflammation, pain, etc.	no problems
astemizole	allergies	no problems
atenolol	high blood pressure	heart evaluation
atorvastatin	high cholesterol	no problems
Avalide high	blood pressure	heart evaluation
Avapro	high blood pressure	heart evaluation
Axid	stomach acid reflux	no problems
azatadine	chest congestion	no problems
Azmacort	asthma	lung evaluation
Azulfidine	ulcerative colitis	gastrointestinal evaluation
Benadryl	allergies	restriction: not within 12 hours of flight
benazepril	high blood pressure	heart evaluation
Benemid	gout, arthritis	no problems
Bentyl	irritable bowel syndrome	requires FAA approval
Betapace	irregular heart beat	heart evaluation
betaxolol	high blood pressure	heart evaluation
Biaxin	infection	no problems
bisoprolol	high blood pressure	heart evaluation
Blockadren	high blood pressure	heart evaluation
bromocriptine	Parkinson's disease	neurologic evaluation
budesonide	allergies	no problems
bumetanide	high blood pressure	heart evaluation
Bumex	high blood pressure	heart evaluation
cabergoline	sickle cell anemia	requires FAA approval
Calan	high blood pressure	heart evaluation
Capoten	high blood pressure	heart evaluation
captopril	high blood pressure	heart evaluation
Cardene	high blood pressure	heart evaluation
Cardizem	high blood pressure	heart evaluation
Cardura	high blood pressure	heart evaluation
carteolol	high blood pressure	heart evaluation
Cartrol	high blood pressure	heart evaluation

Medication	Treatment for	May be approved if
carvedilol	high blood pressure	heart evaluation
Cataflam	pain, inflammation	no problems
Catapres	high blood pressure	heart evaluation
cerivastatin	high cholesterol	no problems
cetirizine	allergies	restriction: not within 12 hours of flight
cilostazol	blood circulation	no problems
cimetidine	ulcers	not until ulcers are healed
cisapride	ulcerative colitis	gastrointestinal evaluation
clarithromycin	infection	no problems
Claritin	allergies	no problems
clonodine	high blood pressure	heart evaluation
clopidrogrel	blood clotting	no problems
Cobenemid	gout	no problems
colchicine	gout	no problems
Cordarone	irregular heart beat	heart evaluation
Coreg	high blood pressure	heart evaluation
Corgard	high blood pressure	heart evaluation
cortef	hormone	evaluation
Corzide	high blood pressure	heart evaluation
Coumadin	blood clotting	evaluation
Covera	high blood pressure	heart evaluation
Cozaar	high blood pressure	heart evaluation
Cytotec	ulcers	no problems
Daypro	inflammation, pain	no problems
Deconsal	allergies	no problems
Demadex	high blood pressure	heart evaluation
Diabeta	diabetes	diabetes evaluation
Dibenzyline	high blood pressure	heart evaluation
diclofenac	pain, inflammation	no problems
dicyclomine	irritable bowel syndrome	no problems
digoxin	irregular heart beat	heart evaluation
diltiazem	high blood pressure	heart evaluation
Diovan	high blood pressure	heart evaluation
diphenhydramine	allergies	restriction: not within 12 hours of flight
disopyramide	irregular heart beat	heart evaluation
Dostinex	sickle cell anemia	no problems
doxazosin	high blood pressure	heart evaluation
Droxia	hormone	no problems
Dyazide	high blood pressure	heart evaluation
Dyrenium	high blood pressure	heart evaluation
Eldepryl	Parkinson's disease	neurologic evaluation
Enbrel	rheumatoid arthritis	no problems
Epivir	HIV	no problems
estrogen	menopause	no problems
etanercept	rheumatoid arthritis	no problems
etodolac	inflammation, pain	no problems
Evista	bone loss	no problems, not for depression
famotidine	ulcers	no problems
felodipine	high blood pressure	heart evaluation
fexofenedine	allergies	no problems
finasteride	prostate	no problems
Flomax	prostate	no problems
flunisolide	asthma	lung evaluation
fosinopril	high blood pressure	heart evaluation
furosemide	high blood pressure	heart evaluation

Medication	Treatment for	May be approved if
gemfribozil	high cholesterol	no problems
glimeperide	diabetes	diabetes evaluation
glipizide	diabetes	diabetes evaluation
Glucophage	diabetes	diabetes evaluation
Glucotrol	diabetes	diabetes evaluation
glyburide	diabetes	diabetes evaluation
Hismanal	allergies	no problems
Humulin	diabetes	diabetes evaluation
hydrochlorothiazide	high blood pressure	heart evaluation
Hydrodiuril	high blood pressure	heart evaluation
hydroxurea	hormone	no problems
Hytrin	high blood pressure	heart evaluation
Hyzaar	high blood pressure	heart evaluation
Imitrex	migraine	restriction: not within 24 hours of flight
indapamide	high blood pressure	heart evaluation
Inderal	high blood pressure	heart evaluation
insulin	diabetes	diabetes evaluation
irbesartan	high blood pressure	heart evaluation
isotretonoin	acne	no problems
isradipine	high blood pressure	heart evaluation
Kerlone	blood pressure	heart evaluation
ketoprofen	inflammation, pain	no problems
ketorolac	inflammation, pain	no problems
labetolol	high blood pressure	heart evaluation
lamivudine	HIV	no problems
Lanoxin	irregular heart beat	heart evaluation
lansoprazole	ulcers	no problems
Lasix	high blood pressure	heart evaluation
Levatol	high blood pressure	heart evaluation
levodopa	Parkinson's disease	neuro evaluation
Lexxel	high blood pressure	heart evaluation
Lipitor	high cholesterol	no problems
lisinopril	high blood pressure	heart evaluation
Lodine	inflammation, pain	no problems
Lopid	high cholesterol	no problems
Lopressor	high blood pressure	heart evaluation
loratidine	allergies	no problems
losartan	high blood pressure	heart evaluation
Lotensin	high blood pressure	heart evaluation
Lotrel, Norvasc	high blood pressure	heart evaluation
Lozol	high blood pressure	heart evaluation
Mavik	high blood pressure	heart evaluation
Maxalt	migraine	restriction: not within 24 hours of flight
Maxide	high blood pressure	heart evaluation
mercaptopurine	leukemia	requires FAA approval
mesalamine	ulcerative colitis	no problems
metformin	diabetes	diabetes evaluation
metoclopramide	stomach acid reflux	no problems
metolozone	high blood pressure	heart evaluation
metoprolol	high blood pressure	heart evaluation
mibefradil	high blood pressure	heart evaluation
Micardis	blood pressure	heart evaluation
Minipres	high blood pressure	heart evaluation
misoprostol	ulcers	no problems
moexipril	high blood pressure	heart evaluation
Monopril	high blood pressure	heart evaluation

Medication	Treatment for	May be approved if
nabumetone	inflammation, pain	no problems
nadolol	high blood pressure	heart evaluation
Naprosyn	inflammation, pain	no problems
naproxen	inflammation, pain	no problems
nicardipine	high blood pressure	heart evaluation
nifedipine	high blood pressure	heart evaluation
nisoldipine	high blood pressure	heart evaluation
nizatidine	stomach acid reflux	no problems
Normodyne	high blood pressure	heart evaluation
Norpace	irregular heart beat	heart evaluation
Norvasc	high blood pressure	heart evaluation
omeprazole	ulcers	no problems
orlistat	obesity	requires 30-day observation period
Orudis	inflammation, pain	no problems
Oruvail	inflammation, pain	no problems
oxaprozin	inflammation, pain	no problems
Parlodel	disease	neurologic evaluation
penbutalol	high blood pressure	heart evaluation
Pentasa	Crohn's disease	no problems
pentoxifylline	blood circulation	no problems
Pepcid	ulcers	no problems
perindopril	high blood pressure	heart evaluation
phenoxybenzamine	high blood pressure	heart evaluation
pindolol	high blood pressure	heart evaluation
pioglitazone	diabetes	diabetes evaluation
Plavix	blood clotting	no problems
Plendil	high blood pressure	heart evaluation
Pletal	circulation	no problems
Posicor	high blood pressure	heart evaluation
Pravachol	high cholesterol	no problems
pravastatin	high cholesterol	no problems
prazosin	high blood pressure	heart evaluation
Precose	diabetes	diabetes evaluation
Premarin	menopause	no problems
Prevasid	ulcers	no problems
Prilosec	ulcers	no problems
Prinivil	blood pressure	heart evaluation
probenecid	gout, arthritis	no problems
Procardia	high blood pressure	heart evaluation
propafenone	irregular heart beat	heart evaluation
propranolol	high blood pressure	heart evaluation
Propulsid	ulcerative colitis	no problems
Proscar	prostate	no problems
Proventil	asthma	lung evaluation
pseudoephedrine	allergies	no problems
Purinethol	leukemia	requires FAA approval
quinapril	high blood pressure	heart evaluation
rabeprazole	stomach acid reflux	no problems
raloxifene	bone loss	no problems,not for depression
ramipril	high blood pressure	heart evaluation
ranitidine	ulcers	no problems
Relafen	inflammation, pain	no problems
Rhinocort	allergies	no problems
ribavirin	infection	no problems
rizatriptan	migraine	restriction: not within 24 hours of flight
Rythmol	irregular heart beat	heart evaluation

Medication	Treatment for	May be approved if
Sectral	high blood pressure	heart evaluation
selegiline	Parkinson's disease	neurologic evaluation
simvastatin	high cholesterol	no problems
Sinemet	Parkinson's disease	neurologic evaluation
spironolactone	high blood pressure	heart evaluation
Sular	high blood pressure	heart evaluation
sulfasalazine	ulcerative colitis	no problems
sumatriptin	migraine	restriction: not within 24 hours of flight
Symmetrel	Parkinson's disease	neurologic evaluation
Tagamet	ulcers	no problems
tamsulosin	prostate	no problems
telmisartin	high blood pressure	heart evaluation
Tenormin	high blood pressure	heart evaluation
terazosin	high blood pressure	heart evaluation
Theo-Dur	asthma	lung evaluation
theophylline	asthma	lung evaluation
timolol	high blood pressure	heart evaluation
Toprol	high blood pressure	heart evaluation
Toradol	inflammation, pain	no problems
torsemide	high blood pressure	heart evaluation
trandoparil	high blood pressure	heart evaluation
Trental	circulation	no problems
triamcinolone	asthma	lung evaluation
triamterine	high blood pressure	heart evaluation
Trinalin	chest congestion	no problems
Tylenol	pain	no problems
Univasc	high blood pressure	heart evaluation
ursidiol	gall stones	liver evaluation
valacyclovir	viral infection	requires FAA approval
Valtrex	viral infection	requires FAA approval
valsartan	high blood pressure	heart evaluation
Ventolin	asthma	lung evaluation
verapamil	high blood pressure	heart evaluation
Virazole	infection	no problems
Visken	high blood pressure	heart evaluation
Voltaren	inflammation, pain	no problems
warfarin	blood clotting	evaluation
xalatan	glaucoma	eye evaluation
Xenical	obesity	after 30-day observation period
Zantac	ulcers	no problems
Zaroyolyn	high blood pressure	heart evaluation
Zestril	high blood pressure	heart evaluation
Ziac	high blood pressure	heart evaluation
Zocor	high cholesterol	no problems
Zovirax	viral infection	requires FAA approval
Zyloprim	gout	no problems
Zyrtec	allergies	not during flight; short-term use only

Medical status changes after certificate is issued

If you feel you have a health problem—whether it is something as simple as a cold or unusual fatigue, or something more worrisome—simply don't fly until it is resolved. Flying while you are ill is not only unsafe, it is also illegal. This is stated in Federal Aviation Regulation 61.53, although it does not define "medical deficiency." If you are unsure, you should visit an AME. Flying with a known deficiency is hazardous, illegal, and will invalidate your insurance.

FAR 61.53
Operations during medical deficiency:
No person may act as pilot in command, or in any other capacity as a required pilot flight crew member while he has a known medical deficiency, or increase of a known medical deficiency that would make him unable to meet the requirements for his current medical certificate.

Getting caught flying without a medical certificate

If you are caught flying without a valid medical certificate—either because it was deferred, denied, expired, or because you simply didn't get around to getting one—you are in big trouble. All of your pilot licenses and ratings may be revoked. A second offense will likely result in a substantial fine, and perhaps even time in jail.

Medical certificate replacement

If your medical certificate has not yet expired, you can get a replacement by writing to:

Manager, Aerospace Medical Certification Division, AAM-300
Federal Aviation Administration
Civil Aerospace Medical Institute
Post Office Box 26080
Oklahoma City, OK 73126-0080

Your request must include:
- A check for $2 made payable to the FAA
- Your full name and date of birth
- The class of your certificate
- The place and date of exam

- The name of your examiner
- The circumstances of loss or destruction of original.

In an emergency, you may fax your request to 405-954-3231, but only for a verification of your certificate. You must still follow up with a mailed request for a replacement. Since your replacement will have the same date as the original certificate, it may be easier just to get another FAA medical exam!

The following is a transcript of an actual radio conversation between a United States Aircraft Carrier and the Canadian authorities off the coast of Newfoundland in October, 1995, released by the Chief of Naval Operations.

USN: Please divert your course 15 degrees to the North to avoid a collision.

Canada: Recommend you divert YOUR course 15 degrees to the South to avoid a collision.

USN: This is the Captain of a US Navy ship. I say again, divert YOUR course.

Canada: No. I say again, you divert YOUR course.

USN: THIS IS THE AIRCRAFT CARRIER USS LINCOLN, THE SECOND LARGEST SHIP IN THE UNITED STATES' ATLANTIC FLEET. WE ARE ACCOMPANIED BY THREE DESTROYERS, THREE CRUISERS AND NUMEROUS SUPPORT VESSELS. I DEMAND THAT YOU CHANGE YOUR COURSE 15 DEGREES NORTH, THAT'S ONE-FIVE DEGREES NORTH, OR COUNTER-MEASURES WILL BE UNDERTAKEN TO ENSURE THE SAFETY OF THIS SHIP.

Canada: This is a lighthouse. Your call.

2

Conditions That May Disqualify You

The following conditions have been singled out by the FAA as disqualifying for the medical certificate. In fact, none of them is absolutely disqualifying. With appropriate medical care and evaluation—and help from a good AME—there is an excellent chance that you can get your certificate despite having almost any of these conditions.

For convenience, the conditions are given with the same letter and in the same order as they appear on the FAA medical certificate application form.

A. Frequent or severe headaches

From 20 to 40 percent of the population complains of occasional headaches. In the United States, it is the second most common cause of days lost from work (after respiratory illnesses). Most headaches are relieved with relaxation and a common over-the-counter pain medication such as Tylenol or ibuprofen (Advil, Motrin, etc.), which is generally allowable for use in flight. More severe headaches may be disqualifying for pilots.

According to the FAA, a severe headache is any headache that causes blurred vision, difficulty breathing, nausea, drowsiness, or other symptoms; any headache that awakens you from sleep; any headache that becomes much worse with exertion; and headaches that just don't go away. If you have any of these, you should see a doctor and find out what the problem is before resuming flight duties.

Migraine headaches

Migraines are vascular headaches, meaning that the problem is caused by a widening of the main arteries of the head, stretching the nerves wrapped around them and bringing extreme pain. There are many variations of migraine headaches. Classic migraines are usually one-sided and cause visual disturbances (such as blank spots, sparks, shimmering) and nausea or other symptoms. Other types of migraine might result in just a headache without visual disturbances or nausea, or a "migraine-equivalent" with visual disturbances or nausea but *without* the characteristic headache.

Migraines are more common in women and in people with other family members who suffer migraines. They may be brought on by emotional or physical stress, lack of sleep, certain foods or alcohol, and menstruation.

Frequent migraines—more than once a month or so—are disqualifying until the condition is brought under control. A number of migraine medications are approved by the FAA, so long as they are well-tolerated and have no bad side-effects. These include Imitrex and Zomig, which act to constrict the arteries and therefore relieve the pain and other symptoms. Pain-relieving medications (e.g., Lortab), muscle relaxants (e.g., Flexeril), barbiturates (e.g., Midrin), or benzodiazepines (e.g., Xanax) are not allowed. All of these medications cause altered mental function and are a safety hazard for pilots.

Cluster headaches

Cluster headaches affect mostly middle-aged men. Their exact cause is not known, although they may be brought on by stress or alcohol. The pain tends to appear in a cluster, every day for a few weeks, especially at night, waking the person for a couple of hours. The pain then goes away, even without treatment, and months can go by without another attack. Along with the headache, there may be a stuffy or runny nose, and teary or reddened eyes.

Most treatments of cluster headache are not very effective. The best strategy is to avoid conditions that produce it, if you are aware of them, and discontinue flying during a period of attacks.

B. Dizziness or fainting spell

Most people have felt dizzy at times, or perhaps fainted, but this will probably not be a medical concern. For example, it is quite common to feel a little dizzy after suddenly standing up, especially during an illness. If you are otherwise healthy and feel dizzy, the underlying reason should be looked at, and flying should be avoided until it is resolved.

Ear problems are quite often the cause of vertigo—the kind of dizziness that gives a sensation of the room spinning. The most common type is *positional vertigo*, a temporary condition of the inner ear that makes you dizzy after abrupt movements of the head. This condition tends to go away after a few days. Because the dizziness can make you feel nauseated or disoriented, you should definitely not fly while you have these symptoms.

Labyrinthitis is a condition of the inner ear that usually causes vertigo, as well as tinnitus (ringing in the ears) and hearing loss. It may occur after a viral infection, such as a cold or flu.

Other inner ear conditions may require lengthy treatment and will probably result in you being refused a medical certificate until you can show that the problem has completely resolved. These conditions include Meniere's syndrome (a more severe type of inner ear problem, with a quick onset of vertigo, tinnitus and hearing loss, that usually lasts 1 to 8 hours) and acoustic neuroma (a tumor on the nerve that connects the inner ear to the brain).

Fainting

Fainting for any reason should be evaluated before you fly. Common causes are anemia, low blood pressure, low blood sugar, dehydration, or a response to stress. You should not fly until these problems are resolved and there is no longer a risk of fainting. If you are not sure of the cause, you should get a medical evaluation to discover the underlying problem. This will include a blood pressure check and an ECG. Even with a complete medical evaluation, however, the cause for about half of all fainting episodes is never discovered. If no obvious problem is found, and it appears that fainting is not a likely occurrence, you should be able to get your medical certificate.

I'm very healthy and active in sports, but one day I just passed out. Does that disqualify me from flight?

You need to find out why you passed out. It could have been dehydration during intense exercise on a hot day—which is a lesson to drink a lot of water (and avoid excessive alcohol or caffeine). Or there could have been a number of other reasons.

Some people pass out from emotional upset, when they give blood (or even see blood), from sudden pain, or when they urinate. All of these involve a sudden drop in blood pressure, so that insufficient blood is sent to the brain, similar to "pulling Gs" during aerobatic maneuvers. You should not fly until you are quite sure of the cause of the problem and can avoid a recurrence.

C. Unconsciousness for any reason

Any unexplained loss of consciousness is disqualifying. Once the cause is known, it can then be reviewed and a plan worked out that will ensure the risk of a recurrence is very low. If there is a significant chance that it will occur again, it is an unacceptable safety hazard in flight.

What are some causes of sudden loss of consciousness? The following have been identified from an extensive review of the problem:

Pilots experienced sudden loss of consciousness after …

- Physical demands
  - Running
  - Standing for a long period
  - Exercise
  - Sitting
  - Hyperventilating
- Needles
  - Injection
  - Vaccination
  - Blood drawn
- Low blood flow
  - High G stress
  - Bowel movement
  - Valsalva maneuver
  - Coughing
  - Urinating
- Emotional shock
  - Threat
  - Questioning

In the week before an unexplained loss of consciousness, the pilot had …

Cold or flu symptoms
Family members with cold or flu symptoms
Stomach or intestinal symptoms
High alcohol intake
Dieted with weight loss
Depression
Insomnia
Used over-the-counter medications
Insufficient sleep
Traveled recently
An emotional event (e.g., death, divorce)

Most of these involve either fatigue or a temporary physical condition with low blood flow, and could be avoided with proper rest and stress management.

Although this survey did not show examples of more serious causes of loss of consciousness, these must be considered before the pilot can take up flight duties. Typically, a medical evaluation will include a blood test, an ECG, and perhaps an EEG (electroencephalogram). If there is a possibility of a risk of seizures, both awake and sleep-deprived EEGs may be done, or a 24-hour EEG.

Head injury

Loss of consciousness from a head injury (a concussion) must be considered carefully. Forget the movie scenes in which someone gets whacked on the head, knocked out, then comes to after a few minutes and goes back into action as if nothing had happened. Real life is not like that. Head injuries that involve a disturbance of consciousness are very serious and may cause symptoms for months or years afterward.

A blow to the head (even when there may be no cuts or bruises) can result in poor concentration, increased irritability, headaches, vertigo, and behavioral changes. This is known as the post-concussive or post-traumatic syndrome. It can last for a shorter or longer time, and requires a neurological evaluation before the pilot can return to flight.

Head injuries can also result in more permanent problems, such as loss of muscular function, impaired thinking, or difficulty speaking or understanding language. Seizures are a common feature of severe head injury, and they can occur at the time of the injury, weeks later, or many years later. Research has shown that 12 percent of patients with a severe head injury experienced epilepsy requiring anticonvulsant medication up to five years after the incident.

On the positive side, pilots can be certified despite head injuries. The FAA requires a thorough neurological evaluation to show that there is no hazard to safety. It recommends that pilots have at least a one-year recovery period after a severe head injury before resuming duties, and the same is true for a single post-traumatic seizure within 24 hours of any head injury. A seizure that occurred more than 24 hours after the injury requires four years of being free of further symptoms and off medication; two or more seizures later than 24 hours after the injury might require ten years of observation before flying duties can be resumed. Overall, medical certification after a head injury depends on its severity and whether there were seizures or other symptoms after the injury.

D. Eye or vision trouble

The number one concern of most pilots is their eyes. Vision provides 90 percent of your sensory perception for flight—knowing where you are, what the airplane is doing, and what is going on outside the airplane. When it comes down to it, an instrument pilot has to learn to ignore almost all the other senses. Your inner ears and the rest of your body might tell you that you are climbing or turning, but if the instruments indicate that you are in a dive, you trust them, and that means using your eyes. Of all the sense organs, the eyes are also the most likely to be affected by fatigue, hypoxia, dehydration, and other physiological problems.

The eyes have it
Vision is the first thing to go when the brain is impaired. Right on the edge of consciousness, it is an odd feeling to experience a "gray out" or "black out" but still be able to hear and smell and have touch sensations.

By far the most common visual problem—one that almost everyone eventually experiences with aging—is being able to focus the eyes. Currently, about 160 million Americans, 55 percent of the total population, are dependent upon corrective lenses to achieve satisfactory vision. In general, this involves an adjustment for nearsightedness, farsightedness, or astigmatism.

The eye focuses light in three ways, using the cornea (at the front surface of the eye), the lens (behind the pupil), and the shape of the eyeball itself (which normally focuses light on the retina at the back). Only the lens can change shape, to actively focus light. The cornea and eyeball are fixed—although, as described below, more and more people are choosing to change the shape of the cornea through surgery to improve their eyesight.

Nearsightedness (myopia) is the most common visual acuity problem. When you are nearsighted, close objects are in focus but distant vision is out of focus. This is because the shape of the eyeball is somewhat flatter than normal, so that distant light doesn't focus on the retina. A temporary type of nearsightedness is space myopia (also called empty field myopia) which can occur when there are no distant objects on which to focus. This can happen when flying at night or in cloud. The result is that there is nothing distant to look at and the eye lens tends to go into a resting state, focusing somewhere between near and far. When you do suddenly need to focus, it might take an uncomfortably long moment to readjust. To prevent this, it is a good habit to occasionally look at something outside the cockpit, such as a wing tip.

Farsightedness (hyperopia) is typically a problem among older people, which is to say, older than about thirty. They are the ones who read a newspaper at arm's length, and can see things in the distance just fine. The lens naturally stiffens with aging, and this cause of farsightedness (presbyopia) eventually affects almost everyone.

Just about the time you can finally afford to buy an airplane, you begin to have trouble focusing on the instrument panel.

With age, there is also a gradual decrease in the amount of light passing through the lens. For this reason, older pilots may have 20/20 vision but still need reading glasses, especially for fine print.

Astigmatism is an irregular curvature of the lens and cornea that distorts focus. For example, a vertical light pole might be in focus but horizontal power lines out of focus. It affects people at any age.

All of these conditions are typically resolved with corrective lenses and pose no problem for medical certification.

Other eye conditions that affect visual acuity are disqualifying until they can be evaluated and determined not to be a safety hazard for flight. Nystagmus is the jerky eye movement seen with some types of dizziness, drug use, or illness. If you have had nystagmus for a number of years, without any change, you may be able to get a medical certificate if you can show that it does not affect your visual acuity and can tolerate low light conditions and acceleration.

Any new changes in vision, such as unusual sensitivity to light, eye injuries, illness or surgery, must be evaluated before flying. Many other illnesses can also affect eyesight, such as diabetes.

Finally, alcohol has a tremendous influence on vision. Most pilots know that eyesight is not the best after a few drinks, but they may be surprised to learn, too, that alcohol can cause a decrease in visual acuity hours after feeling otherwise sober.

Visual acuity requirements

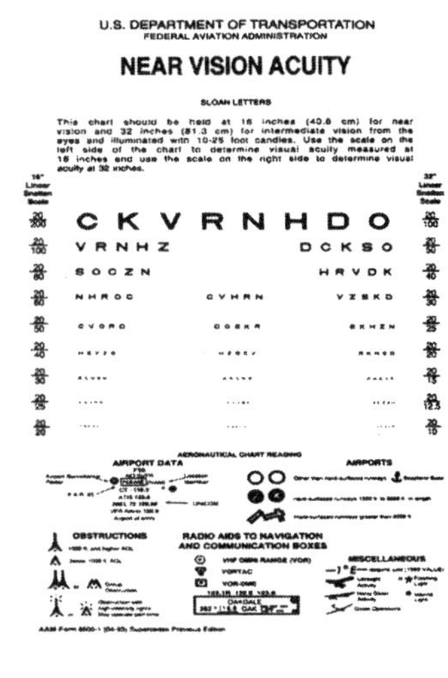

Healthy vision is usually written as 20/20, meaning that you can see at a distance of 20 feet what a person with good vision should be able to see at 20 feet. (Elsewhere in the world, the metric system is used and vision is measured at 6 meters, about 20 feet, and normal visual acuity is described as 6/6.) If, at 20 feet, you can only make out letters of a size that should be seen at 30 feet, your vision is 20/30. If you can only make out huge letters that should be discernable at 200 feet, your vision is 20/200 and you are legally blind.

It is not unusual for pilots, especially younger ones, to have exceptionally good vision—20/10, or even 20/8. This is still no contest to some hawks, which can resolve detail about three times as far. For us to have the same visual acuity, we would need to have eyeballs the size of grapefruit.

The visual acuity requirements for first-class and second-class medical certificates are the same, and require that you be able to see 20/20 or better in each eye, with or without corrective lenses, for distant vision. For near vision, measured at 16 inches, the standard is 20/40. If you are 50 years of age or over, you will also be tested for intermediate vision (at 32 inches), and need to be 20/40 or better in each eye.

For a third-class medical certificate, you need to be able to see 20/40 or better in each eye, with or without correction for distance and near vision. There is no intermediate vision requirement.

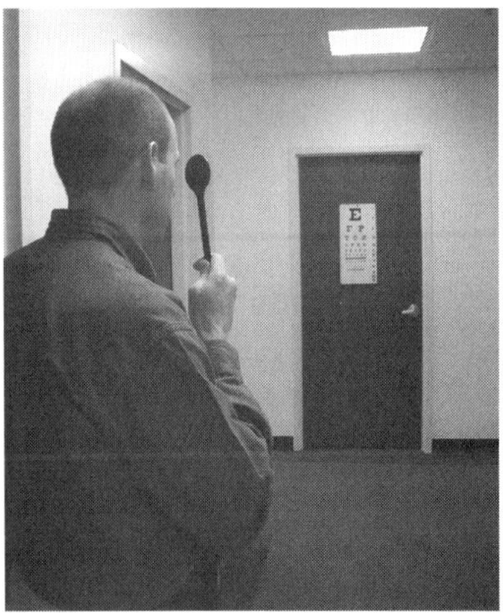

It does not really matter what your vision is without corrective lenses, so long as it meets the standard *with or without* corrective lenses. Your AME will probably check your uncorrected vision anyway, to see what it is. If you need corrective lenses to meet the visual acuity requirement, your medical certificate will show this in the limitations box.

If your eyes are not completely coordinated—if you have double vision, "lazy eye," strabismus ("wall-eye") or other such problems—the AME will defer your medical certificate until your condition can be further evaluated by an eye specialist.

Applications for a second-class or first-class medical certificate will require a test for heterophoria. This condition is somewhat like strabismus, a disorder in which the orientation of the eyes is not well matched. The difference is that strabismus cannot be adjusted by the eye, while heterophoria automatically adjusts when the person focuses on an object. The automatic adjustment still takes some effort, however, and double vision may occur when the person is fatigued or suffering from lack of oxygen. Even if you have heterophoria (measured as greater than 1 prism diopter of hyperphoria, 6 prism diopters of esophoria, or 6 prism diopters of exophoria) you may be certified if you show no sign of double vision or other eye problems.

Eyeglasses and contacts

If you use corrective lenses, either glasses or contacts, the limitations box on your medical certificate will state: HOLDER SHALL WEAR CORRECTIVE LENSES. The statement may be more specific; for example, if the problem is farsightedness, the limitation might be, HOLDER SHALL POSSESS GLASSES THAT CORRECT FOR NEAR VISION.

Is it better to wear eyeglasses rather than contacts? I've heard that contacts are not allowed.

Many pilots prefer frame eyeglasses, but contacts generally give better peripheral vision. The FAA allows the use of contact lenses for correction of far vision only. If you need corrective lenses for near vision, you must have eyeglasses available—but you don't actually have to wear them; you just need to have them handy. This restriction seems to be a holdover from a time when contacts were new and not as reliable as eyeglasses. There is no official record of any accident or incident caused by the use of contact lenses.

In any case, most flight physicians recommend that all pilots who wear contacts or glasses should have an extra set of eyeglasses in their flight bag. Not everyone agrees with this recommendation. To begin with, the chance of losing both contacts is slim, and if you lost one you would have to remove the other one before using your backup glasses. Furthermore, pilots who usually wear contacts have corneal molding to the lenses and cannot easily switch to glasses. You should use your own judgment on this, and try to prepare for possible problems with your corrective lenses.

If you need corrective lenses for both near and distant vision, the limitation will state: HOLDER SHALL WEAR LENSES THAT CORRECT FOR DISTANT VISION AND POSSESS GLASSES THAT CORRECT FOR NEAR VISION. Note again that you can wear either contacts or glasses, but you have to have the frame glasses handy.

The solution for most pilots is to use contact lenses to correct for distant vision, and a pair of glasses dangling around the neck for near vision.

Bifocal glasses have the top part ground for distant vision and the bottom part for near vision. As visual acuity deteriorates with age, it may be necessary to correct for intermediate vision as well, so that you need trifocals. The limitation for this combined defect is: HOLDER SHALL WEAR LENSES THAT CORRECT FOR DISTANT VISION AND POSSESS GLASSES THAT CORRECT FOR NEAR AND INTERMEDIATE VISION. In other words, bifocal contact lenses are OK only if they also correct for distant vision. They are not acceptable if they correct only for near or intermediate vision.

Frame glasses are needed for near or intermediate vision, but possession only is required, because it may be hazardous to have distant vision obscured by the continuous wearing of reading glasses.

What about using one lens in one eye to correct for distant vision, and another lens in the other eye to correct for near vision? That would solve the problem, wouldn't it?

The use of monovision contact lenses (wearing a lens in one eye to correct for distance and a lens in the other eye to correct for near vision) is definitely not acceptable. You are now effectively using only one eye, while the brain ignores input from the other eye because it is out of focus. This combination actually caused an airline accident in 1996.

Sunglasses

Bright light is hard on the eyes, causing eye strain, fatigue, inflammation, and eventually leading to cataracts. Pilots are encouraged to use high-quality sunglasses in bright daylight. If you normally wear corrective lenses, you should get prescription sunglasses. These should not be the only glasses available, however. Sunglasses should not be used in low light conditions. Because they reduce the amount of light by about 85 percent, they cause the pupil to open to bring in more light. The open pupil changes the depth of field, and the eye's ability to focus. For this reason, some pilots will take off their sunglasses even in bright light while landing or maneuvering on the ground.

Cheap sunglasses are made of plastic and scratch easily. You should avoid them and use sunglasses made of glass or polycarbonate. The current standard for sunglasses, ranging from about $15 to $300, is polycarbonate. Glass sunglasses are less common and can be found in the upper half of this range. They are a little heavier than polycarbonate, but have slightly better optics. Standard crown glass has always been thought to give the clearest and least distorted vision.

Glasses that automatically darken in bright light should not be used, because light conditions can change quickly and these glasses don't adjust fast enough. They also tend to block less than 50 percent of light transmission, compared with about 85 percent for high-quality sunglasses.

Should I get polarized sunglasses?

Polarizing sunglasses transmit only light vibrating in a certain direction and absorb light oscillating in other directions. They are not neutral, since they pass more light of certain wavelengths than of others. Polarized lenses are great for glare—light reflected from shiny surfaces such as water, snow, and sand or buildings—since reflected light is itself polarized. They are a godsend for sailing, skiing, and riding a camel through the

Sahara. Flying is a bit different. The problem is that unless you are in an open cockpit, you are seeing light that has come through the windshield, which is usually a plastic laminate with polarizing features. The result is a distortion of the image.

Polarizing lenses have an additional disadvantage. They are made by sandwiching a hermoplastic film matrix of herapthite crystals between layers of glass or plastic. The lamination makes it expensive to produce high-quality curved lenses. Even the best tend to get warped or distorted, especially if they get hot.

What color of sunglasses is best?

Aviation sunglasses should be a toneless color, such as neutral gray. Yellow or amber glasses (blue-blockers) may make it easier to see through fog or haze, but their use has been questioned because they block the blue light used in many panel displays. Ideally, you want as little color distortion as possible. Save the pink lenses for the ski slopes.

Glare

Glare is caused by a large difference in brightness between parts of the visual field. The eyes might be adapted for the darker areas and then irritated by the brighter objects. Snow reflects back 85 to 90 percent of the light falling on it, and white sand, coral, and white clouds may reflect as much as 75 to 80 percent. Grass and forests reflect as little as 10 percent of the light.

Glare is a particular problem for pilots because it usually takes place in the lower field of vision. The human eye is accustomed to see light above and dark below. When, for example, flying above a bright snowfield or cloud layer, the pilot can experience hazy vision and the cockpit panel itself might seem to be in shadow to the degree that instruments are hard to read. White light is considered best to counteract this problem.

Night vision

Adaptation to the dark is a gradual process, taking about 20 to 30 minutes in total darkness for maximal sensitivity. On the other hand, exposure to bright light quickly bleaches the retina, with a complete loss of dark adaptation within 10 seconds. Therefore, it is best to avoid exposure to bright light at night.

The greatest problem affecting night vision is hypoxia (discussed in detail in *Chapter 5: Using oxygen*), and you should make sure you have supplementary oxygen if you need it. There are several other ways to preserve your night vision. As the evening darkens, turn down the cockpit lights, keeping them just bright enough to be clearly seen. Low-level white light is the best. Many pilots use red light in the cockpit (or red goggles) because it preserves dark vision better, but red light also makes it more difficult to shift the focus from near to far vision, and it masks red-colored objects, instrument markings, and maps. Some pilots, if they know a brief exposure to bright light is unavoidable, will cover one eye to preserve its dark adaptation and let the other eye take the hit. This is not really an ideal solution, but can help in a pinch. If you do this, of course, you have only one useful eye, so cover your dominant eye.

Finding your dominant eye
Reach out and point up your thumb. Look at it and then allow your gaze to go to the horizon. Now you will notice a double image of your thumb. One will be a little stronger or more distinct than the other. Your dominant eye is the opposite of the stronger image—for example, if the left one of the double image is stronger, you are right eye dominant.

Color vision

True color blindness is a very rare condition, but many people have some degree of color deficiency. About seven percent of males have some difficulty discriminating red and green. This is an inherited and permanent condition. (The gene for this trait is on the X chromosome; therefore males, with one X chromosome, have a greater chance of color deficiency than females, who have two X chromosomes.)

Other types of color deficiency can be due to aging (as the lens or cornea of the eye becomes discolored), to cataracts, and to drug use (e.g, Viagra). More severe color visual problems can be caused by diseases of the eye, poisoning by lead or alcohol, and from multiple sclerosis or brain injury. These often affect one eye only, whereas genetic color deficiency generally affects both eyes.

Finally, color vision loss is most often caused by hypoxia.

I was told I had red-green color blindness, but I'm sure I can distinguish red and green lights.

Most people with red-green color deficiency can still make out strong red and green lights, such as those used in color light signals. This is the distinction between color deficiency and color blindness. True color blindness is quite rare. If you can show that you can distinguish airport lights, you can be certified.

Why is color vision important? I'm color blind but I can fly just fine.

You might be able to get away with it, since you can use other cues to substitute for color. For example, you might just go by the position of the marker beacon rather than its color, in the same way that color-blind drivers know that the red traffic light is on top and green is at the bottom. However, this deficiency may catch you at a bad moment, and you should be aware of it. Color vision in aviation is needed for:

1. Runway lights (active runway, taxiways, approach lights, and VASI) are in color, and unless you know the airport very well, the specific colors may be the only way to tell them apart.

2. Tower light signals are red and green, indicating the status of the airport.

3. Emergency light signals are red and green.

4. Navigation charts are in color.

5. Increasingly, high-tech cockpits rely on colors in complex instruments.

Actually, "normal" color vision is not a requirement for flying. What is required is, "...the ability to perceive those colors necessary for safe performance of airman duties." In other words, it doesn't really matter what your perception of color is, so long as you can distinguish the major colors used in actual piloting performance. This allows quite a lot of flexibility for pilots to show they can fly safely despite some degree of color deficiency. The standard test for color vision is by reading the numbers on a set of pictures composed of colored dots. This simple test (the Ishihara color plates) is pretty good at detecting color deficiency. Some people might have difficulty making out the numbers because of the lighting in the exam room. If that is the case, you can ask to read the numbers in direct sunlight.

If you do not pass this test, you have several options:

1. You can accept that you are color deficient. This will result in a limitation on your medical certificate that states: NOT VALID FOR NIGHT FLYING OR BY COLOR SIGNAL CONTROL.

2. You can take any of about 15 other tests that are approved by the FAA to check color vision. If you can pass just one of these tests, you may be issued a medical certificate without the night flying restrictions.

   a. The color threshold test uses colored lights at varying intensities. It may show that you are color deficient but meet the criteria for safety. This test is normally done only in the military, and may be difficult to find, but the FAA will accept its results if you can pass the test.

b. The Farnsworth lantern test (FALANT) uses a color light signal. It is also normally found only in the military, but if you can pass it, the results are acceptable to the FAA.

c. An ophthalmologist or optometrist may recommend another color test. Again, if you can pass it, and send the results to the FAA, there is a good chance you will be issued a certificate without color vision limitations.

3. A last resort is to take a color signal light test at an FAA control tower. (This may be the easiest solution if you happen to be based at an airport with a Flight Standards District Office. For more information on FSDOs, see *Appendix I: Further Information.*) The test is given by an FAA inspector. Passing this test will allow the issuance of a Statement of Demonstrated Ability (SODA—see *Chapter 3*), which will also remove the night flying restriction. Practically speaking, the test involves a flight in which you observe the lights flashed from the tower, either while in the air or while stationed at the end of the runway. The inspector will also ask you to read color aeronautical charts. It is important to note that you can only take this test twice. If you fail the color light signal test a second time, you will have the color vision limitations on your medical certificate, and you will not be allowed to use an alternative color vision test. That is why this test is the last resort.

A 48-year-old commercial pilot with 1,750 hours was flying a Beech 18 on instruments at night. To climb above a patch of nasty weather, he climbed to 12,500 and was there for 20 minutes, without oxygen, before returning to 10,000 feet. During his descent, the Receiver Autonomous Integrity Monitoring System (RAIMS) red warning light came on, indicating that his GPS signal had been lost. The pilot was confused by the warning light because it looked "different" to him, and he figured it must mean something else. He motored on, missed his assigned waypoint, and eventually strayed six miles off the airway.

Back on the ground, after getting chewed out by ATC, he discovered what went wrong. His color vision was satisfactory, but he smoked a pack of cigarettes per day and therefore had a lower tolerance for hypoxia (see *Chapter 5: Using oxygen,* and *Smoking,* for more on this)—resulting in a loss of color vision and not recognizing the red warning light.

I'm a little worried about the light signal test. How can I prepare for it?

Call the Aerospace Medical Certification Division in Oklahoma City and request an authorization for the color signal light test. Tell them which FSDO you intend to visit. The FAA will send you an authorization letter and a copy to that facility. After you receive the letter, which is valid for 90 days, call the FSDO and schedule the test.

Then, you should visit the airport and ask the tower controller to flash the color signals in your direction so that you can get a little practice. Have someone with you who has "normal" color vision to confirm that you can correctly identify the colors.

For your actual test, the best time is during late afternoon, or on a cloudy day. It is more difficult to see the lights at midday, when the sun is directly overhead.

Will this work for a first-class medical as well?

Not quite. The light signal test will give you a SODA valid for third or second-class certificates. If you initially had a third-class certificate when you got the SODA, it will usually be upgraded to a second-class without having to take the light signal test again.

For a first-class certificate, the test is more stringent. A medical flight test (check ride) must be successfully completed at various times of day and must include visual verification of the VASI, runways and taxiways, and tower lights, etc.

Can't I use some sort of glasses that correct for color?

Negative. "Color vision correcting" lenses (for example, X-Chrom) are not allowed by the FAA for correcting color vision deficiencies.

Macular degeneration

Macular degeneration is a gradual deterioration of the retina at the back of the eye. In the United States it is one of most common causes of blindness in older people, but it can occur at any age. The visual loss usually affects both eyes, although occasionally just one is involved. It begins with a small blind spot in the center of vision, which may increase until only the peripheral vision remains. The ability to judge distance is not affected.

Severe cases of macular degeneration are disqualifying, but if the defect is small, it is possible to get a third-class medical certificate with a SODA if you can show that you can fly safely. You will need a detailed examination by an ophthalmologist who can support your application.

If the condition is in only one eye, you may also qualify under the monocular vision requirement (see below, *One-eyed pilots*). The opposite eye should not have any illness or defects.

Eye surgery

Eye surgery has become increasingly popular as a way to restore good vision. In 2000, more than 1 million laser procedures were carried out in the United States, and this number is expected to grow rapidly in the next few years. For as little as $300 per eye, according to advertisements, you can get 20/20 vision and throw away those thick glasses forever. Unfortunately, the truth is not quite so simple.

The cornea of the eye is the primary light-focusing surface, and small changes in the curvature of the cornea can cause the focus of light inside the eye to shift forward or backward. If the cornea is made flatter, it causes a backward shift of the focus, which is needed by the nearsighted eye. On the other hand, an increase in the curve of the cornea shifts the focus forward, which helps correct the farsighted eye. Since it is easier to make the cornea flatter than to increase its curve, surgery is more commonly done for nearsightedness.

Presbyopia is a type of farsightedness that is caused by a gradual stiffening of the lens, usually beginning around age 45, and therefore cannot be corrected by surgery.

There are many types of corrective eye surgery, and new variations are appearing almost every year. Currently, the FAA has approved the following types of surgery:

- *RK* (radial keratotomy) changes the corneal curvature by making radial partial-thickness cuts in the surface. This was the first popular corrective eye surgery, but it has fallen out of favor as other, better techniques have become available.

- *CK* (conductive keratoplasty) uses short bursts of radio waves to heat and shrink the collagen fibers in the periphery of the cornea, changing its shape and (hopefully) improving focus. A hair-thin probe is used to target up to 32 sites on each cornea. The contraction of the collagen fibers has a purse-string effect that tightens the cornea's curvature. The whole process usually takes less than a minute, but the final improvement might not appear for several months. CK may result in astigmatism because of the many spots targeted, each of which may react differently.

- *LTK* (laser thermal keratoplasty) also works by heating and shrinking fibers in the peripheral cornea, but it uses a laser beam directed on the surface of the eye. It has several advantages over CK: there are no probes, so nothing touches the cornea, and only 16 spots are treated per eye. The whole process takes place in less than three seconds.

- *PRK* (photorefractive keratoplasty) reshapes the surface of the cornea.

- *LASIK* (laser-assisted in situ keratomileusis) cuts and folds back a flap of the cornea, reshapes the undersurface, and the replaces the flap,

without touching the highly sensitive surface of the cornea. This has become the procedure of choice for most pilots.

Which type of corrective eye surgery do pilots prefer?

LASIK is currently by far the most popular because the recovery time is shorter, there is less discomfort, and fewer complications than with the other techniques. For example, because PRK involves the delicate outer surface of the cornea, it is five times more likely to cause an infection, and 10 to 20 times more likely to cause corneal scarring. On the other hand, LASIK surgery itself has an increased risk of some complications, since it requires a corneal flap to expose the corneal tissue.

Many ophthalmologists recommend CK or LTK for pilots because these techniques are less invasive than LASIK and there are fewer potential side-effects. But if you also have astigmatism, or your farsightedness is greater than 3.0 diopters, LASIK is probably the procedure of choice.

Eye surgery risks

Between 95 and 99 percent of those who have had eye surgery are satisfied, but that leaves up to 5 percent who are not—thousands of people who suffered bad outcomes, ranging from discomfort to blindness. Consider these results before you plan on surgery:

- Overtreatment or undertreatment—you may need more than one surgery.
- With age-related farsightedness (presbyopia)—you may still need reading glasses.
- You may develop visual symptoms—glare, halos, starbursts, etc., preventing night driving.
- You may lose contrast sensitivity—vision could be reduced in dim light.

Will my airline allow me to act as pilot after this surgery?

It depends. Most air carriers have permitted corrective eye surgery for their pilots. Active duty and reserve military pilots do not have this permission at present, and are disqualified after the surgery.

The recovery time after any eye surgery typically lasts from one to six months. Before you can be medically certified, the FAA will want know that there has been a complete recovery and stabilization, with no adverse effects or complications—and, of course, that you have satisfactory vision. When recovery is final, your eye care specialist should complete the Report of Eye Evaluation (FAA Form 8500-7). At the time of your next scheduled FAA medical examination, you should bring this form to give to your AME.

The Report of Eye Evaluation must verify complete healing, stabilization of visual acuity, and lack of significant residual effects that often accompany these types of surgical procedures, including night glare, vision haziness, or eye pain. Complete healing following certain types of refractive surgery is usually accomplished in four to six weeks, but up to 12 months may be necessary in some cases.

Any surgery carries a risk, but eye surgery is particularly worrisome for pilots because it may leave them with visual problems that cause permanent disqualification. These include corneal scarring or opacities, glare, haziness, or another significant worsening of vision. Further treatment or surgery may or may not correct these problems.

Should I have one eye corrected for near vision, and the other for far vision?

Some ophthalmologists recommend that one eye be corrected for near vision and the other for distance. The problem is that this technically results in a person having monocular vision, since at any given distance you only have one eye that is able to focus well (see below, *One-eyed pilots*).

The FAA will allow this option, but requires a six-month period after surgery during which time you must wear eyeglasses or contacts that correct your vision to FAA standards. When you're not flying, remove the corrective lenses so your eyes can adapt to the surgical correction. The six-month period provides the time necessary to learn other visual cues that will re-establish depth perception, just as if you had lost the useful vision in one eye. After six months, you may apply for a SODA to have the corrective lenses restriction removed.

What about cataract surgery?

Any eye surgery is permitted if it results in satisfactory vision. After surgery, you should not fly until the ophthalmologist releases you to resume normal activities and you again meet the vision standard. Ask your ophthalmologist to complete the FAA Report of Eye Evaluation, Form 8500-7, for you to give to your AME at your next medical examination.

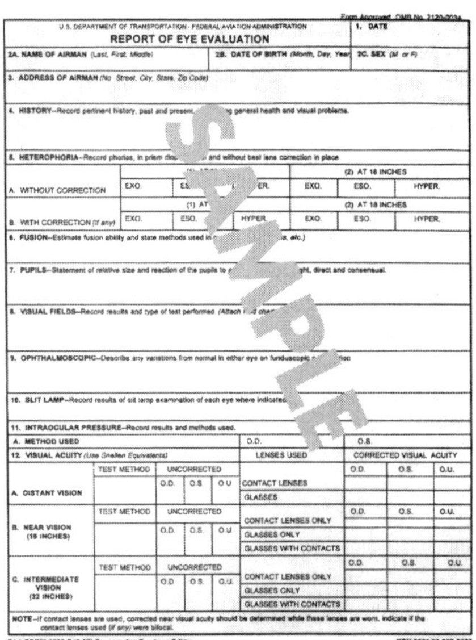

U.S. DEPARTMENT OF TRANSPORTATION - FEDERAL AVIATION ADMINISTRATION

REPORT OF EYE EVALUATION

1. DATE

2A. NAME OF AIRMAN (Last, First, Middle) | 2B. DATE OF BIRTH (Month, Day, Year) | 2C. SEX (M or F)

3. ADDRESS OF AIRMAN (No. Street, City, State, Zip Code)

4. HISTORY--Record pertinent history, past and present, ... general health and visual problems.

5. HETEROPHORIA--Record phorias, in prism dio... and without best lens correction in place.

	(1) AT ...			(2) AT 18 INCHES		
A. WITHOUT CORRECTION	EXO.	ES...	...ER.	EXO.	ESO.	HYPER.
	(1) AT ...			(2) AT 18 INCHES		
B. WITH CORRECTION (If any)	EXO.	ESO.	HYPER.	EXO.	ESO.	HYPER.

6. FUSION--Estimate fusion ability and state methods used in ... s, etc.)

7. PUPILS--Statement of relative size and reaction of the pupils to ... ght, direct and consensual.

8. VISUAL FIELDS--Record results and type of test performed. (Attach ... charts)

9. OPHTHALMOSCOPIC--Describe any variations from normal in either eye on funduscopic ...tion

10. SLIT LAMP--Record results of slit lamp examination of each eye where indicated.

11. INTRAOCULAR PRESSURE--Record results and methods used.

A. METHOD USED	O.D.	O.S.

12. VISUAL ACUITY (Use Snellen Equivalents)					LENSES USED	CORRECTED VISUAL ACUITY		
A. DISTANT VISION	TEST METHOD	UNCORRECTED				O.D.	O.S.	O.U.
		O.D.	O.S.	O.U.	CONTACT LENSES			
					GLASSES			
B. NEAR VISION (16 INCHES)	TEST METHOD	UNCORRECTED				O.D.	O.S.	O.U.
		O.D.	O.S.	O.U.	CONTACT LENSES ONLY			
					GLASSES ONLY			
					GLASSES WITH CONTACTS			
C. INTERMEDIATE VISION (32 INCHES)	TEST METHOD	UNCORRECTED				O.D.	O.S.	O.U.
		O.D.	O.S.	O.U.	CONTACT LENSES ONLY			
					GLASSES ONLY			
					GLASSES WITH CONTACTS			

NOTE--If contact lenses are used, corrected near visual acuity should be determined while these lenses are worn. Indicate if the contact lenses used (if any) were bifocal.

FAA FORM 8500-7 (9-97) Supersedes Previous Edition NSN:0052-00-867-3002

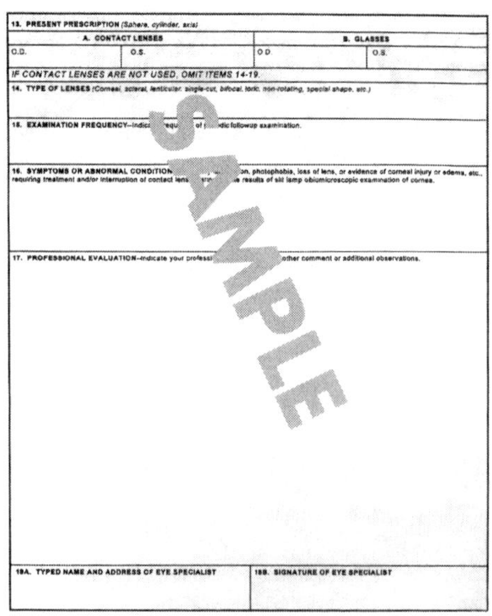

13. PRESENT PRESCRIPTION (Sphere, cylinder, axis)

A. CONTACT LENSES		B. GLASSES	
O.D.	O.S.	O.D.	O.S.

IF CONTACT LENSES ARE NOT USED, OMIT ITEMS 14-19.

14. TYPE OF LENSES (Corneal, scleral, lenticular, single-cut, bifocal, toric, non-rotating, special shape, etc.)

15. EXAMINATION FREQUENCY--Indic... frequ... of p...dic followup examination.

16. SYMPTOMS OR ABNORMAL CONDITION ... on, photophobia, loss of lens, or evidence of corneal injury or edema, etc., requiring treatment and/or interruption of contact lens ... results of slit lamp biomicroscopic examination of cornea.

17. PROFESSIONAL EVALUATION--Indicate your professi... other comment or additional observations.

18A. TYPED NAME AND ADDRESS OF EYE SPECIALIST	18B. SIGNATURE OF EYE SPECIALIST

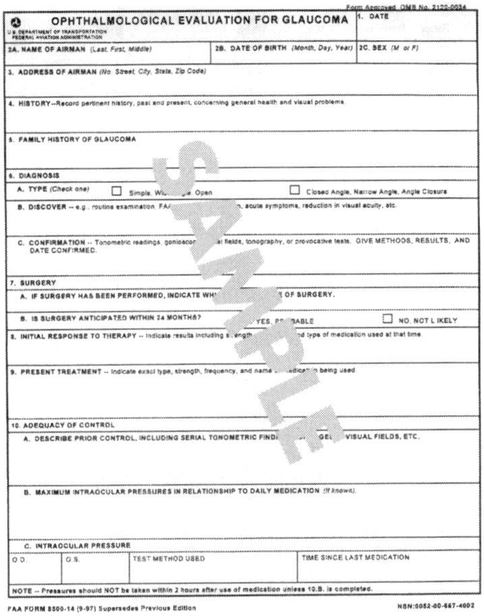

Form Approved OMB No. 2120-0034

U.S. DEPARTMENT OF TRANSPORTATION FEDERAL AVIATION ADMINISTRATION

OPHTHALMOLOGICAL EVALUATION FOR GLAUCOMA

1. DATE

2A. NAME OF AIRMAN *(Last, First, Middle)* | 2B. DATE OF BIRTH *(Month, Day, Year)* | 2C. SEX *(M or F)*

3. ADDRESS OF AIRMAN *(No. Street, City, State, Zip Code)*

4. HISTORY--Record pertinent history, past and present, concerning general health and visual problems.

5. FAMILY HISTORY OF GLAUCOMA

6. DIAGNOSIS

A. TYPE *(Check one)* ☐ Simple, Wi[illegible] Open ☐ Closed Angle, Narrow Angle, Angle Closure

B. DISCOVER -- e.g., routine examination, FA[illegible], acute symptoms, reduction in visual acuity, etc.

C. CONFIRMATION -- Tonometric readings, goniosco[illegible] fields, tonography, or provocative tests. GIVE METHODS, RESULTS, AND DATE CONFIRMED.

7. SURGERY

A. IF SURGERY HAS BEEN PERFORMED, INDICATE WH[illegible] OF SURGERY.

B. IS SURGERY ANTICIPATED WITHIN 24 MONTHS? YES, P[illegible]BABLE ☐ NO, NOT LIKELY

8. INITIAL RESPONSE TO THERAPY -- Indicate results including s[illegible] and type of medication used at that time.

9. PRESENT TREATMENT -- Indicate exact type, strength, frequency, and name [illegible] being used.

10. ADEQUACY OF CONTROL

A. DESCRIBE PRIOR CONTROL, INCLUDING SERIAL TONOMETRIC FIND[illegible] VISUAL FIELDS, ETC.

B. MAXIMUM INTRAOCULAR PRESSURES IN RELATIONSHIP TO DAILY MEDICATION *(If known).*

C. INTRAOCULAR PRESSURE

O.D.	O.S.	TEST METHOD USED	TIME SINCE LAST MEDICATION

NOTE -- Pressures should NOT be taken within 2 hours after use of medication unless 10.B. is completed.

FAA FORM 8500-14 (9-97) Supersedes Previous Edition NSN:0052-00-667-4002

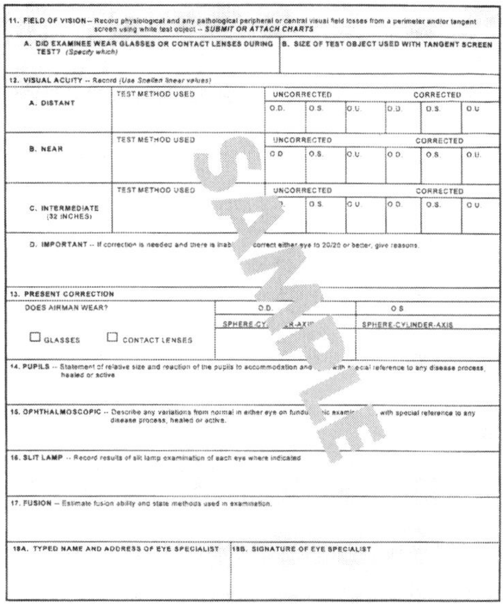

11. FIELD OF VISION-- Record physiological and any pathological peripheral or central visual field losses from a perimeter and/or tangent screen using white test object -- *SUBMIT OR ATTACH CHARTS*

A. DID EXAMINEE WEAR GLASSES OR CONTACT LENSES DURING TEST? *(Specify which)* | B. SIZE OF TEST OBJECT USED WITH TANGENT SCREEN

12. VISUAL ACUITY -- Record *(Use Snellen linear values)*

	TEST METHOD USED	UNCORRECTED			CORRECTED		
		O.D.	O.S.	O.U.	O.D.	O.S.	O.U.
A. DISTANT							
B. NEAR							
C. INTERMEDIATE (32 INCHES)							

D. IMPORTANT -- If correction is needed and there is inab[illegible] correct either eye to 20/20 or better, give reasons.

13. PRESENT CORRECTION

DOES AIRMAN WEAR? ☐ GLASSES ☐ CONTACT LENSES

O.D.	O.S.
SPHERE-CY[illegible]R-AXI[illegible]	SPHERE-CYLINDER-AXIS

14. PUPILS -- Statement of relative size and reaction of the pupils to accommodation and [illegible] with s[illegible]ecial reference to any disease process, healed or active

15. OPHTHALMOSCOPIC -- Describe any variations from normal in either eye on fundu[illegible] examin[illegible], with special reference to any disease process, healed or active.

16. SLIT LAMP -- Record results of slit lamp examination of each eye where indicated

17. FUSION -- Estimate fusion ability and state methods used in examination.

18A. TYPED NAME AND ADDRESS OF EYE SPECIALIST | 18B. SIGNATURE OF EYE SPECIALIST

Glaucoma

Glaucoma is a condition of excessive pressure inside the eyeball, which can lead to worsening of vision or even complete blindness. It can be a painless condition, which may not be noted until the eyes are specifically tested for it. Glaucoma affects two to three percent of the general population and accounts for about 15 percent of blindness in the United States. Open angle glaucoma—the typically painless, unnoticeable kind—accounts for 85 percent of all cases.

Applicants with open angle glaucoma may be certified if they have an ophthalmologic evaluation showing that pressures are under control, that there is little or no visual field loss or other complications, and they tolerate small to moderate doses of allowed medications. Some of these medications cause a constriction of the pupil and may interfere with night vision. Although the FAA no longer routinely prohibits pilots who use these medications from flying at night, it is up to the pilot to make sure that medication does not present a risk to flying. If the AME is concerned, the medical certificate may be issued with the limitation: NOT VALID FOR NIGHT FLYING.

Applicants with other types of glaucoma may also be certified, but require more extensive evaluation.

One-eyed pilots

The reason we have two eyes is for stereo vision, allowing depth perception. With only one eye, depth cannot be perceived and distance must be guessed by familiarity with the size of objects.

Good depth perception was once considered to be important for pilots. There is no longer a requirement for this test, and about 5,000 one-eyed pilots have been certified in United States. A pilot is considered to have monocular vision (in effect, to be legally blind in one eye) if the best-corrected central visual acuity in one eye is 20/200 or worse.

Pilots with satisfactory vision in only one eye may obtain medical certification after showing they can fly safely. This requires a Report of Eye Evaluation (FAA Form 8500-7) after an evaluation by an eye care specialist.

After vision has been lost in one eye, a recovery period of at least six months is needed to adjust to one-eyed vision. During this recovery period, the applicant may get a medical permit with the limitation: VALID FOR STUDENT PILOT PRIVILEGES ONLY, and may not engage in solo flight.

After six months, a medical flight test can be taken to obtain a SODA for monocular vision, and an unrestricted medical certificate can be issued.

Laser blindness

An airline pilot was landing at night. On the long approach, he noticed a green light sweeping back and forth across the sky. While looking outside the cockpit to initiate a turn, the green light flashed again, directly in his face. The pilot immediately felt a sharp pain in his left eye and was blinded. He gave control to the other pilot, who landed the aircraft. By the time they taxied to the terminal, his pain was gone and vision had returned, leaving his eye reddened and feeling gritty.

It was discovered that a powerful laser used for an outdoor light show had flash-blinded the pilot. He recovered fully a few days later.

E. Hay fever or allergy

About nine percent of Americans suffer from pollen allergies, with sneezing, runny nose, and burning eyes. Pilots with these symptoms are more affected by changes in pressure, visual disturbances, and other distractions. You definitely do not want to have a sneezing fit while on final approach in instrument flight conditions.

In general, allergies are not disqualifying unless they are very severe or require medications that interfere with the pilot's performance. If your certification is deferred to the FAA, you may get a letter with approval and the limitation: NOT VALID FOR 24 HOURS AFTER EXPERIENCING SYMPTOMS OR USING ANTIHISTAMINE MEDICATION.

You may fly if your allergies are not affecting your performance, and controlled only by desensitization injections, homeopathy, or other methods that do not require antihistamine medications.

Decongestants

A major problem with allergies is the nasal stuffiness that accompanies the inflammation. When the small openings to the sinuses are blocked, you can suffer from even slight pressure changes, especially during descent. Many pilots carry a nasal spray decongestant in their flight bag just in case they have this symptom. A useful, fast-acting, decongestant spray is Afrin (oxymetazoline). It works so well that some pilots use it regularly and come to depend on it—which is a mistake. Overuse of Afrin causes fast heart rate, high blood pressure, nervousness and tremor, poor coordination, and dilation of the eyes resulting in discomfort with bright light and difficulty focusing. The worst effect, however, is a rebound type of runny nose—a condition called rhinitis medicamentosa—that will not resolve with further medication. If this occurs, you need to stop using Afrin entirely for a few days until your body recovers.

Severe sinusitis or obstruction of the sinuses is disqualifying. Before resuming flight, you need to have this condition treated by medication or perhaps sinus surgery.

Antihistamines

Histamines are components in the blood that react to foreign substances. It is this reaction that produces the symptoms of allergies. Antihistamine medications block histamines. The problem is that these medications also cause drowsiness and sedation, decreased coordination and visual accommodation, dizziness, depression, and may affect the heart.

The first popular antihistamines had a lot of these side-effects. These "first generation" antihistamines, including Benadryl (diphenhydramine), Chlor-Trimeton (chlorpheniramine) and many others, are now quite inexpensive and can be bought without a prescription. The problem is that their side-effects can be quite subtle so that the pilot might not even be aware of them. Poor concentration, for example, is a common side-effect and can last long after the dose, especially if the antihistamine is used regularly.

The newer antihistamines have much fewer of these worrisome side-effects. These "second generation" antihistamines, such as Allegra (fexofenadine) or Claritin (loratadine), penetrate poorly into the brain and therefore cause less drowsiness or diminished concentration. However, even these can cause drowsiness in some people, especially if taken in larger amounts than recommended.

What allergy medications can I use that won't be a problem for flying?

The FAA has approved the following medications, provided the pilot has taken them before and is confident that there will not be problems:

Afrin (oxymetazoline)
Allegra (fexofenadine)
Beconase (beclomethasone dipropionate)
Claritin (loratadine)
Entex (phenylpropanolamine)
Flonase (fluticasone propionate)
Hismanol (astemizole)
Nasalide (flunisolide)
Sudafed (pseudoephedrine)
Vancenase (beclomethasone dipropionate)

With other prescription drugs, your AME will want to see a report from your treating physician including a summary of your condition, a list of the medications, and a statement that you can fly safely with their use. (For a more complete list of allowable medications, see *Chapter 1: Allowable medications.*)

Hives

Hives (urticaria) are a type of allergic response resulting in itchy, red swellings of the skin and lasting for a few minutes to a few hours. Although hives are not disqualifying, the antihistamine used for this condition might be. If you have chronic hives, or hives combined with abdominal pain or diarrhea, your AME may ask for further evaluation to rule out a more serious condition.

Earwax

This doesn't really have to do with allergies, but my ears are often plugged with wax. What can I do about that?

The ear canal naturally secretes a soft wax to help protect it and flush out dust and debris. This wax slowly flows to the outside, where it flakes off or is washed away. Some people produce an excessive amount of wax. This can build up, dry out, and form a solid plug. Impacted earwax (cerumen) is not only a big nuisance and impairs your hearing, it is also disqualifying until removed.

Luckily, removing earwax is quite simple. The worst thing you can do is to try to dig it out using a Q-Tip (or matchstick, toothpick, key, pencil—it's amazing what people will stick into their ears. Didn't your mother ever tell you not to put anything smaller than an elbow into your ear?). Inserting any hard object into the ear just pushes the wax further in, so that it cannot flow out, and carries a substantial risk of perforating the eardrum. The best solution is to use a rubber bulb with warm water to flush out the excess wax. If this is a frequent problem, you may also want to put a few drops in your ears of a solution to soften or dissolve the wax. All of these can be bought without a prescription at any drug store.

F. Asthma or lung disease

Pilots perform their operations in an environment in which changes in pressure, temperature, moisture, and oxygen content occur—often within minutes. Any kind of lung disease is a big concern. Your AME may request additional tests before certification, including a chest X-ray, pulmonary function test, or an evaluation by a lung specialist.

Asthma

Asthma is one of the fastest growing complaints in modern times, affecting almost 10 percent of Americans, and many more who have a milder form of the condition but go untreated. There are many causes of asthma, ranging from air pollution to stress, but why it should be so much more common now is a still a mystery.

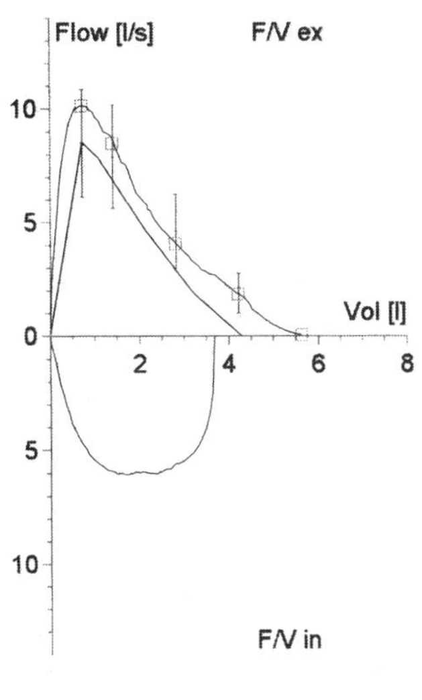

The hallmark of asthma is an inflammation of the airways, especially the small to medium-sized ones, and a greater "twitchiness" of these airways. Both of these features cause the airways to constrict, resulting in wheezing, shortness of breath, and a sense of chest tightness. Many also have a constant cough, and this may even be their only symptom. Some doctors prefer the term "reactive airway disease" for those who have primarily twitchy airways but less inflammation. Military doctors are also hesitant to label a pilot as having asthma, because this will disqualify the pilot. Regardless of the label, however, any form of asthma can be treated and should not be ignored.

Asthma triggers
Allergens (dust, molds, pets, etc.)
Occupational chemicals
Respiratory infections
Food additives
Medications
Cigarette smoke
Stomach acid reflux
Exercise
Cold air
Air pollution
Emotional stress

You can be certified by your AME if your asthma causes only mild or seasonal symptoms. Periodic use of most inhaler medications is also acceptable.

If your asthma is frequent, severe, or has ever resulted in hospitalization, you will need a further evaluation and your application will be deferred to the FAA for review. However, you can still eventually get your medical certificate even with moderate or severe asthma if you can show that your symptoms are well controlled and not likely to pose a hazard to safety. You will need to present a detailed report by a specialist with:

- Recent pulmonary function test results
- Type and dosages of medications required
- Medication side-effects
- Duration of your current therapy
- Nature and severity of any other symptoms
- Details of any hospital or emergency room visits
- Likelihood of having an asthmatic attack.

Even if you do not qualify because of serious concerns, you may be eligible for certification by special issuance (see *Chapter 3: Getting a SODA*), which will allow you to fly with certain restrictions and follow-up evaluations.

Chronic bronchitis and emphysema

Chronic bronchitis and emphysema are forms of chronic obstructive pulmonary disease (COPD), now the fifth most common cause of death in the United States, and a miserable way to go. That's the bad news. The good news, such as it is, is that almost all COPD is due to tobacco smoking—and you can immediately reduce your chances of suffering or dying from this illness simply by avoiding tobacco smoke.

If you already have some degree of chronic bronchitis or emphysema, you will need the same sort of evaluation indicated for asthma. Mild cases are not disqualifying.

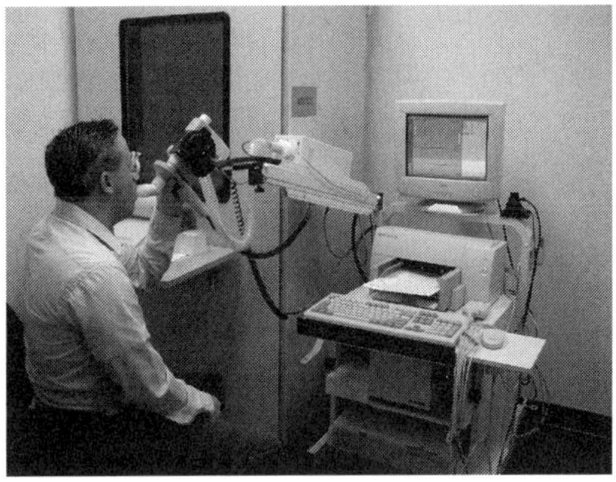

Pulmonary function test

Pneumothorax

Pneumothorax is a condition in which air enters the space just outside the lining of the lungs, causing pain and shortness of breath, and ultimately a collapsed lung. There are many causes of this condition, including illness and trauma to the chest. Some athletic individuals—particularly tall, slender young men—can get a spontaneous pneumothorax that may heal by itself and never come back.

If you have ever had a pneumothorax, you will need an X-ray to show that it has completely healed and there is little risk of recurrence. Repeated episodes of pneumothorax are disqualifying until the underlying condition that caused it is corrected, often by surgery. A recovery period of at least three months is needed before you can get your medical certificate. Once your condition is considered to be resolved, there should be no restriction or altitude limitation on your certificate.

G. Heart or vascular trouble

Heart disease and related problems of high blood pressure and other blood vessel disorders are the number one cause of death in the industrialized world. They are also among the most preventable and treatable illnesses. Changing just a few lifestyle habits—better diet, more exercise, not smoking, and routine health maintenance—would add decades to life expectancy and prevent millions of premature deaths each year.

High cholesterol

Your cholesterol level is not tested as part of the aviation physical, and you will never lose your certificate because of it, but high cholesterol is directly or indirectly responsible for many heart and vascular problems and it is very important to be aware of your cholesterol level.

The National Heart, Lung and Blood Institute estimates that 52 to 65 million Americans have excessively high blood cholesterol, and anywhere from 13 to 36 million people should be on cholesterol-lowering medications. Pilots tend to have somewhat better health than the average person, but their age and lifestyle puts them right into the highest risk group for elevated cholesterol.

In 1936, aviator Charles Lindbergh and Alexis Carrel invented a blood perfusion pump that could maintain organs outside the body—a pioneering step that allowed open heart surgery.

Beginning at age 20 and every five years after, you should have a blood test with a lipoprotein profile—total cholesterol, triglycerides, LDL, and HDL. The last of these is considered the "good cholesterol." It is the smallest and hardest of the fat-carrying molecules in the blood, and it works like a scouring pad to dig out the softer, buttery stuff. That is why many heart specialists consider the ratio of total cholesterol to HDL to be the most important number—it shows the balance between bad and good cholesterol.

On the numbers (mg/dL)

	Desirable	*Borderline*	*High risk*
Total cholesterol:	about 200	200-239	240 or over
Triglycerides:	under 150	150-199	200 or over
LDL:	under 100	100-159	160 or over
HDL:	over 60	40-59	under 40
Cholesterol/HDL ratio:	under 3.5 to 1	3.5-5 to 1	over 5 to 1

Where does cholesterol come from? The liver makes about 80 percent of the cholesterol floating around in the blood, and the rest comes from fatty foods. The total therefore depends on how much you make, how much you eat, and your level of physical activity. Luckily, just a small change in these—especially diet and exercise—can bring a significant reduction in blood cholesterol. And for every 1 percent that excessive blood cholesterol is reduced, your risk of heart disease is lowered by 2 percent.

How do I improve my blood cholesterol?

1. Get more exercise.
2. Eat less food containing saturated fat.
3. Eat more whole grains and vegetables.
4. Drink an occasional glass of red wine (the value of this is debatable, but it is a nice excuse to imbibe—after, not before or while, flying).
5. Use cholesterol-lowering medications as needed.

Heart disease

Almost any kind of heart disease is disqualifying. If you have ever had a heart attack (MI, or myocardial infarction), angina, heart valve replacement, a permanent pacemaker, heart transplant, coronary artery disease, or any heart condition that caused symptoms or required treatment, your AME is not allowed to directly give you a medical certificate. That's the bad news. The good news is that you can still get your certificate by special issuance for almost all heart conditions, although it will take a bit of paperwork. You will also have to wait until you have been free of symptoms for at least six months. The FAA has certified thousands of pilots with previous heart disease, including airline pilots requiring first-class medical certificates.

Risk factors for heart disease
Gender (male)
Family history of premature heart disease
Cigarette smoking
High total cholesterol (>200)
High LDL (>150)
Low HDL (<35 mg/dL)
Diabetes mellitus
Hypertension
Severe obesity (more than 30% overweight)
Presence of arteriosclerosis
Sedentary lifestyle
Low fiber intake

If you have ever had heart disease, the FAA will ask for all of your available medical records. The FAA is particularly interested in three things:

1. Your current functional capacity—are you now fit to fly?
2. Are you completely recovered from your heart disease?
3. What is the likelihood that you will experience further trouble?

The FAA will require the following records:

- Hospital and outpatient treatment records:
  These include all records of any hospitalizations (your admission and discharge summary, operative reports, and daily progress notes) and all records of outpatient treatment. It also includes any pathology, diagnostic test, or cardiac catheterization reports.

A statement (within 60 days) from your treating physician, with the following:

- Your motivation to improve your health, the outlook for your condition, and the risk of incapacitation.
- Operational Questionnaire Form 8500-20.
- Medications you use, or have recently used (specifying their type, purpose, dosage, and duration of use). Any important or unusual diet or regular testing you require.
- A cardiovascular evaluation, describing your personal and family history of heart disease, and a general physical examination.
- The ages and health status of your parents and siblings. If they are deceased, their age at death and the cause of death should be included. It should be noted if any near blood relative has had a heart attack, hypertension, diabetes, or disorder of lipid metabolism. Your habits should be described with regard to smoking, drinking, other recreational habits and physical fitness practices. Any functional limitations should be thoroughly described.

The FAA will also require the results of a number of tests. All tests must be done after the six-month waiting period, and within the past six months. If your test results are more than six months old, you will probably have to repeat some or all of them. These tests include:

- Blood test, including fasting blood sugar and lipid panel (cholesterol, triglyceride, HDL, LDL).
- Urinalysis.
- ECG (electrocardiograph), recorded at rest, lying down, standing, during hyperventilation while standing, and during peak exercise and recovery.
- Exercise stress test (also known as a treadmill test, since it is usually done on a treadmill), to determine how your heart performs under a heavy workload. This test increases stress until your heart rate

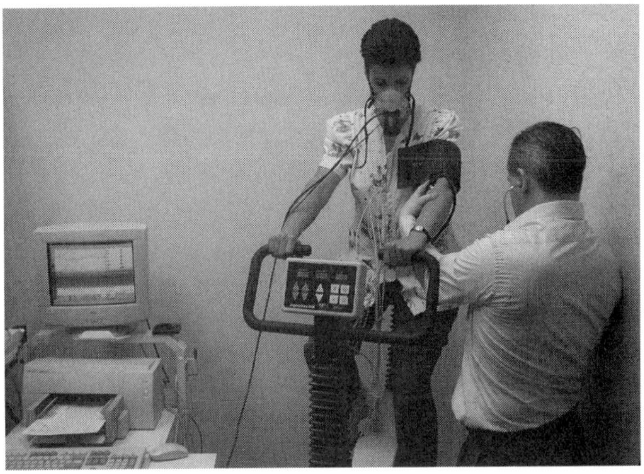

Exercise stress test

approaches your predicted maximum (220 minus your age) for up to nine minutes. If you normally use medications to slow your heart rate, you will be advised not to use them for 48 hours before the test.

If you cannot complete the test because of fatigue, leg cramps, shortness of breath, or chest discomfort, or if the monitor shows high blood pressure or ST segment changes during the test, you will not be considered to have sufficiently recovered to be fit to fly. If the symptoms are mild, the FAA may certify you if you can achieve at least 85 percent of your predicted heart rate.

- Radionuclide stress test may be needed if the exercise stress test results are not clear. This test is similar to the stress test, but also uses an injected dye, such as thallium, to visualize the functioning of your heart and determine whether there is any blockage in its major blood vessels.

- SPECT nuclear cardiology studies may also be done if the ordinary stress test is unclear. These studies use technetium, thallium, cardiolite, or a combination, with sophisticated imaging techniques to detect any heart abnormalities.

- Coronary angiography may be done to examine the major heart blood vessels. For a first- or second-class certificate, you will need coronary angiography and at least one of the radionuclide stress test or SPECT nuclear cardiology studies.

- Echocardiogram (a type of ultrasound, with Doppler color blood flow images) may be done to show blood flow through the heart. This is especially useful for heart valve studies, and it is usually done at rest and within 60 seconds of completion of exercise.

Do you really need all these tests?
Gary Peterson, 55, and a friend bought a 1979 Grumman Cheetah. When Peterson was found to have high blood pressure, the FAA suggested he take a thallium treadmill stress test. Peterson's doctor questioned the need for the test, since it is wrong 25 percent of the time, and costs about $1,400. Would a regular treadmill stress test, at a tenth the cost, be enough? The FAA agreed—but by the time all this paperwork was done, Peterson had to get recertified again.

Irregular heart beat (arrhythmias)

The normal heart beats about 100,000 times a day. A heart that beats too fast (tachyarrhythmia) or too slow (bradyarrhythmia) cannot provide adequate blood flow to the brain and the rest of the body. Even a few seconds of irregular heart beat can cause fainting or other problems. Every year, the Airline Pilots Association (ALPA) reports 5 to 10 pilots who experienced loss of consciousness in the cockpit from this type of heart problem.

Heart rate depends on size
A mouse has a pulse of about 650 beats per minute.
An elephant's heart beats at just 30 beats per minute.
A small person might have a normal rate of 90 beats per minute, while some athletes have an enlarged heart with a resting pulse of 40 or less.

The normal heart rate is considered to be from 60 to 100. Because pilots are often athletic, the USAF chose 50 beats per minute as their baseline. But a slow heart is not always due to athletic conditioning. A good test is hopping up and down for a few minutes. This will cause a normal heart rate to double, or increase to at least 100 beats per minute. If not, you may have heart disease.

Irregular heart beat is generally separated into two categories: those of the atrium (receiving in-coming blood from the body) and those of the ventricle (pumping blood out to the body). In general, the atrial arrhythmias are less worrisome than ventricular arrhythmias.

There are many types of atrial arrhythmias, and they can be due to a wide variety of conditions, including:

hypertension
ischemic heart disease
heart valve disease
cardiomyopathy
congestive heart failure
congenital heart disease
pulmonary embolism

thyrotoxicosis
chronic lung disease
pericarditis
cancer

Normal hearts can also develop arrhythmia from:

alcohol
drugs
caffeine
hypoxia
systemic infection
electrolyte abnormality
stress

Arrhythmia is usually noticed as a palpitation (an awareness of the heart beat, or a sense of a "skipped beat"), but it can also be experienced as weakness, dizziness, shortness of breath, mental confusion, or sudden loss of consciousness.

Ventricular arrhythmias are more worrisome because they prevent blood from adequately reaching the rest of the body. An occasional extra beat (known as a premature ventricular contraction, or PVC) is normal and may be due to stress, caffeine, or stimulating medications such as those used to treat nasal congestion. If they are common, or occur in bursts of more than three at a time, they may be due to some kind of heart disease. If this type of arrhythmia lasts for more than a few seconds, it is a medical emergency.

Your AME is required to deny or defer your application if you have had a significant arrhythmia, but there is a good chance that you will be able to achieve medical certification with a further evaluation that shows you have completely recovered. Even if you still have the arrhythmia, it is not necessarily disqualifying. If there is no underlying heart disease or heart abnormality, you may be approved despite having an arrhythmia such as atrial fibrillation or atrial flutter. Even pilots who have the more worrisome supraventricular or ventricular arrhythmias have been medically certified. Each of these conditions requires an extensive evaluation and may be approved only with limitations. Your cardiologist or internist should provide a statement with the results of a cardiovascular evaluation and the following additional tests:

- 24-hour ambulatory Holter monitor showing acceptable control of the arrhythmia. (If you have atrial fibrillation, this test should show a controlled ventricular response, not a rapid ventricular response.)

- M-mode and 2-dimensional echocardiograms (if a heart abnormality or cardiomyopathy is suspected). This is required in cases of atrial fibrillation or atrial flutter.

Most medications for arrhythmia are acceptable if symptoms are well controlled and there are no adverse side-effects. Drugs such as Tambocor (flecanide) and Cordarone (amiodarone) and other similar medications are now generally considered acceptable in most cases. Some atrial arrhythmias require the use of Coumadin, an anti-coagulant (blood thinner), to prevent blood clots; this is also acceptable on a case-by-case basis. If Coumadin or other anti-coagulant drugs are used, the FAA will require monthly INR (International Normalized Ratio) or PTT (Partial Thromboplastin Time) reports.

Bundle Branch Block

Bundle Branch Block (BBB) is a condition in which the heart has a normal rhythm but part of the heart muscle is slowing the electrical impulses, so that its beat is not entirely coordinated. It may be either congenital or acquired. There are many forms of BBB, some quite normal and others more worrisome. In general, a left-sided BBB presents a greater risk of heart attack than a right-sided BBB.

About 1 in 500 healthy pilots has some type of BBB. In a ten-year study of 372 pilots with right-sided BBB, only one of them went on to develop more serious heart disease. In the USAF, 164 pilots with BBB were evaluated and 83 percent were returned to flying duties. If there are no symptoms, the condition is considered to present no increased risk of incapacitation. If you have a right-sided BBB that was noted previously and you have no symptoms, you may qualify for a medical certificate. Otherwise, your AME will deny or defer your application if you have:

A new right BBB
A left BBB
A second degree or complete heart block.

Cardiomyopathy

Cardiomyopathy is a condition in which the heart muscle is weakened and can no longer contract enough to deliver adequate blood to the body. When this happens, the weak heart muscle often becomes stretched and may develop an irregular heartbeat, with symptoms of shortness of breath, fatigue, or loss of consciousness.

Cardiomyopathy has many possible causes, including bacterial and viral infections, metabolic disorders, drugs and toxins, and connective tissue disorders. It is considered a progressive disease. The extent of the disorder is usually measured by the ejection fraction—indicating the percent of incoming blood that the heart is able to pump out with each stroke. There are a number of medical tests that may be used to determine the heart's functioning, including exercise echocardiography, exercise MUGA, cardiac catheterization, or radionuclide angiogram.

The greatest concern in a pilot with cardiomyopathy is the possibility of developing a sudden irregular heartbeat and losing consciousness. The FAA generally requires an ejection fraction of at least 40 percent, but may allow an even lower level in individual cases if health is otherwise good.

Pacemaker

If you have a pacemaker, you will require a special issuance (see *Chapter 3: Getting a SODA*). You will have to wait at least two months after the surgery before applying for medical certification, to allow adequate recovery and stabilization. When you are ready to apply, you can work together with your AME and cardiologist to send the following documents to the FAA:

- A letter to the FAA requesting special issuance.

- Copies of all medical and hospital records concerning your cardiac condition and the need for pacemaker implantation. Hospital records must include admission and discharge summaries, operative reports, make and model of pulse generator and leads, history and physical exam, daily progress reports, and all ECG treadmill tracings and laboratory work.

- An evaluation of pacemaker function including description and documentation of underlying rate and rhythm with the pacemaker turned "off" or at the lowest setting (pacemaker dependency), programmed pacemaker parameters, surveillance records, and exclusion of myopotential inhibition and pacemaker-induced hypotension (pacemaker syndrome).

- Readable samples of all electronic pacemaker surveillance records over the past six months. The records must include a sample strip with the pacemaker in free running mode and, unless contraindicated, a sample strip with the pacemaker in magnetic mode.

- A current cardiovascular evaluation performed by your cardiologist or internist. This evaluation must be performed after the six-month recovery period and include an assessment of personal and family medical history; a clinical cardiac and general physical examination; an assessment and statement regarding medications, functional capacity, modifiable cardiovascular risk factors, motivation for any necessary change and prognosis for incapacitation during the certification period.

- A report of fasting blood sugar and current blood lipid profile including total cholesterol, HDL, LDL, and triglycerides.

- A current 24-hour Holter monitor including representative tracings.

- A report of M-Mode and 2-D echocardiograms, including film video or any other images resulting from the study.

- A maximal ECG treadmill stress test. All tracings, including a rhythm strip and blood pressure or pulse recordings, must be submitted along with the interpretation. The 12-lead ECG should be recorded at rest, supine and standing; during hyperventilation while standing; one or more times during each stage of exercise; at the end of each stage; at peak exercise; and every minute during recovery for at least five minutes or until the tracing returns to baseline.

- Operational Questionnaire (FAA Form 8500-20). You should note if a lower class of medical certificate than the one you applied for is acceptable.

Heart valve replacement

If you have had heart valve surgery, you will require a special issuance (see *Chapter 3: Getting a SODA*). You will have to wait at least six months after a heart valve repair or replacement before applying for medical certification, to allow adequate recovery and stabilization. If you have had a valve repair rather than replacement, you will need to wait only three months. When you are ready to apply, you can work together with your AME and cardiologist to send the following documents to the FAA:

- A letter to the FAA requesting special issuance.

- Copies of all clinical and hospital records and diagnostic test reports pertaining to the valve replacement. Hospital records must include admission and discharge summaries, operative reports, history and physical exam, daily progress notes, and laboratory work. Also, the make, model, serial number, and implant location of the valve should be included.

- Maximal ECG exercise stress test. All tracings, including a rhythm strip, and blood pressure or pulse recordings must be submitted along with the interpretation. The 12-lead ECG should be recorded at rest, supine and standing; during hyperventilation while standing; one or more times during each stage of exercise; at the end of each stage; at peak exercise; and every minute during recovery for at least five minutes or until the tracing returns to baseline.

- 24-hour Holter monitor with representative tracings.

- Current 2D, M-mode, and Doppler echocardiogram. Include the video of the study.

- If you are on anticoagulant medication, you will also need a letter from your physician stating that you are stable on this medication, without complications, along with the dose schedules, actual prothrombin time (PT) and control determinations, and International Normalized Ratios (INR) that were done at least monthly during the past six months of observation. At least 80 percent of these values must be between 2.5 and 3.5.

Deep vein thrombosis

Deep vein thrombosis (DVT) is the development of a blood clot sticking to the wall of a large vein, especially those of the thighs or legs. The clot (thrombus) is not dangerous in itself, but if it breaks loose it can float downstream to the heart or lungs and cause severe illness or sudden death. The most common symptoms are swelling, pain or discomfort in the legs and, if the clot has broken loose, chest pain, shortness of breath, or irregular heart beat.

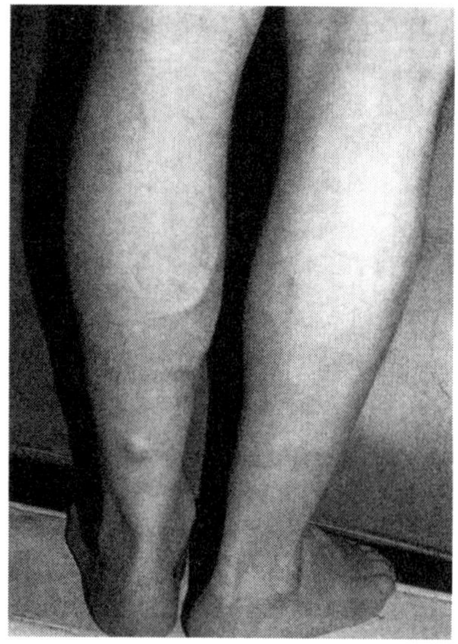
Varicose veins

DVTs were first suspected to be caused by inactivity when they were found in people sleeping on deck chairs in bomb shelters during the London Blitz of WW II. Since then, the condition has been found in about 0.17 percent of the population, often after individuals had spent long periods in a cramped seat on airline flights. For this reason, it has been called "economy-class syndrome" or "travelers' thrombosis," but it is not clear whether immobilization alone is enough to cause a DVT. At the Honolulu International Airport, a study from 1988 to 1993 found 44 cases among the 6 million passengers that come through the terminal each year. All but seven of these cases had one or more risk factors other than immobilization, with most of them having a clotting disorder.

Up to 20 percent of the total population have one or more risk factors that make it more likely for them to develop blood clots. Genetic predisposition to excessive clotting is found in 3 to 5 percent of the general population. The most common are anti-thrombin III deficiency, Protein S and Protein C deficiencies, Factor V Leiden mutation, lupus anti-coagulant (anti-phospholipids), high Factor VIII concentration, hyperhomocysteinemia, and prothrombin 20210A. If you have any of these conditions, you should be especially careful during long flights.

Travel compression stockings

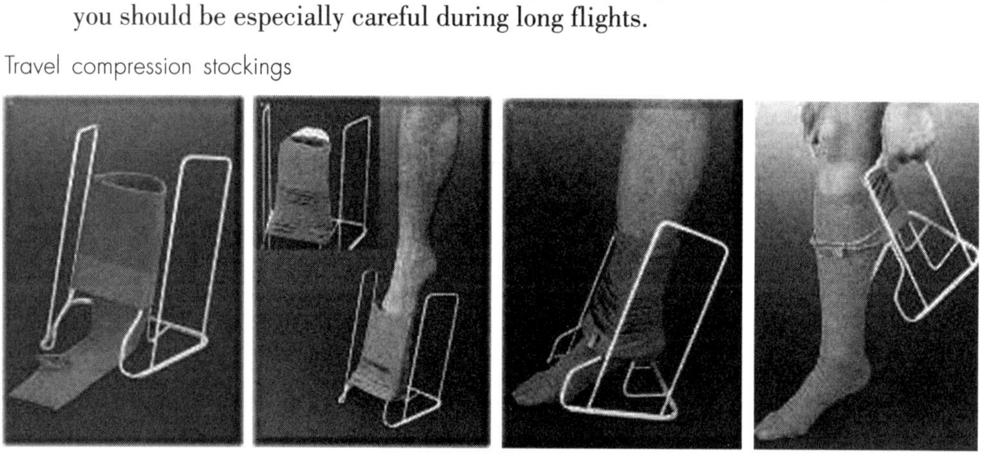

Risk factors for DVT
blood disorder affecting clotting tendency
heart or blood vessel diseases
cancer, either current or previous
recent major surgery
recent trauma to lower limbs or abdomen
personal or family history of DVT
pregnancy
estrogen hormone therapy, or birth control pills
older age, above 40
prolonged immobilization
dehydration
alcohol consumption
smoking
obesity
varicose veins

The best prevention for DVT, if you have any of these risk factors, is to use travel compression stockings. Prices range from $21 to $35 for knee-high stockings. Stockings may or may not prevent DVT—the research is still debatable. These socks are comfortable and not too itchy or hot. Your legs won't look like sausages after a day of flying, but you might get rings around your knees from the elastic band. Mediven travel stockings are available at many pharmacies, or you can contact the company directly (866-223-5234, www.mediusa.com).

If you are on blood-thinning medication (anti-coagulants), you should bring a current report of PTT (Partial Thromboplastin Time) or INR (International Normalized Ratios) tests to your AME. The report from your treating physician should indicate evidence of stability without complications and include dose schedules with INR levels and thrombin times (with control values) accomplished at least monthly during a six-month period of observation.

Raynaud's disease

In 1862 the French physician Maurice Raynaud first described a "cold hands syndrome." There are now two recognized forms of this condition, known as Raynaud's disease and a milder variant as Raynaud's phenomenon. It is usually more of a nuisance than a danger to pilots. Raynaud's affects 5 to 10 percent of people, but is five times more common in women, especially between the ages of 15 and 40. It is most often found in people who live in colder climates and is triggered by cold weather or emotional stress. About 10 percent of Raynaud's phenomenon is due to other diseases or a side-effect of certain medications. The condition causes a sudden constriction of small arteries, usually in the fingers or toes but it may also affect the tip of the nose, lips, or ear lobes.

During an attack of Raynaud's, the fingers may suddenly turn pale and blue with numbness as blood flow is constricted. An attack lasts from about five minutes to an hour, followed by a burning sensation, throbbing and tingling.

The best prevention is to keep the whole body warm, especially during preflight when it is easy to get chilled. Wear gloves, a hat, thick socks, and perhaps earmuffs to avoid chilling the extremities. Some pilots like to keep chemical hand warmers in their pocket. The cockpit should also be kept warm. If symptoms occur during flight, you can hold your hands over your head for a moment and then whirl them around to help circulation. Avoid tobacco use, since nicotine is a vasoconstrictor and will worsen the problem.

Automatic external defibrillators

A common concern of airlines is the possibility of a passenger or crew member having a heart attack. I encountered this myself once on a non-stop flight from Paris to San Francisco. We were somewhere over Hudson Bay in northern Canada when the pilot asked if there was a doctor aboard. I signaled a flight attendant and was quickly ushered to a passenger crumpled on the floor, sweating profusely, his fist clutched to the chest in a classic sign of heart attack. I asked what sort of medical kit they had aboard, and was brought a small bag with a few first aid items and a cheap, throwaway stethoscope. The nearest airport would have been Winnipeg, another three hours away. As luck would have it, the passenger was suffering from indigestion and a few too many cocktails.

What if the passenger had actually suffered a heart attack? Airlines have often considered carrying a defibrillator, but decided against it because the instrument is somewhat complex and the flight crew is reluctant to use it. Recently, a number of automatic external defibrillators (AED) have been developed. Their operation is very simple and intended for use by people without medical expertise.

In 1996, the Food and Drug Administration (FDA) approved a compact AED for treating cardiac arrest on airline flights. By June 1997 American Airlines began to place AEDs on their transoceanic flights. Delta and United Airlines followed in early 1998, and expanded AED use to all flights. The estimated cost for the AED and related equipment is about $3,000 for each unit. Arguments against their use include the very few lives actually saved, and the possibility that airline liability would increase because of higher passenger expectations of successful treatment of heart conditions. A study by Quantas Airlines found that the most common use of the AED was not for actually shocking the patient, but to monitor the condition. The investigators found that "the availability of rhythm monitoring enhanced medical care and improved information on which a decision on whether to divert [the flight] was made."

In the future, AEDs are likely to become more widespread and available both in airplanes and in airports.

H. High or low blood pressure

Hypertension

High blood pressure—hypertension—is the most common cause of pilots failing a medical exam. It is like fuel exhaustion, the most common cause of small aircraft accidents. Both are silent, easily overlooked, and very easily prevented.

> "Hypertension is one of the simplest problems to address."
> —*Ruby Zecher, medical certification consultant*

Many pilots believe that high blood pressure is due to stress, and that the term hypertension refers to people being hyper or tense. In fact, hypertension is a physical condition and, for the great majority of those who have it, the elevated blood pressure is a natural, probably genetic, feature of aging. There are many factors that affect blood pressure, including diet, exercise, smoking, and also psychological stress. But even with the best personal care, you may be one of millions of people who simply need medication to bring your blood pressure into a healthy range.

What is normal blood pressure?

Normal	less than 130/85—you should get regular blood pressure checks.
High normal	from 130/85 to 139/89—you need to get more exercise, lose weight, or quit smoking.
High	140/90 or higher—you should probably be on medication.
Very high	155/95 or higher—you should immediately see a physician for treatment.

What is the cause of hypertension? Basically, it is a matter of plumbing. In any plumbing system, there are three factors: the pump, the pipes, and the fluid pressure. The pressure goes up if the pump is too strong, the pipes are too small, or the fluid level is too high. You can reduce the pressure by backing off on the pump force, widening the pipes, or decreasing the overall amount of fluid. This is how blood pressure medications work: they either reduce the work of the heart (lower pump force), relax the arteries (widen the pipes), or cause the kidneys to release more water, decreasing blood volume. Salt intake causes retention of water, and the extra water will increase pressure. This is a very common cause of hypertension in pilots of African ancestry, who should be especially careful to minimize salt intake, or use medication to increase urination ("water pills," or diuretics). In everyone, arteries tend to stiffen with age and are less able to expand with each pulse of blood from the heart. This is why the first, higher number (systolic) in the blood pressure reading is usually the one that is too high in older people; the second (diastolic) may be normal.

Obesity and lack of physical fitness are also important causes of hypertension. Each pound of fat has miles of additional, tiny blood vessels through which the heart has to force blood. Losing weight takes a huge load off the heart. If you are overweight, decreasing your weight by 10 percent will reduce your blood pressure by 10 percent. Increasing muscle tone also takes a load off the heart, although it might not be so obvious. Every time a muscle is contracted, it squeezes and massages the blood vessels inside and around it. This helps move blood along and does the work for the heart—especially in the legs, where the blood has a long way to go against gravity to get back to the heart. This is why jogging, swimming, and just about every exercise except billiards is so good for you.

To reduce your blood pressure:

Lose weight, if you are above your recommended weight
Get enough exercise; ideally 30-45 minutes of aerobic exercise 4-6 days a week
Avoid foods high in salt or saturated fat
Eat more fruits, vegetables, and high-fiber foods
Avoid a high intake of caffeine (coffee, tea, sodas, weight loss pills)
Avoid a high intake of alcohol
If you smoke or use tobacco, quit immediately
Learn relaxation and stress-management techniques
If you still have elevated blood pressure, use an appropriate medication

Some people get nervous when they are having their blood pressure checked—understandable when you consider that your career and livelihood may depend on those numbers. Their anxiety can cause a rise in blood pressure into the unacceptable range, when it is normally below that value. This condition, called "white-coat syndrome," is quite common. If you think you might have this problem, have your blood pressure checked frequently and bring at least three of these readings (on separate days, both morning and evening, in the last seven days) to the AME. You should also try to schedule your medical examination early in the morning, when blood pressure is normally lower, and absolutely do not drink any coffee or sodas, or take any stimulating food, herb or medicine. Try to arrive at the AME's office about a half hour beforehand. Relax. It will probably be a medical assistant or nurse who will take your blood pressure, so chat with them a bit, and let them know you tend to get a little nervous. They will most likely be very understanding. If the first blood pressure reading is too high, relax some more and have them take it again after a few minutes. Ask them to just record the lowest one. This may help you get your certification, but keep in mind that you clearly have a blood pressure problem and you still need to treat it appropriately.

Curiously, the FAA does not have a regulatory standard on hypertension (requiring a deferral and perhaps special issuance authorization) as it does with other diseases and conditions. This is probably because so many pilots have high blood pressure that it would overwhelm the FAA's ability to handle all the necessary deferrals. Instead, the FAA has issued a somewhat less formal policy. The policy states that your AME may issue you a certificate if you do not take anti-hypertensive medication and your blood pressure is below 155/95. (Note that both the higher and lower values must be below the maximum). If your blood pressure at the time of the examination is slightly high, the AME is allowed to use the previous week's readings.

> "It's a sneaky condition. You may have no idea that you have high blood pressure until the day that you visit your AME for your medical recertification and he says, 'Uh-oh.'"

The aviation medical examination is not the best place to discover that you have high blood pressure. Hypertension does not generally occur overnight. Ideally, you should have routine health care and an increase in blood pressure should have been noted and treated appropriately. That's the ideal. In practice, unfortunately, many physicians ignore or downplay mildly elevated blood pressures and it doesn't become a problem until you see the AME. If your blood pressure is mildly elevated, a good AME will hold on to your application and let you return within a couple of weeks after you have had a chance to show that your blood pressure is under the acceptable limit. (And then he or she should strongly advise you to get appropriate medical care!) If your pressure is still too high, your application will be denied or deferred.

There is a simple way to avoid this possibility: go to your medical care provider before you see the AME. If your blood pressure is too high, treat it appropriately by changing your lifestyle and perhaps getting medication. Bring a record of your acceptable blood pressure readings (see above) and you will likely be issued your certificate.

Blood pressure medications

Once you are on blood pressure medication, you will probably be on it for life. Some people may be able to bring down their blood pressure with aggressive changes in lifestyle, such as quitting smoking or losing weight, to the point where they no longer need medication. Most people, however, will be lucky to avoid worsening the problem and stay on a minimal dose of a single medication.

If you take blood pressure medication, the FAA will require additional documents. Bring these to the AME. Without them, your application will be deferred. You should bring:

- A letter from your treating physician that states:
  - your family history
  - your risk factors for coronary artery disease
  - your blood pressure medications, dosages, and their side-effects
  - three blood pressures (taken on separate days) showing good control

- Blood tests:
  - lipid panel
  - fasting blood sugar
  - serum potassium and creatinine

- ECG

- (If you have heart disease risk factors), a maximal exercise stress test

You will need to do this only once. For subsequent applications, you will simply need a letter from your physician with a status report detailing:

- Your current medications, their dosage, and presence or absence of side-effects
- Adequacy of blood pressure control
- Any end-organ complications of your condition.

You will need an annual examination by your physician to evaluate your condition if you have a first- or second-class certificate. If you have a third-class certificate, you won't need an evaluation until the time of your renewal. The FAA will send you a confirmation letter detailing these requirements.

Virtually all common blood pressure medications are approved for use. The exceptions are medications that act on your central nervous system, such as reserpine, guanethidine, guanadrel, guanabenz, and methyldopa. These medications are typically used only if your blood pressure is very difficult to control or if you have other health conditions. If you take any of these, your application will be deferred, but there is still a good chance that you will eventually achieve certification under special issuance, particularly if you take a low dose and show good blood pressure control.

Low blood pressure

Excessively low blood pressure (hypotension) is less common than high blood pressure, and is usually due to another illness. It is not a fixed number, since some people normally have a much lower blood pressure than others. Hypotension is usually detected when there are symptoms such as weakness, dizziness, or loss of consciousness. The AME will take note of unusually low blood pressure, or any symptoms, and determine if further tests are needed to evaluate the condition.

I. Stomach, liver, or intestinal trouble

A pilot can easily be incapacitated by severe abdominal pain, cramping, vomiting, or the need for a sudden bowel movement. Anyone at high risk of these is therefore likely to be disqualified.

Chronic diseases such as ulcerative colitis, liver cirrhosis, chronic hepatitis, or cancer of the stomach or intestines can bring sudden pain or other discomfort. Each of these is not necessarily disqualifying, however. You will be able to get your certificate if your condition is well controlled and you can show that the risk of incapacitation is low.

Ulcers

When people speak of "stomach ulcers," they are generally referring to peptic ulcer, also known as acid-peptic disease. This type of ulcer usually appears in the small intestine, very close to its attachment to the stomach. It is often noticed by a gnawing, aching, or hunger-like pain that occurs within a half hour to about three hours after eating. The ulcer is then diagnosed by X-ray using a radio-opaque dye (the barium swallow), or by direct visualization during endoscopy.

Ulcers can have a great variety of symptoms, and only about one quarter of people with typical ulcer-like stomach pain actually have an ulcer. On the other hand, many people with ulcers have no pain at all. In fact, about 20 percent of those with the most severe ulcer complications, such as bleeding, have no symptoms—the "silent ulcers." Ulcers tend to come and go for a number of years before they are completely healed. Pilots may be certified if they have ulcers so long as they are healed or have not been active for at least three months. Certification is denied if there is evidence of bleeding or other complications.

In general a rectal examination is not included in aviation physicals. However, your AME may suggest one if you have had recent ulcer symptoms. It will help your application to show that there is no bleeding.

About 10 percent of the American population has an ulcer at some time in their life, with about 500,000 new cases per year and about 4 million recurrences. In the 1970s, the number one prescription drug in the U.S. was the anti-ulcer medication Tagamet (more recently, the number one selling drug has been Prozac, which may say something about the dominant mood in this country). There are now many effective ulcer medications, and the use of most of them is not prohibited for flight.

If you have had ulcer symptoms within the past three months, or bleeding in the past six months, you will need to bring a letter from the treating physician to your AME. The letter should state:

- You have been free of symptoms for at least three months.
- X-ray or endoscopy shows that the ulcer has healed.
- Your medication, dosage, and whether you have side-effects.

Your AME will combine this information and defer your application to the FAA. For this reason, you should allow about 12 weeks before the expiration of your certificate in order to keep flying. The FAA will probably give a limited certification, and may require follow-up reports every six months, for a year, to make sure that there has been no recurrence.

Intestinal disease

Both the stomach and intestines contain a lot of air—the stomach itself is usually filled about one-third with air, and the intestines normally have about one quart of air in them. Air pressure decreases with altitude, causing expansion in its volume. At 10,000 feet, air expands over 50 percent, and at 18,000 feet it is doubled in volume. Therefore, air in the stomach and intestines also expands with ascent and many pilots find themselves burping or passing gas on achieving altitude. This is not normally a problem if the pilot feels comfortable and the cabin has adequate ventilation.

The lining of the stomach and intestines is very slippery, allowing masses of food and air to move around easily. This lining is also very sensitive and can feel painful when stretched. As a result, excessive gas can be quite uncomfortable. Pilots susceptible to forming gas should avoid foods that tend to aggravate this condition.

Chronic inflammatory bowel diseases, such as ulcerative colitis or regional enteritis (Crohn's disease), require full medical documentation to show that they do not pose an excessive risk during flight.

> If stomach gas is a problem you should consider avoiding the foods that are most likely to increase it. These include: vegetables of the cabbage family, dried peas and beans, beer or carbonated drinks, turnips, rutabagas, fibrous raw fruits and vegetables, fatty or spicy foods, and ground beef that contains textured soy proteins. You should also avoid chewing gum, since it promotes air swallowing.

If you have had stomach or intestinal surgery, you should allow at least four months of recovery before applying for a medical certificate. With a favorable report from the treating physician, certification should be no problem. Intestinal surgery often results in an ostomy (colostomy, ileostomy, etc.) in which the intestine is diverted to a hole in the abdomen, with a bag attached for the discharge. Many pilots have been certified with an ostomy, although this requires close work with a supportive AME and regular follow-up reports to ensure good management of the condition.

Medications

Corticosteroid medication (for example, prednisone) is commonly prescribed for chronic intestinal diseases, but can also have mood-altering side-effects. Flying is permitted only if this medication is taken in doses of no more than 20 mg equivalent of prednisone per day.

Lomotil, a medication used for diarrhea and to slow intestinal transit time, presents a special problem. Lomotil is a combination of two different drugs, each of which is normally prohibited for flight. The first, diphenoxylate, is a narcotic and can cause decreased alertness. The second is atropine, a psychoactive drug that may also affect mental functioning. For this reason Lomotil is not allowed. In some cases, the use of small amounts of loperamide (Imodium) has been approved.

Passengers

You should be concerned about any passengers with gastro-intestinal disease. After abdominal surgery, the linings of the stomach and intestines are stickier than normal and may not allow the internal air to move around as readily. The result is increased discomfort and even the danger of rupture of these organs if the expanded air cannot be released and the pressure becomes too great. Passengers recovering from abdominal surgery should not fly for at least two weeks after surgery. If they had excessive complications or bleeding, they should wait until three weeks after recovery. Any type of bowel obstruction can be a severe problem during flight, and before taking passengers with this type of disorder you should have clearance from their physician.

J. Kidney stone or blood in urine

The FAA medical examination includes a simple urine test to screen for a number of common kidney or urinary tract diseases. A paper test strip will show if there is sugar, protein, blood, or other gross abnormalities in the urine. If any of these are present, further investigation will be needed before your medical certificate is issued.

Kidney stones

Kidney stones (nephrolithiasis) are very common and afflict about half a million Americans each year. Most people pass their first stone by age 20 to 40, and men have them four times more often than women. There are five major types of stones, and they have different causes and treatment, so it is important to catch the stone and have it analyzed.

Anyone who has passed a kidney stone will tell you that this is one of the most painful experiences imaginable—second only to what women go through in childbirth. The pain can come on very suddenly, even waking someone from sleep, and be accompanied by nausea, vomiting and doubling over to the point of complete incapacitation. As the stone passes down the urinary canal from the kidney to the urethra, the pain moves with it, causing severe cramping aches in the back, side, abdomen, groin, and often in a man's testicle or woman's labia on the side of the stone. The stone size does not usually match the severity of the pain—an excruciating agony can result from passing just a tiny stone the size of a sesame seed (or, if you're not a cook, figure about the size of a #8 shotgun BB).

Having a pilot suddenly incapacitated with pain is something everyone wants to avoid, and any pilot at high risk of a kidney stone will be disqualified for a medical certificate.

If you passed a kidney stone, but have not had any symptoms for at least one month and your urine looks normal, your AME may go ahead and certify you. Otherwise, the risk of passing another stone needs to be carefully considered, and your medical certification will be deferred to the FAA. You will need to be examined by a urologist who will issue a status report. This report should include the following:

- The dates of your experience with kidney stones.
- The type of kidney stone passed (e.g., calcium oxalate).
- How they were treated.
- Your risk of kidney stones now and in the future.
- The results of recent diagnostic tests to show that there are no further stones, such as a KUB (X-ray of the kidneys, ureters, and bladder), IVP (intravenous pyelogram), or ultrasound.

If this information shows that you do not have kidney stones now, and your risk is low, your certification is very likely.

If the tests show that you still have one or more stones that have not yet been passed, getting a medical certificate is more difficult as the risk of passing the stone is quite high. Your medical is generally suspended until it is clear that you have passed the stone and are free of symptoms.

Kidney stones are affected by diet and fluid intake. People who have passed stones should be careful to avoid becoming dehydrated and should maintain a diet low in sodium and avoid high protein intake. Bran can also help bind some of the excess minerals. If the condition is severe, medication or surgery may be required.

I passed a kidney stone and the IVP and ultrasound showed that there were no more stones—but I still didn't get my medical. Why?

It is likely that you had complicating factors or an unusual type of stone. Even though you passed the stone, you may be at high risk of developing further stones until the underlying metabolic disorder is corrected.

Kidney transplant

Kidney transplant recipients have been medically certified for all classes. If you have had a kidney transplant, you will need to bring complete hospital records and a current status report from your treating doctor. If it is been at least six months since the surgery, your records show good recovery, no organ rejection, and no adverse side-effects from immunosuppressant drugs, you may be able to get a medical certificate.

K. Diabetes

The term diabetes mellitus comes from sweet urine, the result of having too much sugar in the blood. The extra sugar is very damaging to small blood vessels and creates problems throughout the body. Traditionally, diabetes mellitus has been classified as one of two types: Type I is thought to be caused by an immune reaction that destroys the insulin-producing cells of the pancreas, resulting in an inability to manage blood sugar. It typically begins in adolescence and requires insulin for treatment. Type II results from increasing difficulty of the cells of the body to pick up sugar from the blood. It usually begins later in adulthood. While Type I diabetics always require insulin, those with Type II may be treated without medication if the condition is borderline, with blood-sugar lowering medication if it is more severe or, if necessary, with insulin. Recently, doctors have discovered that this classification is overly simple and prefer to distinguish types by whether or not insulin is needed: insulin-dependent diabetes mellitus (IDDM) or non-insulin-dependent diabetes mellitus (NIDDM), but the old terms are still often used.

Type II diabetes is epidemic in modern society. At least 16 million Americans have the condition, and the figure is expected to increase to 22 million in the next 25 years. Diabetes is not only much more common than ever, it is also appearing at younger ages. In the past decade alone, there has been a 70 percent increase in diabetes in young adults, about one third of whom are unaware that they have it. Because diabetes is a slowly progressive disease that may go unnoticed, about half of these people have already suffered serious damage to their eyes, kidneys, nerves and arteries by the time they realize that they have it. Type II diabetes (the most common form) greatly increases the risk of heart attacks and is the major cause of blindness, kidney failure and amputations, killing about 180,000 Americans each year.

Warning signs of diabetes:
You are more often thirsty, hungry, and urinating
You feel sleepy right after a meal
Your vision is a little blurry, or you have headaches after reading
Your blood pressure is higher than usual
Your breath constantly smells like nail-polish remover

Those most at risk of developing diabetes are people who are overweight. The recent rise in diabetes is probably related to the increasing obesity in the American population. The risk of diabetes increases by 6 percent for every 5 to 8 pounds overweight. Type II diabetes used to be seen only in middle-aged or older people, but now is regularly diagnosed even in teenagers, most of whom are obese. Therefore, the very best thing you can do if you are at risk of diabetes is to maintain a healthy weight.

You are at high risk of diabetes if you:
Are overweight
Have a close relative with diabetes
Are Black, Latino, Asian, American Indian, or Pacific Islander
Had gestational diabetes during pregnancy, or delivered a baby weighing more than 9 pounds
Had a blood sugar test that found impaired glucose tolerance
Have heart disease or high blood pressure
Have high triglycerides, or low HDL (the good cholesterol)
Have polycystic ovarian syndrome

What should I do if my urine shows high blood sugar?

If you have discovered this for the first time, it does not necessarily mean that you have diabetes. Some people have kidneys that naturally spill sugar into their urine (a condition called renal glycosuria). However, you should have a blood test to evaluate this condition more thoroughly. This is ordinarily done with a glucose tolerance test, which takes about two hours and involves multiple blood samples after you drink a standard sugar solution. The results show how well your body is able to handle sugar. Your blood sugar level should be below 120 mg/dl at the beginning of the test, and no higher than 160 after you drink the sugar solution.

If your blood sugar is slightly above normal, you may be able to prevent diabetes by losing weight, changing your diet, and getting more exercise. Some studies have shown that just losing 10 pounds has reduced the risk of diabetes by 58 percent! If you are unable to bring your blood sugar level into the normal range with these methods, you will need medication.

If you have diabetes controlled without medication, your AME may be able to certify you directly if you provide the following information:

- A letter from your doctor stating that your diabetes is well controlled and there is no evidence of disease in the heart, blood vessels, nerves, kidneys, or eyes.

- A blood test, within the last 30 days, showing that your
  - Fasting blood sugar is less than 140 mg/dl
  - Hb A_1C is less than 9 percent.

If you require medication to control your diabetes, you may still achieve certification, but your AME will not be allowed to give it to you directly. Your AME will assemble the necessary documents and laboratory test results and defer your application to the FAA.

Oral medication only

Diabetes requiring medication is listed as a disqualifying medical condition. This means that the FAA will issue a medical certificate only under special issuance (see *Chapter 3: Getting a SODA*).

The FAA has long approved the use of oral medications to control blood glucose. You will need a letter from your treating physician and blood tests, as mentioned for applicants with diabetes who do not take medications. The letter from your physician must state in addition that you have been on your medication for at least 60 days and that there is good control of your blood sugar with no significant side-effects or complications, and a hemoglobin A_1C level taken within the last 30 days, with at least three monthly fasting blood sugar readings. After your initial special issuance certification for diabetes, the FAA may authorize the AME to issue future certificates, as long as there are no significant adverse changes. When you return for your medical exam, bring a letter to the AME from your physician documenting your good diabetes control and a current hemoglobin A_1C level.

You will need a follow-up evaluation at least every six months for a first- and second-class certificate, and every twelve months for a third-class certificate. Your AME may request more frequent follow-ups if your condition is unstable.

A major concern with diabetes medication is that it will over-correct the high blood sugar and cause excessively low blood sugar (hypoglycemia). Symptoms of hypoglycemia include tremor, sweating, anxiety, headache, confusion, blurred vision, dizziness, and unconsciousness. None of these are welcome in the cockpit. Note also how similar these symptoms are to hypoxia (see *Chapter 5: Using oxygen*)—which could result in the wrong solution to the problem. If you use any type of diabetes medication, you should always carry some candies or have a sugary drink available in case you feel symptoms of hypoglycemia.

Unfortunately, most people with diabetes also have other health problems that make the condition more complicated. The most common of these is hypertension. Some types of hypertension medication mask the symptoms of hypoglycemia, and are therefore not permitted for flight.

Until 1996, the risk of incapacitation in a pilot using insulin was considered too high to be allowed. As insulin treatment became more sophisticated, the FAA began to certify some applicants who use insulin. The current policy allows only third-class certification, but first- and second-class issuance might be possible in the future.

Insulin

If you use insulin, you will be required to provide the following documents for your initial application for special issuance:

- A complete medical history.
- All records of any incidents or accidents that might have been due to diabetes complications.
- A detailed current clinical evaluation carried out by a diabetes specialist or endocrinologist.
- Two Hb A_1C measurements: a current one and another at least 90 days prior.
- A detailed report of your special diet and insulin regimen, and any other medications you are taking.

- Examinations and tests to detect any kidney disease, peripheral neuropathy or circulatory compromise of the extremities, and perhaps additional tests recommended by the treating specialist.

- Confirmation by an ophthalmologist of the absence of clinically significant eye disease.

- (If you are 40 or older) a maximal exercise stress test.

- Documents that show that you have been educated in diabetes management and thoroughly understand its monitoring.

- A statement from your treating physician, AME, or other knowledgeable person, that you are skilled at using a recording glucometer.

- A statement from your treating physician that you are willing and able to properly monitor and manage your diabetes.

- A statement from you agreeing to immediately report any adverse medical changes to the FAA.

Your records should confirm the absence of any recent significant diabetes-related events and no evidence of significant cardiovascular, kidney, retinal, or other organ disease. You cannot have had, within the past five years, a loss of consciousness, a seizure, or more than one hypoglycemic reaction that occurred without warning symptoms or that required help from someone (for example, a sudden spell of dizziness or weakness, or needing someone to give you glucose). At least one year must have passed after that episode, without further problems. You should have been taking your current insulin regimen for at least six months without problems.

Pilots who are granted a special issuance certificate for insulin use are required to monitor their blood glucose (with an approved glucometer) before the flight begins, periodically during flight, and one half hour prior to landing. They may take insulin during the flight, as needed.

As a pilot using insulin, you:

- May exercise only the privileges of a student, recreational, or private pilot certificate.

- Are prohibited from operating an aircraft as a required crew member on any flight outside U.S. airspace.

- Are required to be in compliance with the monitoring requirements of the insulin use protocol.

- Must have at hand appropriate and unexpired medical supplies for glucose management while preparing for flight and while exercising piloting privileges, including:

  - Whole blood digital glucose monitor with memory
  - Supplies needed to obtain blood samples
  - An amount of rapidly absorbable glucose, in 10 gm portions, appropriate for the planned duration of the flight.

Preflight: Not more than 30 minutes before takeoff, you must establish and document a blood glucose concentration between 100 and 300 mg/dl. If it is less than 100 mg/dl, an appropriate glucose snack (at least 10 gm) may be ingested and a recheck done. If it is over 300 mg/dl, the flight must be postponed.

Inflight: You must monitor your blood glucose one hour into the flight, at subsequent hourly intervals, and within 30 minutes of landing. If it is less than 100 mg/dl, a 20 gm glucose-containing snack should be ingested. If it is greater than 300 mg/dl, you must land at the nearest suitable airport and not resume flight until the glucose concentration can be maintained in the 100-300 mg/dl range.

As always, the first and most important consideration is to *fly the airplane*. Blood glucose measurements are secondary to managing aircraft operations, weather, and air traffic control. You must use good judgment in flight about deciding when to measure your glucose level. If measurement is not practicable, take a 20 gm glucose snack and land at the nearest suitable airport.

Once you are given a medical certificate by special issuance, re-certification is somewhat easier but still a bit of work. You will need a medical evaluation by a specialist every three months. This evaluation must include a general physical examination, a review of the interval medical history, a comment on your daily record of blood glucose measurements,

Hb A_1C, and any other tests recommended by the treating specialist. The evaluation should also have a statement about your continued ability and willingness to monitor and properly manage your diabetes, and whether your condition could reasonably be expected to decrease your ability to safely control an aircraft.

If you have any adverse change in your condition, you are required to immediately stop your piloting activities until you are again cleared by the FAA.

L. Neurological disorders

Injuries and illnesses of the central nervous system present some of the most difficult cases for the FAA to evaluate. The key concern, as with all other medical issues, is the risk of sudden incapacitation of a pilot. Often, there is no clear explanation of a temporary loss of consciousness and it is difficult to determine if the underlying problem is solved or if the condition might return.

In general, you will have your application deferred for further evaluation by the FAA if you have ever had:

- Epilepsy or disturbance of consciousness without a satisfactory medical explanation of the cause.
- A loss of consciousness for more than one hour after an injury.
- A significant nerve problem (numbness or paralysis) anywhere on your body.
- A depressed skull fracture.
- A subdural or epidural hematoma (bleeding in the lining of the brain).

A mild tremor is not disqualifying in itself if it does not impair your functioning. Surgery for a brain tumor is also not necessarily disqualifying. You may get your certificate if the tumor was benign and you have been off medication for at least a year.

For any significant neurological problem, you will be asked for all records of treatment. A report by a qualified neurologist will also be required, with the following:

- Detailed recent neurological examination.
- X-rays, if appropriate.
- Electroencephalogram (EEG) or other tests as determined by the neurologist.

Loss of consciousness

Any episode of loss of consciousness (other than normal sleep) is a concern. There are an enormous number of possible causes for losing consciousness, and sometimes the cause is never satisfactorily determined. These cases may require an extensive cardiac or neurologic evaluation to try to arrive at a diagnosis. If a reasonable diagnosis cannot be made, the FAA will want to see that you have had at least a year without a recurrence of symptoms.

If the unconsciousness, amnesia, or disorientation occurred after an injury and lasted more than an hour, you will need to show that you have not had symptoms for anywhere between one and five years, as determined by the FAA, before you can be medically certified.

Migraine and other headaches

Headaches are very common, and the occasional mild headache that responds to over-the-counter medication is not disqualifying. Use of prescription medication, or the presence of more severe headaches, requires a deferral for FAA evaluation. Severe headaches include:

- Migraine (with or without visual disturbances)
- Migraine equivalent (usually accompanied by nausea)
- Cluster headaches
- Chronic tension headaches
- Conversion headaches
- Trigeminal neuralgia
- Unusual or severe pain in the face.

Epilepsy

A seizure is somewhat like an electrical short-circuit in the brain. Depending on where it occurs, it can affect various muscles, speech, memory or awareness. It can be focal, affecting only one part of the body, or global, affecting the entire body and causing a loss of consciousness.

Epilepsy is a condition in which the brain has recurrent seizures. In about a third of these cases, the cause is not apparent. Others may be caused by head injuries, brain disorders, or other illnesses. For example, about 30 percent of people with bacterial meningitis have had at least one seizure.

Epileptic seizures may be spontaneous or provoked. Triggers that provoke seizures include sleep deprivation, alcohol or medications, and high fevers.

If you have ever had an epileptic seizure of any kind you will be asked for more information about it. You may be certified by the FAA if:

- You had only a single seizure more than four years ago, and have not been on anticonvulsant drug therapy for at least two years.
- You had more than one seizure, but it has been at least 10 years since your last seizure, and at least three years since you used anticonvulsant medication.

If your seizures or anticonvulsant medication were more recent, your application will either be denied or deferred to the FAA. If there is a satisfactory explanation for your seizures and you can show that your risk is minimal, there is a good chance that you will eventually be given medical certification.

The use of anticonvulsant medication, such as phenytoin (Dilantin) or carbamazepine (Tegretol) among many others, is disqualifying. This is true even if these medications are used for other reasons. All anticonvulsants affect the central nervous system, with side-effects such as drowsiness and impaired concentration. Moreover, although these drugs are used to prevent a seizure, they do not guarantee this and the risk remains high.

Stroke

A stroke, properly known as a cerebrovascular accident (CVA), is caused when a part of the brain is starved of blood. This usually occurs because of a blockage in one or more blood vessels. A transient ischemic attack is a "ministroke" that may result from a brief blockage, sometimes only a second or two. Strokes can result in many degrees of impairment, from complete paralysis to complete recovery. Transient global amnesia is a type of stroke in which there is no obvious paralysis or loss of consciousness, but which may result in a partial loss of memory of recent past events. It is often an early sign of future strokes.

If you experienced any type of cerebrovascular disorder, including stroke or transient ischemic attack, or transient global amnesia, you will need at least two years of uneventful recovery and no further symptoms before you can apply for a medical certificate. If you already have a certificate and experience any of these, your medical certification is no longer valid and you will need at least two years of uneventful recovery before you can apply for recertification. Providing a cardiovascular workup is negative, recertification is allowed one year after transient global amnesia.

To apply after the two-year recovery period, you will need a lettter from your treating physician and documentation including:

- A complete cardiovascular evaluation
- An evaluation by a neurologist
- Copies of your previous medical records.

Your AME will collect these and forward them to the FAA for review and, hopefully, issuance of your certificate. In general, medical certification after a stroke is given only by special issuance. This process can take a while to allow time for each case to be reviewed by an FAA neurologist.

The blockage of blood to the brain that causes a stroke is often found in the carotid arteries in the neck—the pulse you can feel just under the angle of your jaw. A common surgery is performed to remove this blockage, known as carotid endarterectomy. If you have had this surgery, you will need to provide the FAA with your hospital records and the results of a post-operative carotid Doppler ultrasound study, or perhaps also a carotid arteriogram.

M. Mental disorders

Mental disorders are as common among pilots as they are in the general population. Indeed, many people (including pilots) think you have to be a little crazy to spend the time and money necessary to fly. Unfortunately, mental disorders are often seen as a personal failure, or lack of willpower, rather than an illness in the same way as any other health problem. Pilots especially should be observant of early symptoms and take care to get appropriate treatment.

In general, medications used to treat mental disorders are psychotropic drugs and therefore impair performance and flying safety. The FAA requires that you have been off these medications for at least 90 days before certification. Herbal medications are a questionable matter. The FAA is taking a closer look at the use of many herbs, not only because they may impair performance, but also because they may hide an underlying disorder. It is best to call the FAA or your AME if you are uncertain whether your herbal medication is allowed.

Mental disorders encompass more than mental illness. For example, if you are very disturbed about a marital or family problem, or just had a crushing setback at work, you should consider whether you are really up to full capacity. If you are furious about a situation, or worried about a dilemma, you may be stuck on the problem and not paying enough attention to the flight. It is better to take time out until the problem is resolved or you feel less distracted.

Ultimately, a pilot is responsible for both the condition of the airplane and the condition of its operator. If either one is not in top form, it is better to delay or cancel the flight. Mental disturbances are no different from physical disturbances. You wouldn't go flying immediately after having a root-canal, and you shouldn't go flying right after being served with divorce papers. Ask yourself: "Can I focus on the flight, and nothing else?" Wait until the answer is yes.

Depression

Depression is one of the most frequent mental disorders, so much so that it is sometimes called the "common cold of psychiatry." An estimated 10 to 20 million people in the United States suffer from it at some time in their lives to the extent that they need medical treatment. In the 1990s, Prozac (fluoxetine) was the number one selling drug in the United States, with 650,000 new prescriptions per month. Since then, it has been joined by many similar medications and herbal remedies. Antidepressant medication has also been found to be effective for pain, menstrual discomfort, and to help people quit smoking.

Common symptoms of depression

Feeling depressed most of the day, often starting in the morning or worse in the morning
Loss of interest in activities that usually bring enjoyment
Tearful episodes
Constant or unusual fatigue
Difficulty sleeping
Frequent feelings of sadness and grief
Changes in appetite
Irritability
Feelings of undeserved guilt, worthlessness, or sinfulness
Difficulty concentrating

Indecisiveness
Illogical thought patterns or misinterpretation of reality
Frequent headaches, stomach aches, backaches, or other complaints
Agitation

All antidepressant drugs affect the central nervous system and are therefore not suitable for pilots. The FAA does not allow the use of any antidepressant medication, even if it is used for another reason, such as to stop smoking.

Pfizer Depression Self-Quiz

1. Do I have little interest or pleasure in doing things?
2. Am I feeling down, depressed, hopeless?
3. Do I have trouble falling asleep, staying asleep, or sleeping too much?
4. Do I feel tired and have little energy?
5. Do I have a poor appetite, or do I overeat?
6. Do I feel bad about myself or feel that I am a failure?
7. Do I have trouble concentrating?
8. Do I move or speak so slowly that other people notice? Or am I too fidgety and restless?
9. Do I think I'd be better off dead or want to hurt myself in some way?

If you answer Yes to three or more of these, you should see a doctor.

If you used medication for only a few days or weeks, you may be certified after having been off the medication for a few weeks. More likely, the FAA will want to see that you have been off medication for at least 90 days to make sure that the drug is entirely out of your system. You will also need a report from your treating doctor summarizing your history of depression, your treatment, and your current mental health status.

I was taking antidepressants a few years ago and lost my medical. I'm off medication now. Can I get my medical back?

If you have been off medication for at least 90 days, and you have a report from your treating physician showing that your mental health problems have resolved, you will have an excellent chance of getting a medical certificate.

Many pilots who are otherwise healthy experience times when they are in a low mood and perhaps even exhibit many of the symptoms of depression. A person in this state has diminished mental capability and may have slow response times or clouded judgment. It is very important to be aware of your own state of mind, and know when to take yourself off flying status. When you feel better, you can return.

> *"Just as an aircraft can stall from too great an angle of attack, too little power, too heavy a load, a person can develop a 'mental stall.'"*

There are a number of good treatments for mild depression:

- The best remedy is physical activity. Many studies have shown that it has as much benefit as psychotherapy. When the body feels good, the mind does too. On a chemical level, exercise releases endorphins, responsible for "runner's high." During long, sustained exercise, problems seem easier to manage. The exercise does not have to be intense—just a long walk will do. Large muscle activity also helps discharge feelings of pent-up anger, frustration, or hostility.
- Avoid the use of alcohol or other intoxicants. Alcohol doesn't help depression and usually makes the problem much worse.
- Anger turned inward is a major cause of depression and fatigue. If you frequently get angry, consider taking anger management classes.
- If you are plagued by shame or guilt, learn to forgive yourself. You simply need to do your best, and no more. You do not need to be perfect.
- Have a sense of humor about the situation.
- Open up about your feelings in a considerate way. By sharing your thoughts and feelings, you will be able to see them more objectively yourself.
- If these methods are not enough, you need treatment. Do not hesitate to consult a professional. You would do that for any other mechanical or physical problem you cannot solve, so you should take the same approach with social or psychological difficulties. Find a competent therapist with whom you can work.

> "My psychiatrist is great, but she's an awfully hard person to talk to." —Not every qualified therapist is suitable.

St. John's Wort is not listed as a prohibited medication by the FAA. Can I use it for depression and still fly?

St. John's Wort (Hypericum perforatum) is an herbal remedy reputed to have some antidepressant properties. It is not regulated by the FDA and is readily available for purchase in supermarkets in a variety of formulations, from pills to tea. Research in Europe has shown that St. John's Wort might be useful to treat mild to moderate depression and anxiety. However, research has also shown that the herb can cause problems in some people, for example, by increasing sun sensitivity.

The answer to the question is Yes and No. Yes, you may use St. John's Wort, but No, you should not fly if you have clinical symptoms of depression. You should be treated properly for your depression, by solving the underlying problem.

Bipolar disorder

Bipolar disorder used to be called manic-depression, indicating the swings from mania (a hyperactive state) to depression. During mania, the mind may seem to be racing, with shortened attention span, unrealistic ideas and poor judgment. During states of either mania or depression, the pilot's judgment and performance are impaired.

Bipolar disorder is a disqualifying condition. However, you may be able to get a special issuance, even if you require medication for the condition. You will need a letter from an accredited psychiatrist describing your treatment and stating that your condition is controlled by medication. You should be stable on your medication, without symptoms or side-effects, for at least three to six months before your application.

Can I fly on Lithium?

Lithium is one of the most effective treatments for bipolar disorder. However, it has a number of worrisome side-effects and may not fully control the condition. It also has a narrow therapeutic range, meaning that the amount needed for improvement is very close to the amount that can cause problems. Therefore, anyone on lithium should have their dosage and blood levels carefully monitored.

The FAA has certified a number of pilots who are on lithium. Your AME will help you gather your documentation and submit it to the FAA for consideration for a special issuance certificate.

Anxiety

At any given time, between two and four percent of the population suffer from an anxiety disorder that requires treatment. The most common cause of mild anxiety is being in a situation in which you have a high level of responsibility but little authority. The result is a sense of urgency, uncertainty, and powerlessness. Remarkably, some jobs that are most demanding are not terribly stressful. People are capable of tremendous accomplishments when they can follow through on what they need to do. The most anxiety-provoking situation is when you have the responsibility for a task but cannot carry it out because you do not have the confidence, ability, or authority or do so.

Common symptoms of anxiety
Irrational fear (phobia)
Shortness of breath
Palpitations (awareness of heart beat, or skipping a beat)
Sensation of choking
Dizziness
Flushing or chills
Trembling
Sweating
Fear of going crazy, or behaving uncontrollably

Anxiety must first be managed with self-awareness. You should analyze the situation, know what you can and cannot do, ask for help when you need it, and refuse a task that is beyond your ability or authority. Anxiety tends to feed on itself and become a learned response. If you learn to recognize your symptoms, you can develop ways to stop your normal reaction to an anxiety-provoking situation and replace it with a manner that is confident and self-assured.

There are many techniques for reducing anxiety, and you should explore them if this is a problem for you. Learning to manage anxiety also has tremendous benefits in other parts of life by increasing a sense of well-being. The one thing you should not do is use medication or intoxicants to control your anxiety. Anxiety-reducing substances will adversely affect flying performance and are not permitted—and they will not do anything to solve the underlying problem. If you are suffering from severe anxiety and require medication, you should discuss this with your AME to determine a suitable time for return to flight after you have resolved the problem and discontinued your medication.

> "The flyer faces not only the stresses of aviation but also the normal stresses of everyday life. Wings on the chest do not protect against acute stress."

Attention Deficit Hyperactivity Disorder

Attention Deficit Disorder (ADD) and Attention Deficit Hyperactivity Disorder (ADHD) are now diagnosed in 5 to 10 percent of American children and an increasing number of adults. The major features of this disorder are trouble with attention and impulsive behavior. In some, but not all, there is also a degree of hyperactivity.

Attention deficit symptoms
Cannot pay close attention to detail
Failure to follow through on instructions and complete tasks
Difficulty organizing activities
Easily distracted by extraneous stimuli
Forgetfulness

Hyperactivity symptoms
Fidgeting of hands or feet
Excessive talking
Difficulty engaging in leisure activities
Impulsive behavior, interrupting or intruding on others

The actual diagnosis of ADD or ADHD is somewhat controversial. At which point is a "high-energy" person considered to have a mental disorder? The easy, though not simple, answer is when this person begins to experience problems because of these traits. For example, a person whose mind is constantly on the move might not be bothered by it—in fact, a lot of people drink coffee just to speed up their mental activity. But it becomes a problem when the mind is so active that it is impossible to concentrate long enough to complete a task or even to read a paragraph. A proper diagnosis will require more sophisticated tests to determine this condition, including at least three of the following:

- Trail Making Test
- Wisconsin Card Sorting Test
- Paced Auditory Serial Addition Test (PASAT).

If significant abnormalities are noted on these tests, a more detailed psychiatric or psychological evaluation may be needed to determine whether medication is useful.

For reasons that are not well understood, the most effective medications for ADD and ADHD are stimulants. In the same way that coffee makes most people jittery but paradoxically helps others to relax, powerful stimulants such as amphetamine can help quiet the mind in sufferers of ADD and ADHD. The most common medication now is methylphenidate (Ritalin), a drug similar to methamphetamine. Unfortunately, the side-effects of methylphenidate are also similar to those of amphetamines, and include insomnia, headache, appetite loss, and blood pressure increase.

If you have been treated for ADD or ADHD, your application will probably be deferred to the FAA for further evaluation. You will need a current psychological evaluation showing that you are without symptoms.

If you took Ritalin or similar medications when you were a child, up to age 16, you will need to have been off this medication for at least 90 days before the evaluation. If you were treated as an adult, you will only need to have been off the medication for three days before the evaluation.

Normally, the use of psychoactive medication such as methylphenidate is disqualifying for flight. However, the FAA has made exceptions for a few individuals who have shown good mental performance and no side-effects from the medication. These people have been given third-class medical certificates under special issuance, and may not use the medication within 24 hours of flight.

Personality disorder

Personality disorders involve a large group of mental disorders that are difficult to diagnose and even more difficult to treat. Psychiatrists like to say that if you scratch deep enough, you will find some sort of personality disorder in everyone. To determine whether these disorders present a hazard to flight safety, the FAA wants to know if there has been "acting out" behavior—in other words, evidence of poor social judgment, impulsivity, antagonism toward authority, or disregard for regulations. The FAA disqualifies applicants with a personality disorder that is "repeatedly manifested by overt acts or psychosis." For example, if you pretend you are Elvis Presley and dress like him, you may get your medical certificate, but if you really believe you are Elvis and demand that people address you as Mr. Presley, you will probably be denied.

Individuals with personality disorders serious enough to come to medical attention usually have other disqualifying conditions or use disqualifying medications. However, you may achieve certification if your condition is resolved or well controlled. A current psychological evaluation showing that you are without symptoms will be required.

A case of gender dysphoria

A 43-year-old male pilot believed he was truly female. This resulted in a string of unfortunate social problems that included "acting out" at work, getting fired from his job, and finally getting arrested for inappropriate behavior. His aviation medical certificate was denied. After psychotherapy, he resolved his interpersonal problems and began taking hormones in preparation for a sex-change operation (gender reassignment surgery). He, soon to be she, was then given a medical certificate under special issuance, with requirements to document emotional changes and make certain that no adverse complications resulted from the medications or surgery.

Psychosis

Psychosis is a severe form of mental disorder in which there are delusions, hallucinations, and grossly bizarre or disorganized behavior. Any evidence of psychosis, or the possibility of psychosis, is disqualifying. Also disqualifying is the use of anti-psychotic medications.

However, you may still be certified if you have had previous psychotic episodes many years ago but are now healthy. A current psychological evaluation showing that you are without symptoms will be required. With a history of psychosis, your AME is required to either deny or defer your application. With deferral, the FAA will consider each applicant on a case-by-case basis and there is a good chance that you will be certified.

A pilot with Alzheimer's disease
A WW II bomber pilot is now 76 years old and continues to enjoy recreational flying. His family is worried and asks the AME to deny his certificate because he is increasingly confused and has got lost while driving his car. His regular physician diagnosed Alzheimer's disease, and put him on doneprezil (Aricept)—a drug approved by the FAA. He wants to keep flying, and insists that he has no problem. What should the AME do?

Alzheimer's disease involves a gradual loss of brain volume—about 2.4% per year compared with the normal aging loss of 0.4% per year. Along with this loss is a gradual decrease in mental ability, particularly memory and reasoning. As long as the pilot can perform well on mental status tests, he will be able to be certified and keep flying. His family might, however, encourage him to fly with a co-pilot for extra safety.

Psychiatric and psychological evaluation

The key to certification for applicants with current or previous mental health disorders is a thorough evaluation by a qualified psychiatrist or psychologist. A psychiatrist is a physician specializing in mental health, and often treats patients with medication. A psychologist is a non-medically trained specialist in mental heath, and usually focuses on non-drug treatment, such as counseling, psychoanalysis, or behavior modification. "Qualified" in this case is important. A psychiatrist is expected to have a license to practice medicine in your state and to have completed specialty training recognized by the American Board of Psychiatry. A qualified psychologist should have a state license and a Ph.D. in Clinical Psychology from an accredited institution. Unlike most other medical professions, there are many practitioners of psychiatry or psychology who are inadequately trained or not fully competent. Some physicians switch to psychiatry without having the appropriate training, and there are many psychologists who have only mail-order degrees. You must make sure you find a qualified individual, since the FAA will reject your application otherwise.

All records covering prior psychiatric hospitalizations or other periods of observation or treatment should be submitted. These records must be in sufficient detail to permit a clear evaluation of the nature and extent of any previous mental disorders. The current examination and evaluation should be thorough and give special attention to the demands of piloting an aircraft. A summary statement alone is not enough.

Psychological tests should include:

- Revised Wechsler Adult Intelligence Scale (WAIS-R)
- Minnesota Multiphasic Personality Inventory (MMPI)
- Any three or more of the following (or their equivalent) as appropriate:
    - Trails Making Test
    - Category Test
    - Wechsler Memory Scale
    - California Verbal Learning Test
    - Rey Auditory Verbal Learning Test
    - Rorschach Test
    - Sentence Completion Test
    - Personality Assessment Inventory
    - Millon Clinical Multiaxial Inventory (MCMI)
    - Beck or Hamilton Scale (for depression)
    - MAST (for alcoholism).

With a favorable evaluation, you have an excellent chance of achieving certification.

N. Substance dependence or abuse

Substance dependence is not the same as substance abuse. Dependence, often thought of as addiction, is characterized by the following:

- Increased tolerance
- Withdrawal symptoms
- Impaired control over use
- Continued use despite damage to health
- Impairment of social, personal, or occupational functioning.

Of these, the most important feature is the last one. If you are continuing to use a substance that is causing harm to your life, you have a problem. Dependence can refer specifically to physical dependence (having increased tolerance to the substance and suffering withdrawal symptoms when use is stopped, such as a caffeine addiction) or psychological dependence (a craving for the substance, or compulsive behavior regarding its use, such as nicotine addiction).

The FAA is concerned about both physical and psychological substance dependence because they affect judgment and overall ability to function. Even if the substance itself does not noticeably diminish performance, the physical and mental aspects of the addiction can be a safety hazard.

Substance abuse is a somewhat separate issue. The FAA defines abuse as one or both of:

- "Use of a substance in a situation in which that use was physically hazardous."
- "Verified positive drug test result acquired under an anti-drug program."

Legally, "substance abuse" refers to use of any drug (or other material used to achieve the same effects as a drug) in a way that is prohibited or not recognized as an appropriate use. For example, nitrous oxide has many legitimate uses, such as the relief of pain and anxiety during dental work, and to pressurize canisters of whipped cream and other foods. But sniffing nitrous oxide to become intoxicated is abuse of this substance.

In general, any use of an illicit drug within the past five years is disqualifying. However, you may have your application deferred to the FAA and eventually approved if you can show documented recovery and abstinence for at least 24 months prior to the application. This documentation requires a psychiatric evaluation and a completion of a special protocol outlined by the FAA.

In summary, you can be certified by:

- Your AME, if you have been abstinent from substance dependence and not used any illicit substance for at least five years.
- The FAA, if you can document abstinence for 24 months.
- The FAA by special issuance, if you can document abstinence for 12 months.

Drug conviction

Under FAR 61.15, conviction of the violation of any federal or state statute relating to the growing, processing, manufacture, sale, disposition, possession, transportation, or importation of narcotic drugs, marijuana, or depressant or stimulant drugs or substances is grounds for:

- Denial of an application for any certificate or rating for a period of up to one year after the date of final conviction.
- Suspension or revocation of any certificate or rating.

Transporting intoxicated passengers or drugs

Pilots are responsible not only for themselves and the airplane, but also for their passengers and cargo. FAR 91.17 states that a pilot may not allow a person to be carried in his or her aircraft "who appears to be intoxicated" or "demonstrates by manner or by physical indications" that he or she is under the influence of drugs. Note that this regulation does not require actual intoxication, but just the *appearance* of intoxication. To the surprise of many passengers, the airlines often enforce this rule. There is an exception for transporting a medical patient under proper care, or in an emergency. It is also illegal to carry prohibited drugs: FAR 91.19(a) states that "no person may operate a civil aircraft within the United States with knowledge that narcotic drugs, marijuana, and depressant or stimulant drugs or substances as defined in federal or state statutes are carried in the aircraft." The only exception is if the pilot has specific authorization to carry these substances.

Penalties for illegal drug transport can be very severe and often include the loss of the vehicle. The DEA has hangars filled with aircraft confiscated from drug traffickers. You can sometimes get a good deal on these planes when they are auctioned off, or resold by dealers. A clue to the bird's previous life is if the advertisement says something like "Previous ownership unknown" or "Incomplete logbooks." Ah-huh.

O. Alcohol dependence or abuse

An estimated 90 percent of adult Americans drink alcohol and about 75 percent do so on a regular basis. About 10 percent of them experience problems from drinking or have alcoholism. Abuse of alcohol means that there have been physical, psychological, social, or legal problems stemming from the use of alcohol. In other words, abuse means a manner of drinking that causes any kind of problem whatsoever. Common sense would suggest that anyone who experiences problems related to alcohol would avoid it. This is where alcohol dependence becomes an issue. Dependence means that there is either physical dependence (increased tolerance to alcohol, and withdrawal symptoms when drinking is stopped) or psychological dependence (a craving for alcohol), or both. It is not really important to make a distinction between dependence and abuse—the point is, you have a problem.

As long as alcohol is used in a manner that does not cause difficulties, the occasional drink may be a healthy and perhaps even beneficial practice. There is some evidence that one or two drinks a day (about an ounce of alcohol) may protect against heart disease. However, in amounts greater than this, the liver has trouble metabolizing the alcohol. The result is damage to the liver and heart, and ultimately almost every other part of the body.

Alcohol is absorbed quickly on an empty stomach. Carbonation or sugar in the drink increases absorption. Food, especially fatty or greasy food, binds alcohol and slows its entry into the blood. The result is a less intense but more spread out intoxication.

The reason most people drink alcohol is for a sense of well-being. Initially, a drinker might feel a slight increase in energy and is more talkative. Larger amounts bring relaxation, a diminished awareness and concern, and eventually sleepiness. With even a small amount of alcohol, there is a detectable loss of fine control of muscles and physical skills. Memory, concentration, and touch discrimination are reduced. The sense of balance and orientation is impaired. Because alcohol weakens judgment and awareness, the drinker is usually completely oblivious to these effects, and might strongly deny that he or she is impaired. With a level of 0.04 percent, well within the legal driving limit, there is a markedly decreased ability to do an ILS approach. Research shows that blood alcohol concentration as low as 0.02 percent—an almost undetectable amount—can result in impaired performance. Even after the blood alcohol level returns to zero, the individual can be shown to have a slowed reaction time and diminished ability to monitor multiple sensory inputs or to switch rapidly from one task to another. These performance measures were affected 14 hours after drinking, with the pilots completely unaware of any impairment.

The physical effects of alcohol also persist after intoxication. Once it is absorbed into the bloodstream, alcohol is converted into acetaldehyde and then to acetone. The process takes place at a steady rate of about one-third ounce of alcohol per hour, in the average-sized person. The metabolites then persist for up to 48 hours until they are flushed out of the system. In the meantime, the pilot is dehydrated and has a poorer response time, alertness, and tolerance for acceleration. Another effect following alcohol ingestion is Positional Alcohol Nystagmus (PAN), a jerky movement of the eyes that occurs with abrupt head turning or exposure to acceleration. PAN is thought to be due to changes in the inner ear fluid, and can affect a pilot up to 44 hours later.

While I was in medical school, an obviously drunk, loud-mouthed man smelling of alcohol arrived by ambulance at the emergency room. Clutching his chest, he insisted he was having a heart attack, and denied having had any alcohol. Naturally, we couldn't take any chances and hooked him up to a heart monitor. After asking him a few more times, "Are you sure you haven't had any drinks?" he angrily said, "I told you, NO!" and we stepped out of the room. He probably rolled over and pulled off the wires, because the nurse outside the room saw the monitor line go flat. She figured he was having a heart attack and immediately called the emergency resuscitation team. They burst into the room, slapped the paddles on his chest and shocked him. THAT got his attention. He jumped up and yelled, "OK! OK! I did have a couple of drinks!"

A large dose of alcohol puts a heavy burden on the body to metabolize it, resulting in a hangover—tremors, thirst, nausea and vomiting, heartburn, sweating, dizziness, headaches, irritability, anxiety, and mental depression. All of these have a negative effect on flying performance.

The only cure for alcohol intoxication or a hangover is time—up to 36 hours of rest, a proper diet, and plenty of fluids to make up for the dehydration. Caffeine can make a person feel better, but all this does is cause a more jittery intoxication or hangover. It may actually be more dangerous, by fooling a drinker into thinking that he or she is now sober.

Don't you get drunk more easily at higher altitude?

Alcohol intoxication affects judgment, memory, and slows interpretation of data. These effects are also seen with hypoxia experienced at high altitudes (see *Chapter 5: Using oxygen*). Extreme altitude is often described as a "drunken" feeling. In fact, the way each of these affects the brain is quite different. Despite the popular belief that you get more drunk at higher altitude, there is no difference in alcohol intoxication.

Alcoholism

Alcoholism is a somewhat old-fashioned term. It loosely refers to a "drinking problem" and not only addiction. The preferred term now is substance dependence, recognizing that people can develop unhealthy habits of using a large variety of other substances besides alcohol.

How do you know if you are a problem drinker? It takes an unusually self-aware person to acknowledge that his or her drinking is out of control. The key feature of alcohol abuse is denial. Less than 10 percent of the requests for treatment come from the drinkers themselves; the majority come from their family, concerned friends, business partners, flying colleagues, or supervisors. Everyone seems to be aware of the problem except for the drinker. Ask anyone how much he or she drinks and you will probably get an underestimate, and the more they drink the more misleading the answer will be.

Physicians diagnose alcohol abuse by using a standard questionnaire. There are many such questionnaires and an enormous amount of research has made them very sophisticated. Some are highly specific, in-depth, and quite accurate. But I always like the simple CAGE questions, because the test is quick and gets right to the point:

Are you an alcoholic?

C Have you ever tried to cut down on your use of alcohol?
A Has anyone ever become angry because of your drinking?
G Have you ever felt guilty about your drinking, or your actions because of it?
E Do you ever take an "eye-opener"—a morning drink to relieve a hangover or to feel better?

1 Yes answer: You had better take a very close and honest look at your drinking and give some serious thought to the role of alcohol in your life.
2 Yes answers: You definitely have a problem. There is a 50:50 chance you are an alcoholic. Time to stop drinking, or seek counseling, before you get into trouble.
3 or 4 Yes answers: You are more than 90% likely to be an alcoholic. If you doubt it, you are in denial.

Alcohol and pilots

The rate of alcohol abuse among commercial pilots is not known, but it is believed to be about the same as the rate among other professionals in the United States—in other words, about 5 to 10 percent. Flying while intoxicated, however, is quite rare. This may be because the penalties are very harsh. Commercial or air transport pilots who are found to have used alcohol while on duty generally have their licenses revoked permanently. There is no opportunity for reinstatement.

Alcohol use among all pilots

	1st class	2nd class	3rd class
One alcohol offense	4,694	3,934	10,318
Two alcohol offenses	440	443	998
Three or more offenses	111	129	242
Alcohol abuse, but not addiction	975	656	1,812
Alcohol addiction	981	221	381

Alcohol is involved in 6 to 8 percent of all general aviation accidents, and 10 to 30 percent of fatal accidents. In comparison, airline accidents due to alcohol are very rare.

The FAA has several overlapping regulations regarding alcohol use. A person may not act as a pilot (or required crewmember) of an aircraft:

1. Within eight hours of consuming any alcoholic beverage, regardless of whether he or she is under the influence of alcohol.

2. If he or she is under the influence of alcohol, no matter how long ago that alcohol was consumed.

3. If the blood alcohol concentration is 0.04 percent or greater.

The FAA does not conduct tests for alcohol on people other than FAA employees. The FAA does require, however, that a pilot submit to an alcohol test if requested by a state or local law enforcement officer. The law enforcement officer must be authorized to request the test, and must have reasonable suspicion that a violation of the law has occurred. The test must be administered within four hours after the person acted, or attempted to act, as an aircraft crewmember. The test must also indicate the blood alcohol concentration.

While the FAA sets the blood alcohol concentration standard at 0.04 percent, most airlines use a more restrictive requirement that there is no detectable amount of alcohol in the blood. In practice, this means about 0.02 percent blood alcohol. For this reason, the US military increases the 8 hour post-drink time to 12 hours, and most airlines require 24 hours "bottle to throttle."

How to get a medical certificate after recovery

It used to be that someone who had ever been an alcoholic, even if it was 25 years ago, would not be medically certified. Now the FAA regulations are much more compassionate and it is possible to be certified with total abstinence in as little as two years. A few first- and second-class certificates have been granted after just six months under special issuance.

The key feature of alcoholism is denial, and the most important first step in recovery from alcoholism is to recognize that there is a real problem. Some problem drinkers are astute enough to see that they are getting into trouble and manage to stop drinking before they have a violation. Once you have an alcohol violation, it is necessary to convince the FAA that you have completely recovered before you will be eligible for certification.

Most recovery programs involve a lengthy period of attendance at Alcoholics Anonymous (AA) meetings. You will have a "sponsor," typically a former alcoholic who has recovered and can meet with you frequently to discuss problems and progress.

Your application will be deferred by your AME to the FAA for evaluation. You should write a letter to the Federal Air Surgeon stating that you have been treated for your alcohol (or other substance) abuse, and had at least one full year of complete abstinence. Although the FAA requirement is two years of complete abstinence, they will consider your application after one year. You will need to submit a record of your treatment. If you were admitted to a residential facility, you will also need to submit your discharge summary. Finally, you will need to provide a thorough evaluation by an addiction specialist, such as a substance abuse counselor, psychologist, psychiatrist, or other physician with training in addictive disorders. This evaluation should include enough information to determine whether an addiction problem still exists, and comments about your character and behavior addressing the following features:

- **Personal**
  - Anxiety, depression, insomnia
  - Suicidal thoughts or attempts
  - Personality changes
  - Loss of self-esteem
- **Social**
  - Isolation
  - Family problems
  - Marital separation or divorce
  - Irresponsibility

- Child or spouse abuse
- Separation from family or friends

Legal
- Alcohol-related traffic offenses
- Public intoxication
- Assault and battery

Occupational
- Absenteeism or tardiness at work
- Reduced productivity
- Demotions
- Frequent job changes
- Loss of employment

Medical
- Blackouts
- Memory impairment
- Stomach, liver, or cardiovascular problems
- Sexual dysfunction

Economic
- Frequent financial crises
- Bankruptcy
- Loss of home
- Lack of credit

Alcohol use
- Alcohol tolerance
- Withdrawal
- Loss of control
- Preoccupied with alcohol use
- Continued use despite consequences

The FAA may require a program of random drug tests, liver function tests, or other tests. They will also want a list of charges, dates, and states of occurrence for all court convictions previously undeclared to the FAA, if any.

By January 1996, 1,500 pilots recovering from alcohol abuse had regained their medical certificates under special issuance. John Denver, a gifted musician and actor, was not among them. He died on October 12, 1997, shortly after departing on an illegal solo flight from Monterey, California.

Studies show that relapse rates after even the best treatment for alcohol abuse are about 7 to 15 percent within the first year. Because of this, medical certificates for recovering alcoholics are usually given for just 6 months. The FAA will likely require a monitoring program for 24 months, with a final evaluation of recovery by the Federal Air Surgeon. If you were in a residential facility, you will need to submit an aftercare plan and monthly reports from your treatment coordinator beginning 30 days after discharge. The reports describe your participation in therapy sessions or AA meetings, your continuing progress and, of course, your abstinence from further alcohol or substance abuse.

"We can't solve problems by using the same kind of thinking we used when we created them."—Albert Einstein

P. Suicide attempt

Any indication of attempted suicide, suicidal gestures, or other self-destructive behavior will require a psychological evaluation. Your AME will probably defer your application to the FAA for review and recommendations for further evaluation.

People change. A self-destructive gesture when you were a teenager does not mean you are barred for life from getting a pilot's license. If you feel confident that you have resolved the issues related to that event, and are no longer at risk for any such behavior, you should pursue your goal. Like anything else of value, this will take time, patience, and determination.

The recent, highly publicized events of suicide by pilots have heightened public concern and politicians have demanded that the FAA take more caution in approving flying privileges. That means you might have to do a bit more work to get certified, but the fundamental regulations have not changed.

Q. Motion sickness requiring medication

Motion sickness has been a common problem ever since the beginning of vehicle travel thousands of years ago. It was well known during Biblical times as "camel sickness"—the gentle swaying caused nausea in many riders (in fact, Lawrence of Arabia was often sick to the point of incapacitation from his long camel journeys). When traveling by sea became widespread, the name changed to seasickness. The word nausea actually comes from the Greek "naus" meaning ship. More recently, we have carsickness, airsickness, space motion sickness, simulator sickness, and virtual reality motion sickness.

Motion sickness is not a disorder. It is a normal response to an abnormal stimulus. All types of motion sickness are due to the same basic problem:

a disagreement between the information you get from your eyes and the information from the vestibular organs of your inner ears—between what you see and what you feel. The result is a confusion in your brain's normal sensory awareness processing. Something doesn't feel right. This is the same sort of sensory disturbance that might result from eating toxic or spoiled foods. The body is programmed in this case to get rid of the food as fast as possible. This is why motion sickness causes vomiting.

Airsickness is the main concern for pilots. Surveys show that incapacitating airsickness occurs in 29 percent of airline pilots. Motion sickness is even more common when using a flight simulator, and up to 70 percent of pilots are affected. Surprisingly, the best pilots are the most susceptible. This is probably because they are more familiar with how the simulator should act, and when it doesn't, the difference between visual and vestibular senses is more obvious.

Motion sickness is familiar to most people: it begins with an uncomfortable sensation that is often called "stomach awareness." This leads to increased salivation, swallowing and burping. Sometimes, there is less stomach discomfort and more of an overall sense of feeling drowsy or tired, with perspiration, difficulty concentrating, and mental confusion. All of these feelings can quickly progress to outright nausea and vomiting. That usually makes the person feel slightly better, but the unfortunate ones who are most affected go on to repeated bouts of retching and diarrhea.

There is no way to predict who is going to become motion sick. A number of factors increase your likelihood:

- Youth: susceptibility to motion sickness begins at about age two, increases to a peak in adolescence, and then steadily diminishes with passing years—a minor blessing of old age.
- Females tend to be more susceptible than males. This is especially true during menses or pregnancy, or if they use birth control pills.
- Athletes are more susceptible. Why? Probably because people who are fit tend to have highly tuned senses and are more likely to notice sensory conflict.
- Anxiety and stress increase motion sickness.
- Large meals, especially those high in salt, protein, or dairy products.

- Alcohol.
- Smoking.
- Bad odors; it is best to get cool, fresh air.
- Abrupt head movements; it is best to move slowly rather than sharply bobbing or swiveling the head.

Because motion sickness is caused by a conflict of senses, it tends to go away as the person becomes accustomed to this conflict and accepts it as natural. This is why seasickness usually resolves within a day or two. The problem with flying is that pilots rarely stay aloft that long.

Once people experience motion sickness, they are much more likely to get it again. They will quickly recognize the uncomfortable sensation and they know what is coming next. Some pilots who have often become airsick will start to feel nauseated even if they just look at an airplane or smell aviation fuel. By that point, it takes a lot longer to reverse the tendency to airsickness.

Simulator sickness

Simulator sickness is slightly different from the usual airsickness. The most often reported symptoms are eyestrain, blurred vision, difficulty focusing, and visual flashbacks, with occasional headache and difficulty concentrating. Some pilots, even those who never have any problems during flight, get a little unsteady on their feet after being in a simulator for several hours. The FAA recommends that pilots do not fly, or even drive, for a few hours after an extended session in a simulator. If the simulator is a very high-quality cockpit substitute, the effects are more severe and the FAA recommends delaying actual pilot-in-command flight for 12 hours.

Motion sickness medications

All standard motion sickness medications cause drowsiness or other mental impairments. They also have many other side-effects, such as visual disturbances and dry mouth. Because of this, the FAA does not allow the pilot in command to use motion sickness medication. (The military makes an exception, and may allow pilots to use a combination of scopolamine and dextroamphetamine, "scop-dex.")

The most common motion sickness medications are antihistamines, including diphenhydramine (e.g, Benadryl), meclizine (Antivert), dimenhydrinate (Dramamine), cyclizine (Marizine), and buclizine (Bucladin-S). In general, they cause some drowsiness but are otherwise relatively safe and can also be used by children. They are available without prescription, but none of them are allowed by the FAA.

The most effective motion sickness remedy is scopolamine, usually taken in the form of a patch placed behind the ear. This medication works slowly as it leaches into the skin and the effects continue for a long time—a single patch will last for about three days. Scopolamine also has the worst side-effects, with visual problems and even severe mental effects in some people. Users must also take great care in handling the patch. If the hands are not washed immediately after, touching an eye can result in a horrendously enlarged pupil. Scopolamine (Transderm Scop) patches are available only by prescription.

Other very effective motion sickness medications include the anti-nausea drugs promethazine (Phenergan) and trimethobenzamide (Tigan). These are available by prescription, and may be combined with ephedrine to minimize drowsiness, but are not allowed by the FAA.

Airsickness medications can be very useful while training since they allow the pilot to become accustomed to the sensations of flight without becoming ill. However, they may be used only when accompanied by an instructor pilot or so long as you are not acting as pilot-in-command.

Airsickness medication can be very useful while training, but may not be used by a solo pilot.

If you are worried about becoming airsick, it is useful to experiment with medication during your training flights. Once you feel comfortable flying while using medication, begin flying without the medication but only on calm days and doing only mild, gentle maneuvers. Then gradually increase exposure to more extreme maneuvers. The best way to combat airsickness is to take it easy. You must condition your body to accept the sensory disturbance as a normal feeling.

How about those acupressure wrist bands?

Many people claim that acupressure relieves motion sickness. Elastic wrist bands and an electrical stimulating device are available. The point to be stimulated is on the front forearm, about 1.5 inches from the wrist crease, called the P6 point in acupuncture. A number of studies have been undertaken to see if stimulating this point is effective in preventing motion sickness. The results have not been impressive. On the other hand, the practice does not cause any harm, so if it works for you, great, but I wouldn't count on it.

Does ginger root work? Does the FAA allow it for pilot use?

Ginger root has long been used in traditional Chinese medicine to prevent nausea. There is some evidence that it can alleviate motion sickness. It is taken as a powder, in tea, or as candied ginger. Some people even chew the fresh root, although it has a very sharp taste. The FAA does not specifically prohibit the use of any herbal remedy, but prohibits use of any medication, substance, or supplement that might impair performance. Since ginger is unlikely to cause any side-effect, it is allowed.

In summary, ginger root appears to be safe and may be helpful for some people. You should inform your AME if you are taking ginger for this purpose, or any other supplements or herbal remedies.

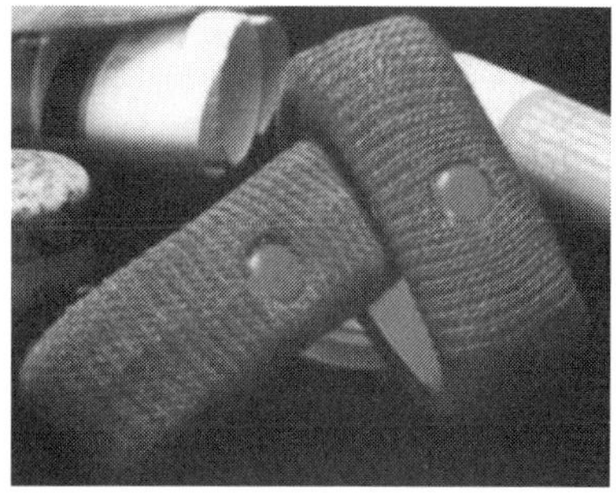

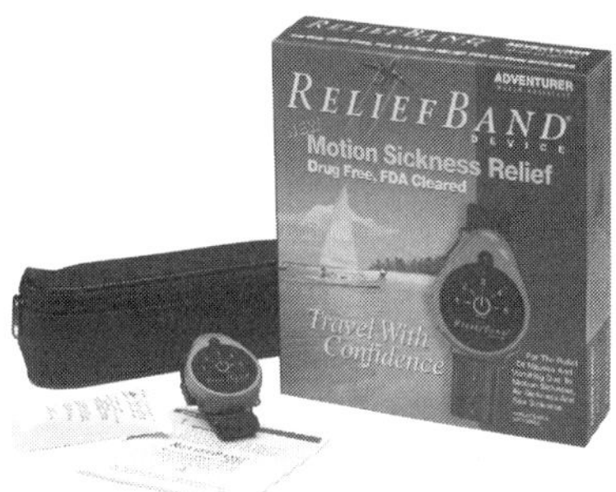

How to prevent airsickness without medication

With enough sensory disturbance, everyone will eventually experience some degree of motion sickness. The best way to avoid it is by minimizing the sensory conflict, and by a process of adaptation so that the conflict is less bothersome. The military uses a program of "G Awareness Maneuvers" to prepare candidates for aerobatics and dogfighting. They do this with a series of brief flight maneuvers, gradually increasing in intensity, never progressing until the pilot is comfortable with the milder maneuver. In this way, a steady accommodation is allowed. You can do the same with training flights or by hitching a ride as a passenger.

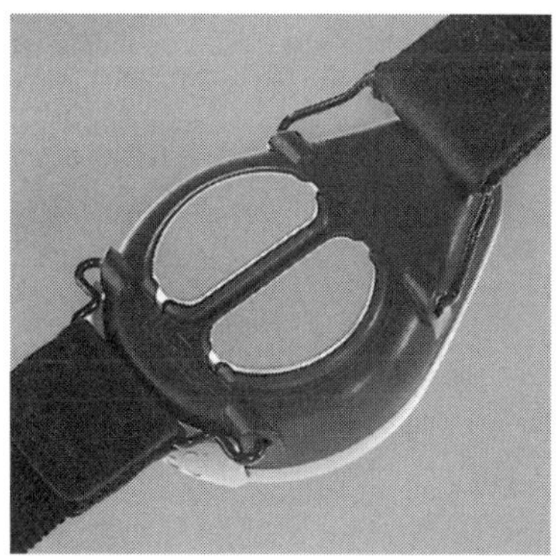

Acupressure wrist bands and Relief Band: Resembling a sports watch, the Relief Band is worn on the underside of the wrist, sending electrical pulses to the median nerve.

To prevent motion sickness before flight:

- Eat a light, non-spicy snack 2-3 hours before flight. Avoid large or spicy meals, or a completely empty stomach. Also avoid alcohol.

- Do not smoke.

- Become familiar with the planned flight, where you will go and what maneuvers will be done. Do not do aerobatics with another pilot without fully briefing each other before takeoff.

- Wear light, loose clothing that allows free movement.

- Relax. Try to deal with any anxiety about the flight or other conditions by resolving problems or discussing them with your instructor. Try to get to know your instructor on a personal level so that there is trust, understanding, and good communication.

> Lucy loved flying but got airsick on all of her five training flights. She worried that she would never get over it and went to an AME in desperation. Her physical examination showed no abnormalities. On the contrary, she was in great shape and had been a college gymnast. Lucy described herself as a competitive person, one who tackled physical problems head-on. To handle the stress of gymnastic contests, she had learned some relaxation techniques. The AME encouraged her to use these techniques, eat lightly before flying, and do a thorough preparation for each flight during which she would visualize the flight maneuvers—just as she used to do for her gymnastic meets. She discussed this with her instructor, and they decided to keep initial flights to early morning and evening when the air was calm. Lucy overcame her airsickness, became comfortable in rough air, and earned her pilot certificate.

To prevent motion sickness during flight:

- Concentrate on flying tasks, keeping the aircraft straight and level or in a precise turn. It is especially useful to keep pitch and vertical changes to a minimum.

- Focus on the horizon, if you have one. If in instrument flight, pay even more attention than usual to the Attitude Indicator, with its artificial horizon.

- Open the vents to get some fresh, cool air on your face.
- Use supplemental oxygen if it is available.

Flicker vertigo

About 1 in 4 pilots have been annoyed or distracted by flicker at some time in their careers. This happens most often with helicopter pilots, but also occurs in propeller aircraft on the ground with the engines idling, or with flashing or rotating lights reflecting off cloud or other surfaces. Some people are abnormally sensitive to low-frequency flashing lights and may even suffer epileptic seizures. Most people simply feel a sense of annoyance or discomfort, with pain in the eyes, headache, a sense of movement, spinning, nausea, or drowsiness. Studies show that from 4 to 6 percent of helicopter pilots have abnormal brain waves during low-frequency light flashes, but do not show any problem in performance. About 1 in 20,000 has a more severe reaction and should not fly.

A medical helicopter pilot told his AME about a disturbing problem. While facing the setting sun, the rotors produced a strong flicker and he suddenly felt very dizzy, nauseated, and disoriented. The AME recommended that the pilot try to avoid this kind of flight condition by turning away from the light source or changing the RPM. The AME also suggested that if the pilot had to fly in such a condition, he should use sunglasses or a sunshade and frequently glance away or briefly close his eyes to avoid gazing at the flicker.

R. Military medical discharge

A military medical discharge does not disqualify you, but the underlying reasons need to be examined. You should bring records of your discharge to the AME, showing the dates and circumstances surrounding the discharge, and whether you are receiving disability compensation. If you are on a veteran's disability, you should show your claim number and service number. This information will be assembled by the AME for submission to the FAA. Your initial medical certificate may be deferred to the FAA, but will ultimately be approved if you have no other problems.

For recertification, your initial letter of approval from the FAA will be enough to get your certificate.

S. Medical rejection for military service

A medical rejection for military service does not disqualify you, but the underlying reasons need to be examined. You should bring records of your medical rejection to the AME. The records should include the place, cause, and date of rejection; it is also useful to have copies of any other military documents. This information will be assembled by the AME for submission to the FAA. Your initial medical certificate may be deferred to the FAA, but ultimately approved if you have no other problems.

For recertification, your initial letter of approval from the FAA will be enough to get your certificate.

T. Rejection for life or health insurance

A rejection for life or health insurance does not disqualify you, but the underlying reasons need to be examined. You should bring records of your rejection to the AME. The records should include the place, cause, and date of rejection. This information will be assembled by the AME for submission to the FAA. Your initial medical certificate may be deferred to the FAA, but ultimately approved if you have no other problems.

For recertification, your initial letter of approval from the FAA will be enough to get your certificate.

U. Admission to hospital

For each admission to a hospital, you should bring your complete hospital record. This should include:

- Address of the hospital or clinic
- Date of admission
- Diagnoses
- Duration of hospitalization
- Treatments
- Name of the attending physician
- Discharge summary.

This is only necessary once. For each subsequent medical examination, you may state "PREVIOUSLY REPORTED, NO CHANGE".

V. History of traffic conviction

It is long been noted that pilots who have a bad driving record are also far more likely to be involved in an aviation accident. This is especially the case with pilots who have convictions of driving under the influence (DUI). A DUI is essentially the same as the older term Driving While Intoxicated (DWI), but does not require actual intoxication. Studies show that a private pilot with just a single DUI has twice the likelihood of being involved in an aircraft accident. A study in Florida found hundreds of pilots who couldn't drive to the airport because they had lost their driver's license because of DUI convictions, but were legally flying!

The problem is especially worrisome because a key feature of alcohol abuse is denial. An alcoholic is less likely to admit any other kind of problem on an FAA application. The Office of Inspector General (OIG) of the United States Department of Transportation carried out a seven-year study in which the FAA medical files of 711,648 active pilots were compared with state records of alcohol- and drug-related traffic offenses. They found that 3.4 percent of the pilots had at least one DUI conviction. Of these pilots, about 75 percent did not report this information to the FAA.

The National Driver Register (NDR) keeps track of all motor violations recorded in the United States. In the past 10 years, more than 4 million names of pilots have checked in the NDR and over 100,000 pilots found to have drug-related or alcohol-related motor vehicle violations. The FAA has investigated each of these, and handed out more than 8,300 enforcement actions. About 3,000 pilots have lost their medical and airman certificates for failing to notify the FAA of their motor vehicle violations. That accounts for almost one third of all revocations by the FAA, and it is the most common reason for a pilot to lose a certificate. Pilots lying about their traffic convictions used to be quite common, but do so less since word got out about the NDR. According to Mark Sweeney, manager of the Compliance and Enforcement Branch of the Civil Aviation Security Division, the number of violations has fallen significantly since the program was put into place.

What kind of motor vehicle violation do I have to report?

You must report every:

- Conviction, under any federal or state law, of operating a motor vehicle while intoxicated by alcohol or drugs.

- Denial, cancellation, suspension or revocation of your driver's license for driving while impaired by drugs or alcohol.

- Refusal to take a breathalyzer test, when suspected of driving while impaired by drugs or alcohol.

> Some pilots have been advised by their lawyers that a report to the FAA is not required if the case was dismissed, or plea-bargained to a lesser charge. This is not correct. If your driver's license is suspended (or canceled, or revoked) you must report it.

I had a DUI. When, and how, do I report it to the FAA?

You have to do two things:

- Write a letter to the FAA within 60 days of the DUI (see *Sample DUI Report Letter*).

- Report the DUI on Form 8500-8 at your next medical application.

You must do both. Neither one will substitute for the other.

According to FAR 61.15(e), any DUI must be reported to the Aviation Security Division within 60 days. You should send the letter by certified mail with a return receipt. There is no printed official form on which to report motor vehicle actions, which is odd since there is an official form for almost everything else.

What happens if I don't report an alcohol-related motor vehicle action to the FAA?

When you sign your medical application, you are authorizing the FAA to access your data on the National Driver Register. If the FAA finds that you falsified your application by omitting information, they can suspend or revoke any or all of your certificates for a year. The usual penalty is a 30-day suspension of your airman certificate.

> The most common cause of losing an aviation certificate is failing to report a DUI motor vehicle violation.

I had a DUI and I reported it. What happens next?

A single DUI conviction will not affect your FAA certification. If you have had two within three years, or more than three in any period, the FAA may revoke or deny your medical certificate. The denial is usually for one year following the most recent violation, but may be longer. It depends largely on the results of a substance abuse or mental health evaluation.

I have a student pilot certificate, but haven't soloed yet. Do I still have to report a DUI to the FAA?

Yes. The regulation holds for all aviation certificates.

Sample DUI Report Letter

Your address
Date

FAA Civil Security Division
AMC-700
PO Box 25810
Oklahoma City, OK 73125

Dear Sir:

I am sending this letter to report a motor vehicle action as required by FAR 61.15. My address is printed above. My date of birth is __________ and my certificate number is __________.

The type of violation with which I was charged on __________(date) was __________(driving under the influence), which resulted in __________(action or conviction). The date of this action was __________. The state that holds the record of this action is _________. This is my first and only (or whatever number) violation of any kind regarding 61.15. I have had ________actions against me at any time regarding this FAR.

If you require any further information in this matter, please notify me and I will respond immediately.

Respectfully,
Name (signature and print)

How can I get a copy of my NDR file?

You must submit a written, notarized request to:
DOT
NHTSA
NTS-24
400 7th Street, SW
Washington, D.C. 20590-0001

Just write on a sheet of paper, "I would like a copy of my NDR file." Include your name, address, and driver's license number. It is also helpful to include your social security number and date of birth. You should then take the letter to any notary public (most banks and other institutions have a person who can act as a notary public; they may charge you a small fee for the service). The notary will ask for picture identification, ask you to sign the letter, and then put a stamp of verification on your letter that you signed it.

I had a DUI. First my license was suspended and then I was convicted. Do I have to report both the suspension and conviction, even though it was the same incident?

Yes, each event must be reported. However, the FAA will recognize that this involved a single incident and will not penalize you for two events.

I was charged with a DUI and my license was suspended. The charge was eventually dropped. Do I still have to report this to the FAA, even though my record is clear?

Yes. Any suspension of your license must be reported, even though the charge was dropped and your license reinstated.

I had not been drinking, but was asked to take a breath test anyway. I refused, since I consider this a violation of my civil liberty. The FAA then revoked my certificate. How can they do this, since I did not commit any alcohol violation?

Refusal to take an alcohol test when appropriate is also considered a violation, even if you had not consumed alcohol.

W. History of non-traffic conviction

If you have been convicted of any crime, you should report this and give details. Report the charge, the date of the conviction, and the state or other jurisdiction where it took place. This information will not disqualify you in itself, but will be reviewed by the AME and FAA to evaluate your application.

Failure to report any conviction is a serious offence. More pilots lose their certificates because of falsifying their application than for the actual conviction. Therefore, it is very important to list any convictions. Once this has been done, and you receive your certificate, you may simply state, "PREVIOUSLY REPORTED, NO CHANGE" on future applications. Of course, if you have any new conviction since your last examination, you will need to report it.

X. Other illness, disability, or surgery

Any illness or surgery that presents a possible hazard to flying will be carefully reviewed. In the vast majority of cases, you will have recovered from the problem by the time of the medical examination. If you had a serious illness or surgery, you should bring a copy of your medical record to the AME. It is possible that the AME will have to defer the application to the FAA. This is not a denial, but a *deferral*—it simply means that the FAA wants to ensure that the condition is resolved, or at least poses little risk, before certification. Deferral means, "Let's take a closer look and make sure everything is OK." As anyone who has had any experience with the government knows, this closer look can take plenty of time, involve a seemingly endless amount of paperwork and phone calls, and quite a bit of frustration as well. This is where a good AME can be invaluable, and where it pays to be well prepared.

It is really just a matter of common sense. You, the AME, and the FAA all want to be reasonably certain that you are fit to fly. This can be done in an endless run-around in which everyone is exasperated and you finally give up in frustration. Or it can be done in a straightforward process—describing the problem, doing the necessary tests or examinations to show that the problem is resolved (or at least controlled), and forwarding the proper documentation to the appropriate individuals. Simple.

> While you are sick with any kind of illness, however mild, you should avoid flying—a temporary "self disqualification."

How sick do you need to be?

For the purpose of your aviation medical examination, you should report as illness anything that is more than a cold, flu, or mild pain that went away after a few days and did not require anything more than over-the-counter medications. Illness, in this case, also does not include routine dental work such as cleaning. It does, however, include mental or emotional issues that require visits to a mental health professional, social worker, or counselor.

Surgery

Any major surgery—more than just a few stitches for a cut or a mole removal—will require a letter from the surgeon and deferral to the FAA for evaluation. The FAA will want all medical records, including the admission history and physical examination, the discharge summary, and the pathology and operation reports. Normally, these are included in a single packet in your medical record, and getting a copy of this record should be easy.

Arthritis, muscle, or skeletal problems

The pilot population is aging. There was a time when almost all pilots were young males. The typical flying school student was a line-boy with dreams of an airline career, or a recently discharged soldier taking the opportunity to learn to fly with his Veteran's benefits to pay for the lessons. That is no longer the case. The majority of new students, and the flying population as a whole, are now more likely to be middle-aged professionals—men and women—flying for work, pleasure, or the convenience of independent travel. Along with increasing age comes arthritis, a gradual erosion of the joints that eventually afflicts everyone if they live long enough.

Arthritis is not a disqualifying condition if it causes no severe symptoms. If it is treated only with non-prescription medications, you may be certified by the AME. A more severe case will require a letter from your treating physician describing your medications and the absence of problematic side-effects or other conditions that might affect flying performance.

A previous experience of other bone or joint diseases, such as degenerative disc disease, may also be certified by the AME, if:

- There has been complete recovery.
- There is no need for further medications.
- There is no neurological deficit, such as pain or numbness or loss of muscle strength.

If any of these are present, it will be necessary to provide a report from the treating physician, and this will be forwarded to the FAA for evaluation. Even with quite severe residual problems, it is still possible to be certified.

I twisted my ankle, but I feel fine now. I told my AME, and he kept me from flying for another three weeks. I'm angry and wonder if I shouldn't have told him!

You were right to tell the AME, and it could have been a costly mistake to hide any illness or injury. A sprained ankle is a good example. The initial sprain may stop hurting after a few days, and feel like it has healed, but it is still weak for weeks or even months depending on the injury. You may feel fine and not notice the weakness until the day you are caught in a strong crosswind landing and you push hard on the rudder pedal and your ankle gives out. Then, my friend, you have a problem.

Your AME is looking out for you. Hiding information is about as useful as not telling your mechanic about a glitch in the airplane. It is better to be a little extra careful than take the risk.

Sleep disorders

Sleep disorders are a very common problem (see *Chapter 5: Fatigue*) and an increasing number of pilots report using medication or mechanical aids to help them sleep. Any medication or sleep treatment must be reported at the time of application. If there has been medical treatment for a sleep disorder, two basic reports must be provided:

- A sleep study
- A maintenance of wakefulness test.

Once these are done, follow-up reports will normally only need to include a status note from the treating physician.

A sleep disorder is usually treated in four ways:

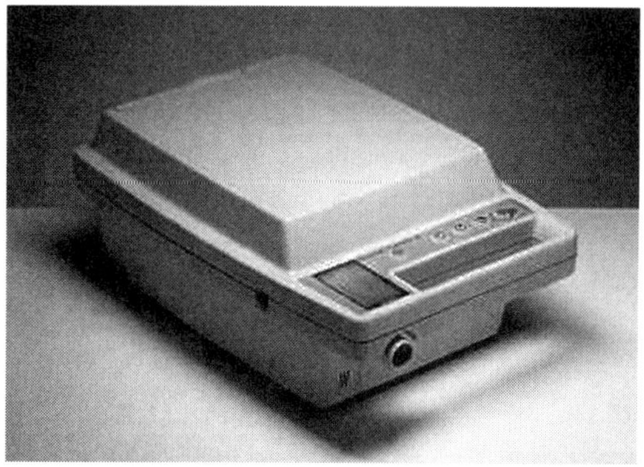

The ResMed SULLIVAN VPAP II (Variable Positive Airway Pressure) delivers quiet, comfortable, bilevel therapy with customizable pressure transitions. The VPAP II is suitable for spontaneously breathing patients with sleep-disordered breathing.

1. Improving "sleep hygiene": avoiding alcohol and stimulating substances, a better sleep arrangement, relaxation techniques, etc. These require only a brief description and may be certified by the AME.

2. Mechanical sleep aids, such as mouthpieces or nasal devices, ranging up to CPAP or BIPAP machines for obstructive sleep apnea. The AME must defer certification, and a report will be required from the treating physician showing that the disorder is controlled.

3. Surgery, including the removal of obstructive nose or throat tissue to allow breathing during sleep. Once the initial reports show that the treatment was successful, without complications, no further reports are required.

4. Medication, including "sleeping pills." In general, most sleep medications have an extended influence on mental alertness and are therefore disqualifying for flight duties. Once these are discontinued, however, flying may be resumed and certification is achievable.

Cancer

If you had a low-grade cancer and present very good documentation of it being resolved, your AME may be able to certify you directly after getting approval with a phone call to the Regional Flight Surgeon or Aerospace Medical Certification Division in Oklahoma City. In most cases, however, a diagnosis of cancer will require that the AME defer your application to the FAA for further evaluation.

If you were admitted to a hospital, you will need to provide a copy of all medical records, including the admission history and physical examination, the discharge summary, and the pathology reports. If you had chemotherapy or radiation therapy, you will also need a letter from the oncologist and radiation therapist. All of this, plus a recent (within 30 days) status report from the treating physician. Whew! That's a lot, but your doctor should be able to assemble these fairly quickly so that you can be well prepared for your visit to the AME. The application will still need to be deferred, but the process will be greatly speeded up with all of this documentation.

If you have completed all chemotherapy or radiation treatment, and there is no evidence of metastatic disease, you should be eligible for a medical certificate for a specified period—usually a year. The FAA will most likely require an annual status report to ensure no further complications have occurred.

I had skin cancer recently. Can I get certified?

The FAA has the same basic requirements for all types of cancer. Your treating doctor should write a report detailing the type, location, and extent of the malignancy. The report should also indicate any surgery or treatment regimen used (for example, radiation or chemotherapy). The dates of your treatment and the doctor's prognosis should also be included. The FAA will consider certification after 60 days have elapsed from the date of surgery or treatment.

The FAA certification decision depends on the type and location of the cancer. In general, common skin cancers such as basal cell or squamous carcinoma are more readily approved than melanoma.

Some cancer treatments require chemotherapy on and off for a few days every month. If you have no side-effects and recover well from chemotherapy, you may be able to fly as soon as 72 hours after your course of chemotherapy has been completed. On-going oral chemotherapy may be allowed on a case-by-case basis. In general, intravenous chemotherapy is disqualifying, but the FAA has in fact certified pilots on continuous chemotherapy infusions.

Cancer of the breast or lung, or melanoma skin cancer, requires a specific evaluation. If the melanoma tumor is greater than 0.75 mm on the Breslow Scale, you will need to have a current MRI of the brain to show that there is no spread of the cancer. When cancer spreads to the brain, the chance of a seizure is quite high and you will probably be disqualified for flight. If there is no evidence of cancer in the brain, you may be given a:

- Third-class certificate if you have a repeat MRI of the brain and status report *every year* for at least five years.

- First- or second-class certificate if you have a repeat MRI of the brain and status report every *six months* for at least five years.

If you have ever had metastatic cancer of any type, you will need to show at least one year of stability before your application. If you had metastatic cancer of the brain, lung, or melanoma, you will need a current MRI of the brain, to be repeated annually, and you will need to show at least three years of stability. If you have ever had cancer (of the breast, lung, or melanoma) spread to the brain or central nervous system, you will need to show at least five years of stability before your application, and a current MRI of the brain, to be repeated annually.

HIV

The treatment of HIV infection and AIDS is progressing rapidly and each year brings newer and more effective medications. The FAA now regularly issues medical certificates to pilots who are HIV positive or who have had an AIDS-defining illness. Your AME will not be able to issue you the certificate directly, but will defer the application to the FAA for further evaluation. To facilitate your application, you should bring the following documents to your AME:

- An examination report by a physician who is knowledgeable in the treatment of HIV-infected individuals. This report should include a detailed medical history with your symptoms and treatment, listing medications and whether there have been side-effects.

- A "viral load" determination by polymerase chain reaction (PCR).

- A CD4+ lymphocyte count.

- A complete blood count (CBC).

- A panel of liver function tests.

- An initial assessment of cognitive function by COGSCREEN (or similar test).

At the time of your application, your viral load must not exceed 1,000 copies per milliliter of plasma, and cognitive testing must show no significant deficit that would affect safety.

Every three months, you should have follow-up lab tests reporting viral load by PCR, CD4+ cell count, and other tests as suggested by your doctor. These results will need to be submitted to the FAA every six months to continue your medical certificate under special issuance. Cognitive testing must be done every year for a first- or second-class certificate, and every two years for a third-class certificate. This will continue as long as you do not have a severe worsening of your condition, cognitive changes, or an increased viral load beyond 5,000 copies/ml.

In general, all HIV or AIDS medications that are approved by the FDA are also approved by the FAA. Acceptable protocols are described in *Guidelines for the Use of Antiretroviral Agents in HIV-Infected Adults and Adolescents*, developed by the Department of Health and Human Services Panel on Clinical Practices for Treatment of HIV Infection.

Amputations or paralysis

Pilots with almost any physical handicap may be certified after an FAA review of medical records and a satisfactory completion of a special medical flight test. This is usually done by special issuance and may include a number of restrictions or, in some cases, additional aircraft equipment. Many pilots have been certified despite amputations, paraplegia, muscular dystrophy, myasthenia gravis, and many other conditions (see *Chapter 3: Disabled pilots*). In each case, the initial application will be deferred by the AME to the FAA for review.

3

Getting a SODA

What does it mean to be disqualified?

In addition to the general health requirements, the FAA regulations list 15 medical conditions that are specifically disqualifying for a medical certificate. In practice, it is possible to obtain certification despite having even quite severe health problems or almost any of the listed conditions. If you have a significant health problem, the certification process may take a long time and a lot of paperwork, and probably involve extra testing and perhaps even a flight test. In the end, the chances of success are very good if you are highly motivated and have the support of a competent AME.

What is the difference between "deferral" and "denial" of my application?

If you have a disqualifying condition, your AME has two options: either deny your application, or defer it to the FAA for further evaluation. The choice is really up to you. If you feel that you are unlikely to get your medical certificate, you may decide to abandon the effort. This does not mean you can't fly (see *Chapter 1: Can I still fly, even though my medical was denied?*).

A better option is to ask the AME to defer your application to the FAA. This process may take anywhere from a few days to a few months, but in the end you may well be approved.

If you are disqualified for any reason, you may apply to the FAA for a medical certificate by authorization for special issuance, or by a statement of demonstrated ability (SODA). Neither of these can be issued directly by your AME. However, your AME can be a great help in the process by collecting the necessary information and forwarding the package to the FAA. The certificate may then be granted by the Federal Air Surgeon, the Manager of the Aerospace Medical Certification Division of CAMI, or by any Regional Flight Surgeon. The key to getting the FAA to approve your medical certificate is to show that your medical disorder is not a hazard to flight safety, and that you can handle all of the demands of the certificate you have applied for. Expect about 8 to 12 weeks before you get a response.

You should keep a copy of everything you send to the FAA. If an original document is important, keep the original and send a copy to the FAA. Normally, your AME will handle this for you. However, if you prefer to send the records yourself, use the following address:

Federal Aviation Administration
Mike Monroney Aeronautical Center
CAMI Bldg
Aerospace Medical Certification Branch, AAM-300
P.O. Box 26080
Oklahoma City, OK 73126-0080

Make copies of everything you give to the FAA.

The FAA is like any busy bureaucracy: records can be misdirected or lost and you may be asked to provide another set before the case can be resolved.

Is it better to use the Regional Flight Surgeon's office than the FAA in Oklahoma City?

The Aerospace Medical Certification Division office in Oklahoma City can be overwhelmed with complex applications. If your medical disorder is relatively straightforward, as most are, and you require only a third-class certificate, you are better off to direct your request to the Regional Flight Surgeon. That office may be able to give you a certificate within a few days rather than the months often taken by the FAA. (For a list of Regional Flight Surgeons, see *Appendix I: Regional flight surgeons.*)

Special issuance authorization

About one percent of all medical certificates, around 4,600 per year, are granted by an authorization of special issuance. Authorizations have been granted for all classes of medical certificates and for almost all disqualifying conditions.

More than 25,000 pilots have been given a special issuance certificate, including more than 1,100 airline pilots.

A special issuance certificate is not an automatic right. It is given at the discretion of the Federal Air Surgeon (or a representative), in recognition that the applicant is able to function safely as a pilot despite having an otherwise disqualifying health condition. The issuance of the certificate depends on further evaluation by the FAA, and occasionally a special flight test. Typically, the information first submitted will not be enough and additional tests or documents will be required, resulting in some back and forth communication between the FAA and you or your AME. This process can be quite lengthy. However, the most common cause of delays is a failure of the applicant to respond to requests for more information.

After all necessary documents and reports are submitted, the FAA may take as long as two to three months before making a decision. The possible results are:

- Medical certificate is denied because the information is inadequate.
- Medical certificate is denied because the disorder is considered a safety hazard.
- Medical certificate is approved with specific limitations.
- Medical certificate is approved without unusual limitations.

By regulation, a special issuance certificate has a shorter period of validity than the normal certificate, and requires specific, periodic follow-up medical tests, examinations, or evaluations to assess the stability or progression of the medical condition. There may also be an operational limitation, such as limiting a commercial pilot to carrying passengers for hire only when acting as part of a qualified two-pilot crew.

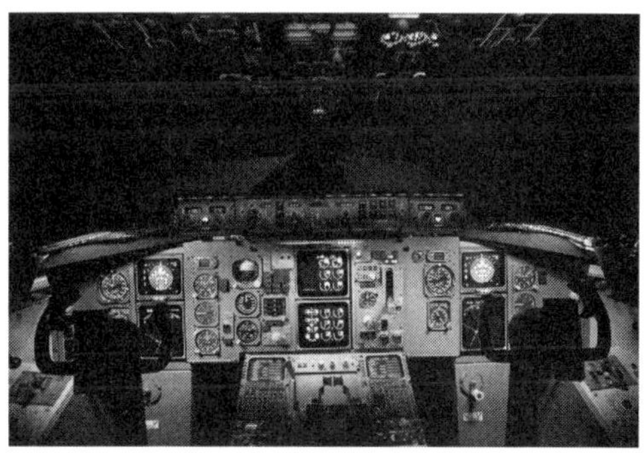

To renew an existing certificate, the applicant must again show the ability to perform safely by submitting the required documents or test records. This can involve as little as a letter from the physician who is treating you for the condition, or as much as a whole new set of diagnostic tests and examinations.

The special issuance authorization has a separate time limitation from your medical certificate, although they are often the same. For example, the required re-examination for your special issuance may be every six months, while a second-class medical certificate requires renewal every 12 months. Regardless of your special issuance, the date of renewal of your FAA medical application and physical examination does not change.

Example of an FAA Authorization of Special Issuance letter

Dear Mr. Piper: PI# 100111

I have reviewed the information submitted by you in support of your request for an airman medical certificate. The medical evidence reveals a history of myocardial infarction and coronary artery disease requiring coronary artery bypass surgery. You are ineligible for third-class medical certification under Section 67.111(a) (1) (3), 67.211(a) (c), and 67.311(a) (c) of the Federal Aviation Regulations (FARs).

However, based on the complete review of the available medical evidence, I have determined that you may be granted authorization for special issuance of third-class airman medical certification under Section 67.401 of the FARs.

Your Aviation Medical Examiner is authorized by this letter to issue you a third-class medical certificate bearing the limitation "NOT VALID FOR ANY CLASS AFTER APRIL 30, 2003" provided you are found to be otherwise qualified.

This Authorization expires on April 30, 2003.

Consideration for a new Authorization will be contingent upon the following, performed in accordance with the enclosed specifications:

On or about March 1, 2003:

A current cardiovascular evaluation and current lab work.

A current radionuclide scintigraphy exercise stress test.

If there have been no significant adverse changes in your medical status, you have complied with all conditions of certification described in your Authorization, and I am satisfied that the duties permitted by our medical certificate can be performed without endangering public safety, the Medical Appeals Branch may then grant you a new Authorization for an additional time. You will still be required to have your regular third-class physical examination at the frequency prescribed under the provisions of CFR 61.23.

In order to avoid a lapse in certification, the necessary testing should be completed near the date noted above and forwarded in one package to the following office.

Medical Appeals Branch, AAM 320
Aerospace Medical Certification Division
FAA Civil Aeromedical Institute
Oklahoma City, OK 73126-0080

You must promptly report any adverse changes in your medical condition to the FAA Medical Appeals Branch, AAM 320.

Use of the above reference number and your full name on any reports or correspondence will aid us in locating your file and expediting a reply to you.

Sincerely,

Warren S. Silberman, D.O.
Manager, Aerospace Medical Certification Division
Civil Aeromedical Institute

Note that you are assigned a specific PI number, which appears at the top of the letter. You should use this number for all correspondence.

You can send your renewal information up to 90 days before the expiration of your special issuance authorization. The FAA letter might indicate 60 days, but you may want to take the full 90 days to make sure all the necessary information was received.

Status reports

A special issuance authorization will generally require periodic re-examination reports from your treating physician. There may also be a request for an additional test, especially in cases of heart disease, such as an exercise stress test or radionuclide perfusion scan.

The status report from your physician should include:

- Your disqualifying condition
- Current symptoms
- Recent treatment
- Current medications
- Prognosis
- Recommended lifestyle changes or new diet
- All existing and new limitations.

Withdrawal of special issuance

The FAA can withdraw the special issuance certificate at any time if there is evidence of:

- Worsening of your condition
- Failure to comply with any functional or operational limitation
- Failure to provide requested information
- Falsification of information
- A danger to public safety.

If a special issuance authorization is withdrawn, the FAA will send the pilot a letter of withdrawal, stating the reason for the action. You can request a review of this decision, but must do so in writing not later than 60 days after you receive the letter. Within 60 days of your request for review, the FAA must issue a final decision either affirming or reversing the decision to withdraw. If your certificate is withdrawn, it becomes invalid and you must legally surrender it to the FAA upon request.

Denials and appeals

If your application is denied, you can appeal the decision. The majority of these appeals are successful, and ultimately only about 0.1 percent of applications are given final denial of certification for medical reasons. By far the greatest number of denials result from simply not providing the requested information.

You may want to prepare for the appeal by getting further medical and perhaps legal advice to support your claim that you can fly safely despite your medical condition.

You can request an appeal by writing to the Aerospace Medical Certification Division manager, who will provide the initial reconsideration of your application.

Federal Air Surgeon
Attn: Manager, Aerospace Medical Certification Division, AAM-300
Federal Aviation Administration
Civil Aerospace Medical Institute
Post Office Box 26080
Oklahoma City, OK 73126-0080

If this initial review still results in a denial, you can appeal all the way to the National Transportation Safety Board (NTSB) for a review. You must do this within 60 days of your final FAA denial, by writing to:

National Transportation Safety Board
490 L'Enfant Plaza, East SW
Washington, DC 20594-0001

While you are waiting for your medical certificate, you can still fly so long as there is another qualified pilot aboard. In fact, continuing to fly in this way shows that you are dedicated and sincere in your quest to get your certificate. The FAA looks very favorably at this, and it is worthwhile mentioning your flying activities in your letter.

There is no limit to the number of times you can apply for special issuance. Persistence may eventually pay off, especially if you continue to produce further evidence of your ability to fly safely.

Statement of demonstrated ability

A statement of demonstrated ability (SODA), which used to be referred to as a waiver, is different from a special issuance authorization. A SODA is issued by the FAA to certify pilots who have a static defect that is not likely to change. For example, a medical condition such as heart disease might require a special issuance authorization, but an amputation would require a SODA.

SODAs typically require a medical flight test to demonstrate that the applicant can safely operate the aircraft. In some cases, such as color vision deficiencies, the applicant may need only to pass a special color signal light test. Getting a SODA is a one-time process and it becomes part of your medical certificate. For subsequent AME examinations, you just need to show your letter (and previous medical certificate) indicating the SODA.

If you are going to get a SODA, you should do so for the highest certificate you think you will ever need. The reason for this is that a SODA for a third-class medical certificate is not valid for a second- or first-class certificate.

Functional limitations

SODAs for second-class certificates often include functional or operative limitations. For example, there may be a limitation against flying at night, carrying passengers for hire, or a requirement for additional installed equipment in the aircraft. Limitations may be stated as "NOT VALID FOR CARRYING PASSENGERS OR CARGO FOR COMPENSATION OR HIRE," or "VALID ONLY WHEN SERVING AS A PILOT MEMBER OF A FULLY QUALIFIED TWO PILOT CREW." A limited second-class certificate usually allows full third-class operations.

Old SODAs

Since a SODA is issued for a condition that is considered permanent, it does not expire, unlike special issuance authorizations. (Like authorizations, however, SODAs can be withdrawn at any time.) What happens if there is a change in the conditions that require a SODA? For example, what if you got a SODA for hearing impairment and then had surgery that improved your hearing to the normal range? The easiest way to handle this is by informing your AME at the next examination why you no longer need the SODA. You should ask the AME to attach a letter to your application requesting that the SODA be removed from your FAA medical file. This may even occur automatically, when the AME submits your medical application with the resolved condition.

IMPAIRMENTS AND DISABILITIES

The terms disability and impairment are often misleading or used incorrectly, but they are better than the old-fashioned "handicapped." Disability refers to loss of function. Impairment is a physical loss. A person can be disabled but not impaired, or impaired but not disabled. If you have a limb amputation, or hearing loss, etc., but you can carry out flight duties, you have an impairment but are not disabled for this activity. Disabled has become the common term to refer to both disability and impairment, but it is important to remember that your ability, not your physical state, is what counts. If you can carry out flight duties, you should consider yourself a fully functioning pilot. This is the purpose of the SODA—it is a recognition by the FAA that you have the ability.

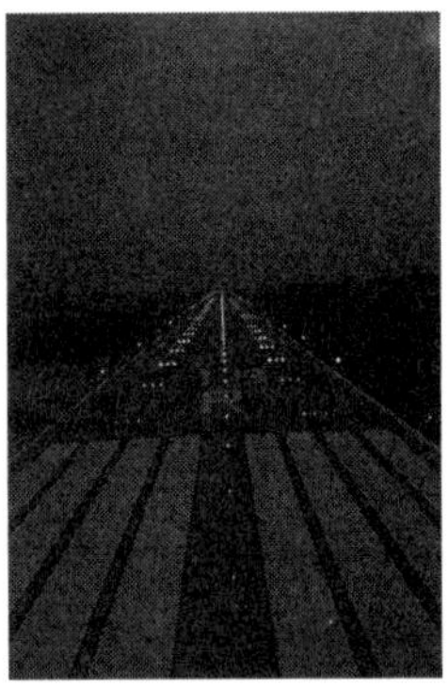

Pilots with almost any physical impairment may be certified after an FAA review of medical records and a satisfactory completion of a special medical flight test. The final license may include a number of restrictions or, in some cases, additional aircraft equipment. Many pilots are certified despite amputations, paraplegia, muscular dystrophy, myasthenia gravis, and other conditions. In each case, the initial application is deferred by the AME to the FAA for review. Note that a certificate based on a medical flight test is valid only for the model of aircraft used for the test. For any other aircraft the applicant wants to fly, a separate medical flight test must be conducted.

Clyde Smith, a deaf pilot, founded the International Deaf Pilots Association to help others with a similar condition achieve their goals. There are now many hearing-impaired pilots, and even an FBO and aircraft dealership owned and operated by deaf pilots.

> "You need to stay lean and mean; watch your diet and stay healthy. You need to be a bit of an athlete climbing in and out of a plane."
> —*Richard Logan, paraplegic pilot*

Richard Logan, after losing the use of his legs, was the first pilot to become a CFII using a hand control. Mike Penketh, a former American Airlines pilot who lost both hands, went on to become one of the world's top aerobatic pilots. Disabled pilots should consider joining the International Wheelchair Aviators, an association that deals with all types of disability and can provide advice and support (see *Appendix: Further Information*).

For pilots with amputations or paraplegia, the aircraft may need to be specially fitted to allow control with the remaining functional limbs. In this case, the initial medical certificate will be valid only for student pilot privileges—regardless of other certificates the pilot may already hold. This initial certificate will allow the completion of special flight training with the modified aircraft.

> Any modification to the aircraft will require a Form 337 signed off and submitted by the aircraft mechanic.

At least two months before being signed off for the flight test, the pilot should request an authorization for a medical flight test in the modified aircraft. The FAA will then issue an authorization letter that is valid for 90 days. When this letter is received, the pilot should arrange the flight test at a Flight Standards District Office (FSDO), and show the letter to the FAA inspector at the time of the flight test. The purpose of the medical flight test is to demonstrate that the pilot can:

- Reach and effectively operate all controls.
- Perform emergency procedures such as stall recovery, or engine-out procedures for multi-engine aircraft.
- Lift power levers for reversing thrust (in turboprop aircraft).

With successful completion of the flight test, the FAA flight inspector is authorized to issue a medical certificate with a SODA. The certificate will show any necessary limitations, such as the installation of special equipment in the aircraft.

Disabled pilots (by Capt. Sheri Coin Marshall)

When I was three years old, an accident caused the amputation of my right arm. Growing up in a two-handed world, I learned to innovate. You get used to making adjustments. But when I went to ask about flying lessons, as a teenager in Fullerton, California, I was told to forget it. Ten years later I was living in Washington, and decided to try again. I asked the local FAA safety inspector about it, and he said, "Go fly." The flight school, at Felt's Field Aviation in Spokane, was a little less sure about it. They said they had never had any experience with this situation, and the whole process

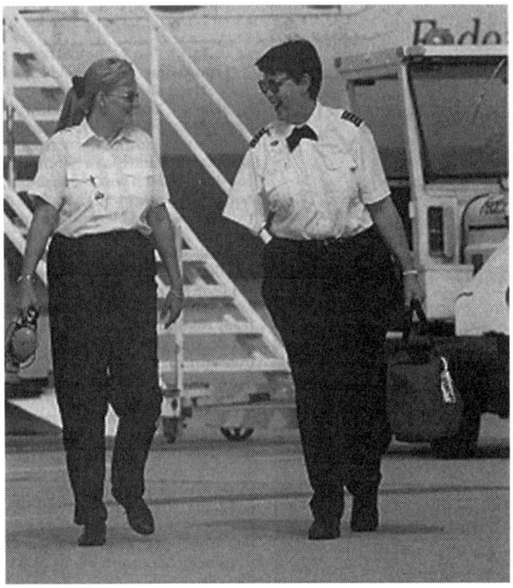

was mired in mystery. They were doubtful that I could get a medical, much less actually fly the airplane, but decided to let me go as far as I could.

I was given a list of AMEs to choose from, and eventually went to the doctor my own flight instructor used. During the physical I passed all the normal requirements—blood pressure, eyesight, etc. Then the doctor suggested that I give up my dream of ever flying. A pilot himself, he figured I'd never be able to handle an aircraft in an emergency situation, and he told me so. "Just think," he said, "there's no way you'll be able to land at Mead (a small, 35 ft wide strip north of Spokane) in the constant crosswind." I just listened to him and said, "Well, can I try?"

He begrudgingly issued me a third-class medical certificate with the restriction, FOR STUDENT PILOT PURPOSES ONLY. I found out later that this medical certificate would allow my flight instructor to allow me to solo, which I did at 20 hours—and would have even sooner if I wasn't plagued by the typical Washington weather. The actual practical check ride for my private certificate would also be a third-class medical check ride for my SODA. Seven months after I started, I had my license.

Years later, I found out that I could have taken the check ride for the SODA at any time. It made sense to the flight school, however, that I do the ride at the same time as my practical flight test because the maneuvers required by the FAA for the private certificate are the same as for the SODA. Later, I took a separate check ride for a SODA at the second-class level. In 1994, I combined the check ride for the first-class SODA with the practical flight test for the ATP.

Now, let's fast forward to the present. I mentor students from all over the world who have some sort of physical impairment and want to learn how to fly. This is what I tell them:

1. Learn how the FAA system works. This includes how to get a medical certificate, being a student pilot, how to choose a flight school and a

flight instructor, the Practical Test Standards, personal performance standards, difficult maneuvers, aircraft types, prosthetic devices, and the check ride with the FAA.

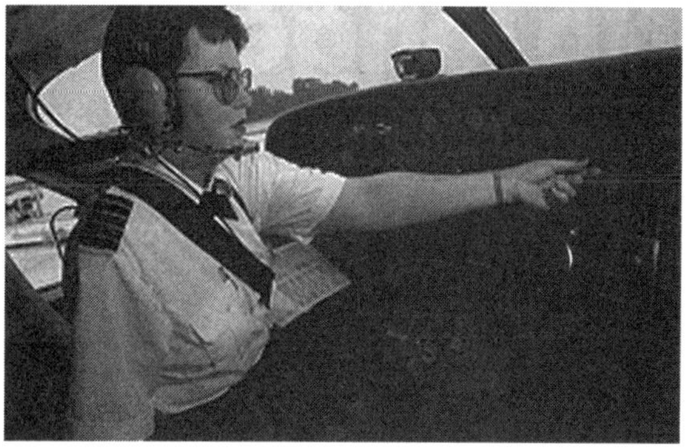

2. Try to establish a relationship through your CFI with the local FSDO General Aviation Safety Inspector, so you know who you will be riding with before the actual SODA check ride.

3. I emphasis that you must be able to do better than the standards on all areas in the Practical Test Standards. Is this fair? No. But don't be offended by this extra scrutinizing by the FAA. They ultimately have public safety to be concerned about, and are very sensitive to potential hazards. I am not saying an impaired pilot is any more dangerous than a "whole" pilot, just different. The FAA wants to give the student their blessings. The aviation community wants the FAA blessing as well. The higher standard may be harder to achieve, but it will make you a better pilot. It is worth the extra work to allay any concern others might have and for your own self-confidence.

4. Flight instructors/schools bristle when they see a physically impaired student walk through the door because they:

    a. Have not had a student like that before.

    b. Have worked with an impaired student who didn't do well (probably taking more time, which is often considered a bad sign).

    c. Do not want to spend the time and effort to find out what procedures are required for the impaired student's certification.

5. Be patient and persistent with the medical/SODA process. I have worked with students that get impatient or don't want to undergo the lengthy FAA required medical process. I've explained on more than one occasion that the FAA is very procedurally bound. If you do exactly what they ask, including all of the required paperwork, and do it within their time frame, then you'll have success.

6. Don't get caught in a time crunch. When the time is near for the practical test, notify the safety inspector. The FAA authorization letter is valid for 90 days. During this time, the FAA examining inspector must receive all the paperwork and arrange and administer the flight test. This is why it's important to have that established relationship with the inspector.

The key to success is persistence. Don't be surprised if you encounter resistance or skepticism. If anyone along the way suggests that you won't be able to do it, just be polite and say, "Well, can I try?"

4

Flying High: Drug-Testing Programs

The long, strange history of drug abuse

Recreational drugs have been used for thousands of years, not only during leisure time but also while on the job. Workers have used drugs for stimulation, for extra strength, for relaxation, to numb themselves against pain, or just to relieve boredom and help pass the time. The only difference today is the much wider variety of drugs available.

Drugs are commonplace in almost every type of work. The most widespread is caffeine, although it is so familiar that most people don't even think of it as a drug. Alcohol and tobacco are the second most common, with a huge impact on worker safety and productivity. Other drugs may be used less openly but are pervasive in many occupations. For example, during the Second World War, soldiers, pilots and factory workers were given amphetamines to increase performance. Amphetamines continued to be popular after the war, to the extent that they eventually accounted for 20 percent of all prescriptions. Many new stimulants have joined the amphetamines and drug use is now more common than ever. A current study of long-distance truck drivers found that 62 percent reported at least occasional illicit drug use while driving.

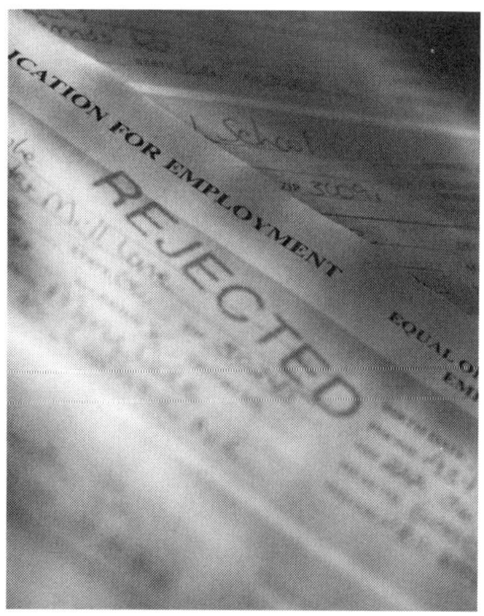

While people's right to use recreational drugs is controversial, most agree that there is no excuse to use illegal drugs at work or while operating complex machinery. Drug use by workers, however, continues to be a huge problem in the United States. In 1997, the National Household Survey on Drug Abuse found that there were 6.3 million illicit drug users among the 81.8 million people in

U.S. workforce. In an average month, 5 percent of employed people age 20 to 40 had used cocaine.

Concern about drug use in the workplace reached a peak in the 1980s. It is debatable how much of this was due to a genuine increase in worker drug use, and how much was simply driven by the federal government's overall anti-drug program. The emphasis on worksite drug control was considered a useful way to increase drug awareness and decrease use, both in and out of the workplace. For example, there is no evidence that there has ever been a commercial airline accident because of pilot drug use. Strict drug monitoring of pilots was instituted anyway, largely to enhance the public's sense of safety.

On September 15, 1986, President Ronald Reagan signed an Executive Order requiring federal agencies to establish an employee drug-testing program. In response, a comprehensive program was developed by the Department of Transportation (DOT) and the United States Coast Guard (USCG). Each of the DOT administrations expanded the program in their operations: the Federal Aviation Administration (FAA), which oversees pilots and air traffic controllers; the Federal Highway Administration (FHWA), which oversees professional drivers; the Federal Railroad Administration (FRA); the Federal Transit Administration (FTA); and Research and Special Programs Administration (RSPA), which regulates pipelines. The Nuclear Regulatory Commission (NRC) uses more stringent standards.

In 1988, the follow-up Drug Free Workplace Act required all federal grantees and contractors having a contract for property or services of $25,000 or more to have programs for a drug-free workplace. Now, almost all major companies and federal agencies have drug monitoring programs in place. Drug screening is done not only for airline pilots, but most occupations that are related to the transport industry, including mechanics, baggage handlers, and anyone that might get their wages from government contracts.

Refusing a drug screen is entirely legal, but will probably result in the loss of the employee's job or position. If a person is fired for refusing to take a drug test, it is virtually impossible for him or her to collect unemployment benefits.

Drug use and aircraft accidents

Pilots are human and it should not be surprising that a number of them use illicit drugs. Because of the high level of performance needed for flight, drug use in aviation is scrutinized very closely. The results of extensive studies show that drug use is actually quite uncommon among pilots. In

1999, just 14 accidents showed evidence of the possible involvement of alcohol, illicit drugs, or unapproved medications. In each of these, other factors were also involved. Because drug use among pilots is so rare, the cost-effectiveness of drug monitoring programs has come into question. The FAA has found that about 0.06 percent of pilots and air traffic controllers have a confirmed positive drug test, which works out to a cost of about $45,000 per positive result. However, the programs are likely to continue because of public worries about safety.

In January 1988, a crash of a Colorado commuter airline flight killed two crewmembers and seven of the 15 passengers. The aircraft captain was found to have used cocaine before the accident.

Drugs found in investigation of 2,326 aircraft mishaps

Substance	*Number testing positive*	*Legal use?*
Salicylates	109	Yes
Acetaminophen	61	Yes
Cannabinoids	54	No
Ethanol	51	No
Opiates	18	No
Chloroquine	6	Yes
Barbiturates	5	No
Amphetamines	2	No
Benzodiazepines	1	No
Chlorpheniramine	1	Yes
Cocaine	1	No
Diphenhydramine	1	Yes
Furosemide	1	Yes
Hydrochlorothiazide	1	Yes
Lidocaine	1	Yes
Phencyclidine	1	No
Total	**314**	

A highly skilled pilot experienced engine failure due to contaminated fuel, and managed to land on a frozen lake. He had 20,000 hours of flight time, was an FAA pilot examiner, president of a major pilot organization, the winner of a U.S. National Unlimited Air Race, and had received a Three Million Mile Safe Pilot Award.

Despite his successful landing, he and his companion died of exposure even though they had fuel, matches, ski clothing, and food. What went wrong? The answer might be found in the traces of amphetamine and cocaine in the urine of the pilot.

Most airlines have drug abuse policies that are separate from, and in addition to, the FAA regulations. Any employee with a substance abuse infraction will probably be given the option to attend a treatment program, during which he or she is removed from safety-sensitive operations but does not suffer any disciplinary action. If the rehabilitation program is successfully completed, the employee may return to full duty. If there is a second infraction, the employee is disciplined or employment is terminated.

Federal regulations: the NIDA 5

Other than alcohol, the federal regulations require tests for only five types of drug. These were recommended by the National Institute of Drug Abuse (NIDA) as the most common and worrisome drugs of abuse, and have come to be known as the NIDA 5:

- Marijuana
- Opiates (codeine, morphine, and heroin)
- Cocaine
- Amphetamine and methamphetamine
- PCP (Phencyclidine).

There are really two types of tests: screening and confirmation. The screening test is supposed to be quick, easy to administer, and cheap. It is intended to pick up anyone who *might have* used drugs. If the screening test is positive, the same sample goes on to a second, quite expensive and specific, confirmatory test. If this test is positive, it confirms that the person *did in fact* use the drug. A drug test is reported positive only if the confirmatory test is positive.

Under the federal drug testing programs, the laboratory methods use immunoassay for the initial screening and gas chromatography/mass spectrometry (GC/MS) for confirmation. All cutoff levels are in nanograms per milliliter (ng/mL), which is approximately one part per billion. If a screening test is positive for opiates, the confirmation test will look for the specific type of opiate: morphine, codeine, or 6-AM (indicating heroin). If a screening test is positive for amphetamines, the confirmation test will look specifically for amphetamine and methamphetamine.

The federal drug test regulations require testing only for the NIDA 5, and not the hundreds of other possible drugs of abuse. Individual airlines and companies may add further tests, at their discretion.

Federal drug testing cutoff levels

Initial test cutoff levels	*(ng/mL)*	*Confirmatory levels*	*(ng/mL)*
Marijuana metabolites	50	Marijuana metabolite*	15
Cocaine metabolites	300	Cocaine metabolite**	150
Opiate metabolites	2000		
		Morphine	2000
		Codeine	2000
		6-AM	10
PCP	25	PCP	25
Amphetamines	1000		
		Amphetamine	500
		Methamphetamine	500

* Confirmation for marijuana is by testing for the THC metabolite 11-nor-delta-9-THC-9-carboxylic acid.

** Confirmation for cocaine is by testing for the cocaine metabolite benzoyl-ecgonine.

On February 11, 2000, a Mitsubishi MU-2B-60 was destroyed when it landed a mile short of a county airport. Cleared for the ILS 26 approach, the aircraft was in sight of the tower in clear weather and light winds. The pilot reported dual engine flameout. On post-mortem screening, the pilot was positive for dihydrocodeine, hydrocodone, and diphenhydramine. How was it possible that he had passed the required drug screen?

A subsequent investigation showed that years earlier the pilot had taken some codeine tablets from his wife's prescription for back pain. It supposedly made him "feel good." He began taking them regularly, up to eight a day. He realized he had a problem and successfully completed a substance abuse program. Afterwards, he was monitored by random tests by a standard DOT drug screen—but this tests for only the NIDA 5 drugs, and not the other drugs he had taken.

Americans with Disabilities Act

All employees, whether staff or management, fulltime or part-time, are usually included in the drug-testing program. A "mature minor," typically at least age 15, can agree to the test without parental consent.

The Americans with Disabilities Act (ADA) was enacted in 1990 to protect people with disabilities from discrimination in the workplace. It applies to government agencies and all employers with 15 or more employees. Most people think the disabled are those who are blind, paralyzed, or have other obvious impairments, but disabilities also include psychological conditions, such as depression and schizophrenia—and drug addiction. It is estimated that about 45 million people, or 1 out of 6 Americans, are considered disabled.

Under ADA, drug addiction *in the past* is considered a disability and protected, but current illicit drug use is not. Therefore, employers are prohibited from asking about your former drug or alcohol use, but can ask about and test your current use. They can also ask about your criminal record.

Questions an employer *cannot* ask during a job interview

- What prescription drugs do you use?
- Have you ever abused drugs or alcohol?
- Have you ever been in drug or alcohol treatment?
- Have you ever had a driving under the influence (DUI) charge?

Questions an employer *can* ask during a job interview

- Do you drink?
- Do you currently use illegal drugs?
- Have you ever been convicted for a drug offense?
- Have you ever had a driving under the influence (DUI) conviction?

Under ADA, job candidates may not be discriminated against by a medical examination. Urine testing for alcohol is defined as a medical examination, and is therefore not allowed. But the testing for illegal drugs is not considered a medical examination, and is allowed. For that reason, most pilot job offers include a drug screen but not an alcohol test.

Drug surveillance programs

The FAA requires six main types of drug-monitoring tests, which apply to all employees occupying safety- or security-sensitive positions (Testing Designated Position). TDPs are subject to:

Pre-employment or *pre-placement*
A pre-employment drug test is given after an applicant has been considered for a job, but before the employment offer has been made. This practice has been questioned legally. Most companies now use a pre-placement test, which is given after an offer of employment has been made. The offer of employment is made conditional upon passing the drug screen. This is also called a post-offer test.

Reasonable suspicion, also known as *reasonable cause* or *for cause*
A reasonable suspicion test is given to an employee who is suspected of using a prohibited drug. In DOT-regulated programs, "reasonable suspicion"

occurs when a supervisor (some DOT programs require two supervisors) has observed conduct or appearance suggesting drug use. In non-DOT programs, the basis for reasonable suspicion may be defined by state law, company policy, or by company agreements with the employee's union.

Post-accident or *post-incident*
Many companies have a policy in which a drug test is automatically given to any employee involved in an accident or other serious incident.

Random
A test is given to employees selected at random, without warning.

Return-to-duty
A test given to an employee who has previously had a positive drug test or has previously refused to submit to testing (and was therefore removed from work), before he or she returns to work.

Follow-up
Testing done on a frequent, unannounced schedule after an employee has passed a return-to-duty test. Most DOT programs require a minimum of 6 follow-up tests in the first 12 months, and continue follow-up testing for up to 5 years.

Non-TDP employees are subject only to reasonable suspicion, post-accident, and follow-up testing.

How are people tested for drugs?

Drug use can be determined by testing almost any tissue in the body. For example, fatal accident victims are often tested by analysis of the vitreous humor inside the eyeball. Some bodily tissues can be tested for toxic substances after a period of months or even years—such as the bones or hair of historical figures who died hundreds of years ago.

In current testing programs, the following body substances are used:

- Urine testing is by far the most common. It is easy to collect, can be collected on the job site, and is a good indicator of recent drug use. Urine is tested in most workplace programs, as well as treatment and correction programs. Almost all drugs can be detected in urine; an exception is methaqualone.

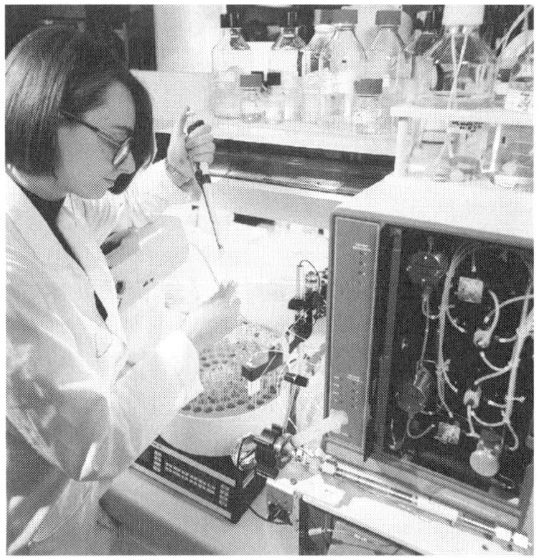

- Hair testing is preferred by the gambling industry for pre-employment screening because it is easy to do without special facilities. It is also used for investigations when other tests are not available, such as criminal cases or deaths. Hair can be tested for most drugs.

  The advantage of testing hair is the long period of detection: the life span of a typical hair ranges from about four months for hairs from the eyelashes or armpit, to four years for hair from the scalp. Hair grows at a rate of about one quarter to one half inch per month. Drugs enter the hair while it is growing and therefore present a record of drug use during the entire period of growth.

  For drug testing, hair samples are usually taken from the back of the head. In a bald person, hair from another part of the body may be used. For people without hair, or who have shaved themselves completely, fingernails may be used.

  Hair testing is less accurate than other methods because of contamination from shampoo residues, hair treatments, smoke, air pollution, and other environmental effects. Another disadvantage is that people have different types of hair, which may affect the readings in the analysis. Dark-haired people such as Hispanics, Asians, and African Americans have a higher concentration of melanin, which incorporates and retains drugs to a higher degree. The result is that a dark-haired person can be ten to fifty times more likely to test positive than a lighter-haired person who used the same amount of drugs. Because of these concerns, most federal programs do not engage in hair testing.

- Blood testing is most commonly done for clinical, diagnostic, and drug overdose purposes. It is routine in hospital emergency rooms. Blood testing can be done even with a severely intoxicated, injured, or dead person, and is therefore favored for post-accident investigation. Almost all drugs can be tested in blood, although THC (marijuana) is particularly difficult to measure.

- Sweat testing is commonly used in the criminal justice system for monitoring parolees and prisoners. The PharmChek patch is a waterproof adhesive pad about the size of a playing card. It is worn like a bandage for about one week. It is then removed and sent for analysis to PharmChem Laboratories in Menlo Park, California. Sweat testing can be done for cocaine, morphine, 6-AM (heroin), codeine, amphetamine, methamphetamine, THC, PCP, and methadone.

- Oral fluid (saliva) testing is done only for private insurance evaluations, since the technique is not considered reliable enough under federal guidelines. A swab is rubbed on the inside of the cheek and then placed in a sealed container and sent off for testing. Saliva will show amphetamines, barbiturates, cocaine, marijuana, opiates, and PCP. Oral fluid testing is more efficient than urine at detecting recent use but is less effective after three days. Advantages include the ease of collection and difficulty of adulteration or substitution, and this form of testing may soon become standard.

Chain of custody

Since a positive drug test can have a devastating effect on a pilot's livelihood, and future prospects for a job, it is critically important that great care is taken to ensure that the testing process is secure and confidential. To do this, the testing specimen is handled in a very precise way, called the "chain of custody."

Most drug testing is carried out by collecting a small amount of urine—about one ounce. The chain of custody is the process of documenting the transfer of the urine specimen from the donor to the collector, from the collector to the courier, from the courier to the laboratory, and within the laboratory from one person or department to another. Each collection procedure is documented on a custody and control form (CCF), also known as a chain-of-custody form (COC). Most programs use a standard seven-copy federal CCF, also known as the NIDA Form.

Tampered specimens

Urine specimens are collected in a controlled setting, such as a designated collection booth or bathroom. If it is suspected that the specimen has been tampered with, a special collection may be authorized in which the donor is actually observed urinating into the cup. Tampering is suspected when:

- The urine specimen is outside the allowable temperature range, which is within 1 degree C (1.8° F) of the donor's body temperature. Since the urine supposedly just came out of the body, it should be the same temperature as the donor. If it is not in the allowable temperature range, the urine sample will be suspected as falsified.

- The donor is observed attempting to submit a substituted or adulterated specimen. Most drug testing bathrooms will have a blue die in the toilet water to prevent the donor from adding water to the urine.

- The urine specimen is too diluted (see below, *Diluted urine*).

- If the laboratory cannot analyze a specimen because of contamination, a "Specimen unsuitable" report will be sent back to the collecting site, and the donor will be suspected of tampering with the specimen.

The "shy bladder" excuse

Some pilots try to avoid a urine test by simply saying they have no urge to urinate, or cannot urinate because they are shy. When "shy bladder" occurs, the donor will be expected to drink up to 40 ounces of fluids and wait for up to three hours. If he or she still cannot urinate, it will be considered a refused test.

Laboratory analysis

Drug-testing laboratories must be extremely reliable and legally precise to avoid falsely accusing someone of taking drugs. A negative test may be wrong, but a positive test must be a hundred percent accurate. To ensure that a drug detected in a sample is not from accidental exposure, a certain amount of the drug must be present for the sample to be considered positive. This amount is termed the "cutoff value" and is established for each type of drug assay. If the specimen's drug concentration is at or above the cutoff, the result is positive; if the specimen's drug concentration is below the cutoff, the result is negative. "Negative," in this case, does not mean that no drug was detected, but simply that the amount of the drug (if any) was not high enough to meet the established cutoff concentration for that assay. After a laboratory receives the specimen, it checks the Custody and Control Form for completeness and accuracy. The specimen is then examined for evidence of tampering. If everything is in order, the drug testing takes place.

Screening tests

There are two steps to laboratory testing: screening and confirmation. A screening test is used to "rule out" drug use. It should be quick, cheap, and easy to perform on large groups of people. It is not necessarily very accurate. A typical screening test might use immunoassay. Immunoassay tests give a simple "yes" or "no" answer. They are sensitive to very minute quantities of a drug but not very specific for it, so that a positive result could be to due to the presence of a related substance. For example, it is very easy to do a screening test for amphetamines, but a great many substances will give a falsely positive test. If the screening test is negative, nothing more is done. If it is positive, a second, confirmation test is done.

Confirmation tests

Confirmation tests are extremely accurate, but they also tend to be time-consuming, expensive, and not very practical for large groups of people. Their purpose is to "rule in" drug use. Confirmation cutoff levels are set individually for each drug. It is almost impossible to fool a confirmation test; however, many small companies or organizations do not bother with this expensive additional procedure.

For a confirmation test, the laboratory takes a further sample from the specimen and starts a new internal chain-of-custody form for that sample. Confirmation testing uses two analytical techniques: gas chromatography and mass spectrometry (GC/MS). Gas chromatography is used to physically separate the different substances present in the specimen. Mass spectrometry can then be used to identify these individual substances. With GC/MS, the specific molecule that corresponds with a drug or drug metabolite can be identified.

Specimens that test negative for drugs are discarded. Specimens that test positive are frozen and stored for at least 12 months in case they need to be tested again or used as legal evidence.

Can drug tests be fooled?

Not surprisingly, many people try to fool the drug tests. Some of their methods interfere only with immunoassays and not with GC/MS, which may be effective because the sample can clear the screening process and never reach the confirmatory level. If the laboratory has any reason to suspect adulteration, however, the confirmation test will usually show the true amount of the drug.

Adulteration products

There are many products advertised in magazines or on the Internet that claim to fool drug tests:

Klear or *Whizzies*

These products contain nitrite, which interferes with the GC/MS assay for THC. The specimen may screen positive for marijuana, but the marijuana metabolite used for confirmation cannot be detected by GC/MS. Unfortunately, nitrite also removes the substance used by the laboratory as an internal standard for detection of the marijuana metabolite. If the laboratory fails to recover this substance, it will test for nitrite by GC/MS.

Naturally high urine nitrite levels can be caused by urinary tract infections and by eating foods such as beef jerky, which can cause urinary nitrite concentrations as high as 300 ng/mL. However, using Klear (potassium nitrite) or Whizzies (sodium nitrite) will produce a urine nitrite concentration greater than 500 ng/mL, and the laboratory will report the sample as adulterated.

Mary Jane's Super Clean

This product contains alkylphoxysulfonate, which is also present (and much cheaper) in Joy and other dishwashing detergents. If this is added to urine, it may cause an apparent decrease of marijuana metabolites when tested by immunoassay. The results of GC/MS analysis will not be changed.

In theory, the product works as a surfactant, by forming tiny droplets which trap drug molecules and make them "invisible" to the antibodies used in immunoassay tests. Adding Visine eye drops to urine has the same effect. Current laboratories have a number of methods to detect this type of adulteration, making it less effective than in previous years.

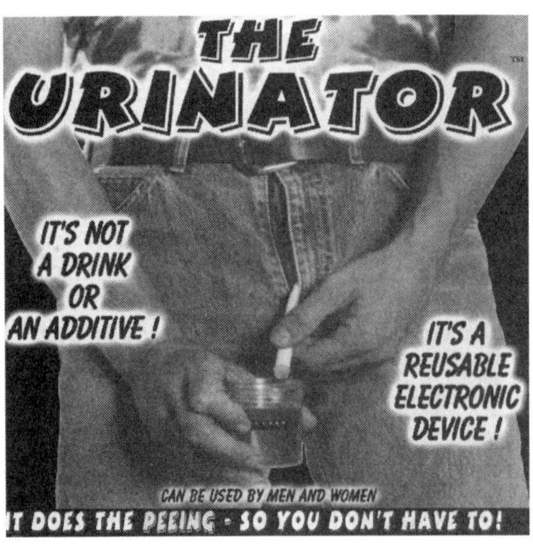

Attempts to avoid urine drug testing can be quite creative. This product might work—unless a special collection is authorized. If caught, the donor could face severe penalties for trying to falsify a drug test.

Salt

Sodium and chloride are normally found in urine but occur in especially high concentrations when salt has been added as an adulterant. High concentrations of salt can cause a decrease in the apparent concentrations of many drugs when tested by immunoassay.

UrinAid, Clear Choice, or *Glutaraldehyde*

These products contain glutaraldehyde, which interferes with immunoassays of all NIDA 5 drugs. When glutaraldehyde is added to a urine specimen, it makes the immunoassay uninterpretable. It does not interfere with GC/MS results. Gluteraldehyde is not found in normal urine. If the laboratory finds glutaraldehyde in the specimen, it will be reported as adulterated.

Urine Luck

Besides a clever name, Urine Luck uses a clever process to fool marijuana tests. It contains the salt pyridinium chlorochromate, which dissolves in urine to form pyridine and chromate. The effect of chromate is similar to nitrite by interfering with the detection of marijuana. If the laboratory cannot recover the marijuana metabolite standard, it may test the specimen for pyridine by GC/MS and report it as adulterated.

Diluted urine

The easiest and simplest way to fool a drug test is by diluting urine. Some people try to add water to the urine sample, but this may be difficult in a proper testing location. The most common way is to drink a lot of fluids beforehand, and avoid early-morning urine (which has the highest drug concentration).

Some "beat the drug test" products that act by diluting urine

Clear Choice Herbal Detox Tea
Detoxify Carbo Clean
Eliminator
HealthTech Pre-Cleanse Formula
Naturally Klean Herbal Tea
Quick Tabs
Quick Flush Capsules and Tea
Ready-Clean
Test Free
Test Pure
THC Terminator Drink
The Stuff

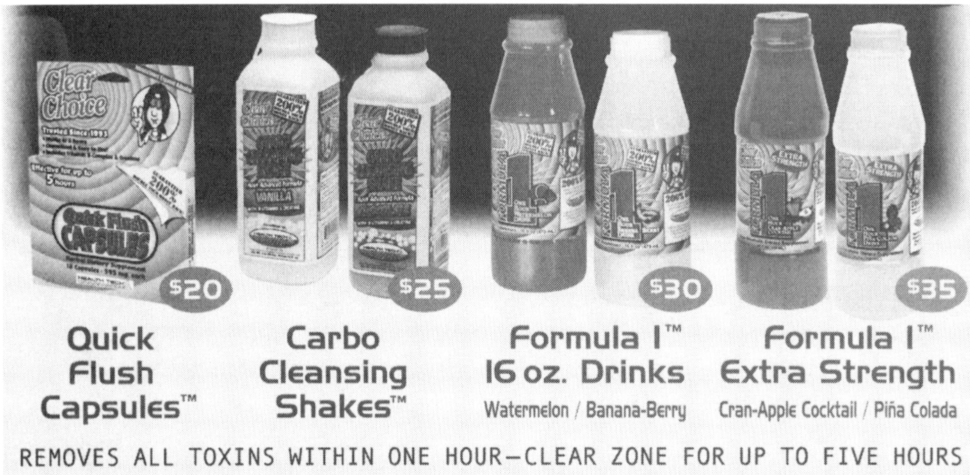

Urine is more dense than water. It should have a specific gravity greater than 1.003 (the specific gravity of water is 1.000). Urine also contains a certain amount of creatinine, which is produced by the muscles of the body. Normal urine has a creatinine level greater than 20 mg/dL. Testing urine for specific gravity and for creatinine prevents donors from fooling the drug tests by pouring water into the sample, or drinking enormous quantities of water to dilute their urine and therefore also dilute any drugs that might be present.

To a certain extent, diluting urine does increase the chance of beating a drug test. Some drug-using employees will take furosemide (Lasix), a prescription diuretic that produces a very dilute urine. To avoid the problem of having their urine rejected because of a very low creatinine, they will eat a lot of red meat beforehand. It is questionable whether this strategy works. Drinking large quantities of water, or taking Lasix, can dilute urine as much as tenfold and therefore lower drug concentrations. But this can also reduce the specific gravity below 1.003, in which case the laboratory reports it as a dilute specimen, and it is rejected. If the specimen is at or below 1.001, this is very close to water and the laboratory report will state "Specimen substituted: Not consistent with normal human urine."

The solution to pollution is dilution.

Dilute urine that looks very pale or colorless will arouse suspicion. Some donors take Vitamin B complex beforehand to give a deep yellow color to the urine.

There are many products that claim to cleanse the system of drugs, or at least help the user escape detection. Most of these products are supposed to be taken with large amounts of water, and they work by simply diluting the urine. In general, they do not actually interfere with the drug test. Some also contain vitamin B complex to make the urine more yellow, so that it doesn't look so diluted.

In general, products that claim to beat the drug tests are a waste of money and give the user a false sense of confidence. In some states, these products are illegal. The manufacture, sale, or use of adulterants is a misdemeanor crime in Nebraska, Pennsylvania, and Texas.

Legal medications that can cause positive drug tests

A positive drug test may be caused by many legitimate prescription medicines.

Illegal drug	Legal medication
Amphetamines	Adderall tablets Atapryl tablets Biphetamine capsules Carbex tablets Desoxyn Gradumet tablets Dexedrine tablets and capsules Dextrostat tablets Didrex tablets
Barbiturates	Anolor 300 capsules Arco-Lase Plus tablets Axocet capsules Bellatal tablets Bupap tablets Donnatal tablets, capsules, and elixir Esgic and Esgic-Plus tablets and capsules Fioricet tablets and capsules Medigesic capsules Nembutal capsules, solution, and suppositories Pacaps capsules Phrenilin tablets and capsules Quadrinal tablets Repan and Repan-CF tablets and capsules Seconal sodium capsules Sedapap tablets Tenake capsules Tuinal pulvules

Cocaine	cocaine hydrochloride (used in ear, nose, throat, or dental surgery) TAC (Tetracaine, Adrenaline, and Cocaine preparation used in emergency rooms to numb the skin) Brompton's Cocktail (contains cocaine and morphine or heroin, for extreme pain in dying patients).
Marijuana	Marinol Capsules Marijuana approved for medical condition
Methaqualone	none
Opiates	Acetaminophen with codeine Amogel PG Brompton's Cocktail (see above) Brontex Butalbital, aspirin, caffeine, and codeine capsules Capital and codeine suspension Codimal PH syrup Deconsal C expectorant and syrup Diabismul Dimetane-DC and Dimetane DX cough syrup Duramorph injection Fioricet with codeine capsules Fiorinal with codeine capsules Fiortal with codeine Infantol Pink Infumorph solution Kadian capsules MS Contin tablets MSIR capsules, solution, and tablets MS/L and MS/S Nucofed expectorant, syrup, and capsules OMS concentrate Oramorph SR tablets Paragoric Parepectolin suspension Pediacof cough syrup Phenaphen with codeine capsules Phenergan VC with codeine Poly-Histine CS syrup Promethazine hydrochloride and codeine phosphate syrup RNS suppositories Robitussin A-C and Robitussin-DAC syrup Roxanol and Roxanol 100 solution Ryna-C liquid Ryna-CX liquid Soma compound with codeine Triaminic expectorant with codeine Tussar-2 and Tussar SF and syrup Tussi-Organidin NR and SNR liquid Tylenol with codeine (#1,2,3, or 4)

What happens when a drug test is positive?

A Medical Review Officer (MRO) is a specially certified medical doctor with training in the interpretation of positive drug tests. Under federal guidelines, a worker testing positive must have an opportunity to talk about the results with an MRO or appropriate physician to see if there might be another explanation besides drug use. In fact, the MRO may not declare the test positive unless there has been an attempt to contact the specimen donor. Most MROs try to call the employee by telephone. If a "reasonable attempt" to contact the employee is unsuccessful, the MRO may declare the drug test a verified positive. In other words, it is up to the employee to convince the MRO that there might have been another reason why he or she tested positive.

The MRO interview
"Hello Mr. Smith, this is Dr. Murphy at Bay City Medical Center. I'm calling because your drug test came back positive for amphetamines. Your company doesn't know this yet. I wanted to call you first, to see why this happened. Are you taking any medicines, or do you know of any reason why your test might be positive?"

The most common excuse for a positive drug test is that the employee did not personally take drugs but was at a party where others were using drugs. This rationalization is often used for marijuana: "I was in a bar where people were smoking up … I couldn't help inhaling it." In the 1980s, more than a dozen experimental studies on passive inhalation were published. Some of these researchers were able to cause a positive drug test among people passively inhaling the smoke, but only when the exposure was extremely intense and unrealistic. They concluded that it was almost impossible for someone to test positive because others nearby smoked marijuana.The government decided that this excuse would not be allowed.

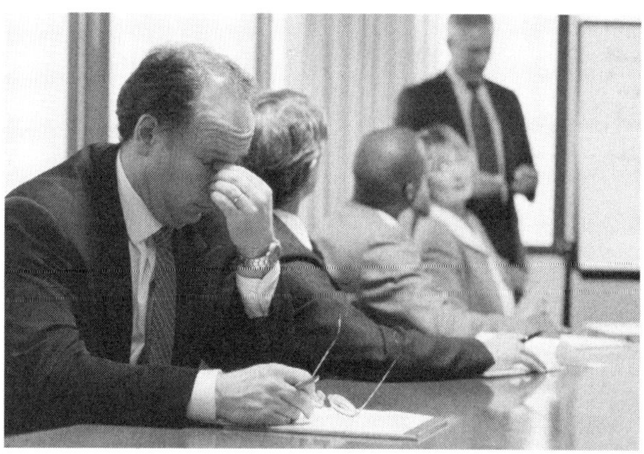

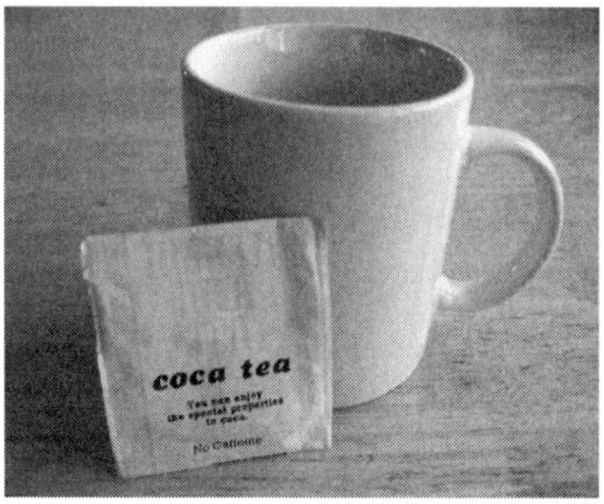

In the early 1980s, some health food stores sold a tea made from coca leaves called *Health Inca Tea*. The tea was supposedly made from "decocainized coca leaves." A study in 1986 showed that this tea contained detectable amounts of cocaine and could cause a benzoylecgonine-positive urine test result. The tea is no longer available.

Other excuses have included inhaling cocaine powder when sitting beside someone cutting cocaine, or seemingly innocent exposures. The government has determined that these types of exposures are not enough to cause a positive drug test, and has not accepted such excuses.

Positive drug test?
A woman denied using cocaine. She claimed that her positive test was due to her body absorbing cocaine from the semen of her boyfriend. The government did not accept the excuse.

5

Cleared for Flight

Taking care of yourself

A survey of the armed forces during World War II found that the pilots in the Army Air Corps ranked at the very bottom in physical fitness. If that comes as a surprise to most people who think pilots are healthier than average, the truth is that the level of fitness among pilots is now even worse.

The main reason why pilots, like the rest of the population, have poor health is their lifestyle. As in the general population, about 70 percent of all health problems are due to smoking, obesity, drug and alcohol abuse, lack of exercise, and a poor diet with too much fat and sugar. The good news is that, with a little bit of effort, these factors can be changed quickly.

Health does not mean the absence of disease. True health is being able to function at the best of your abilities with an overall sense of well-being. To maintain good health, all you really need to do is use common sense to take care of yourself, get appropriate medical check-ups, and keep a positive attitude to life. The rest of this chapter concerns pilots' most common health problems.

Back pain

Low back problems are the most common cause of disability in people under age 45. About 50 percent of working-age people admit to back symptoms yearly. Pilots are especially at risk. Sitting puts the greatest load on the spine, even more than standing, and sitting for long periods in a narrow airplane seat may be the worst.

Percent of adults who have pain

Daily	42
Weekly (ages 18 to 34)	66
Weekly (ages 65 and older)	75
At least once a month	89
Caused them to miss work in the past year	27
Caused visit to physician in past 3 years	51
Think pain is "just something you have to live with"	60

People who have never had severe back pain should be eternally grateful. The pain can be so intense that it feels like a broken back or life-threatening disease. In fact, the first thing a doctor will do is rule out the four serious, but thankfully rare, conditions that cause back pain:

- Infection
- Tumor
- Cauda equina syndrome
- Fracture.

If you have any of these, you won't be flying for a while.

By far the most common cause of back pain is a compression or rupture of a cushioning disk between the vertebral bones. Normally, these disks are very tough—even stronger than bone. If you have a severe blow to the back, you are more likely to have a burst fracture of the vertebra than a disk problem. That is little comfort to the millions of people suffering from a degenerative condition of the disks, in which the disks slowly become thinner and less elastic. The result is that the spine begins to settle like an old house. Parts of the disk may squeeze out or break off and push on the nearby nerves—the condition known as a herniated disk.

The spinal disk is a fluid-filled wafer wrapped by about 90 layers of a tough shell called the annulus fibrosis. It is the largest structure in the body that does not have a blood supply. That means the disk keeps its cushioning ability by absorbing fluid from the nearby blood vessels. Anything that decreases the blood flow to the area—dehydration, smoking (nicotine constricts the vessels), or poor conditioning—will eventually produce a thinner, stiffer disk. By the time people are 20 to 30 years old, the disks have begun to degenerate. This process tends to increase with age, and by the time people are 60 years old, 46 to 93 percent of them have severe degenerative disk disease. The majority of these, surprisingly, do not complain of any back problems. In others, the weakened disk may leak, crowd the spinal nerve, and then cause all sorts of pain and other symptoms such as weakness or numbness in the back, buttocks, thighs, legs, and feet. The disks most likely to be affected are those that carry the greatest weight: the disk between the fourth and fifth lumbar vertebrae (L4-L5), and the disk between the fifth lumbar and first sacral vertebrae (L5-S1). The herniated disk causes inflammation in the surrounding area, which in turn greatly increases the pain. If the nerve to the bladder is impinged, the result can be difficulty urinating or even incontinence.

Spondylolysis is a break in the side-bones of the vertebra that connect them to each other (the spinal laminae). It does not always cause problems; in fact, 1 to 2 percent of NFL football players have this condition. When both sides are broken, the vertebrae can slip aside from each other (spondylolithesis). This condition also may not cause problems and is quite common in younger males. If the slippage is severe, it may pinch the spinal cord and require treatment.

What is the best help for back pain?

Unfortunately, research shows that there is no specific therapy that reliably cures back pain. That includes chiropractic, physical therapy, ultrasound, trigger point injections, epidural injections, and even surgery. All of these have benefited some individuals, but studies show that people tend to heal gradually no matter what they do. The long-term use of back braces, or narcotic drugs, is especially discouraged because they may actually slow healing. Even with the best drugs, 75 percent of people will still have pain after one year.

So what should you do? Everyone will benefit from quitting smoking, losing weight, and increasing aerobic exercise. A common cause of back pain is weakness in the paraspinal muscles, providing less stability to the spine. The solution is to strengthen these muscles. Perhaps the very best exercise for this is yoga, which is becoming popular for its many health benefits. Gently and gradually increasing flexibility will provide more blood flow to your spine and speed natural healing.

Dehydration

At altitude, air tends to be dry, and this is especially so in pressurized aircraft where the cockpit humidity approaches 10 percent within 20 to 30 minutes after takeoff. Most pilots do not drink enough water to balance this loss. Even worse, pilots tend to drink coffee or sodas. Although you are taking in liquids, the body actually loses fluid because the caffeine acts as a diuretic and increases urination.

For every cup of coffee, you lose two cups of body water.

Dehydration can be very subtle. Long before you feel thirsty, your performance may be diminished by inadequate water. The usual symptoms are fatigue, headache, dizziness, nervousness, irritability, decreased coordination, and narrowed span of attention. Chronic dehydration can also lead to kidney stones, which are quite common among pilots.

Caffeine is a strong stimulant, and too much can present problems. Some people experience headaches, nervousness, and anxiety or panic. In women, it tends to worsen premenstrual syndrome. Over-stimulation of the heart can cause irregular or skipped beats. If a person is used to a high caffeine intake, sudden withdrawal can also produce miserable feelings, often with headache and difficulty concentrating.

> How do you know if you are dehydrated? There is a simple test. Weigh yourself before and after the flight. Every pound you lost was a pound of body water. For future flights, you should plan to drink 16 oz of water for each pound lost.

The solution? Drink plenty of water before and during the flight. Water can be a little bland, and you may prefer to flavor it by mixing in a little fruit juice. Juice by itself is usually too sweet to supply your fluid needs. Reduce your caffeine drinks to 1 or 2 cups or cans a day. Try to avoid caffeine before or early in the flight, so you won't be distracted by the need to urinate while you are on the gauges. Save your drink until the last hour of the flight, when the demand for alertness is highest and you will be on the ground when the diuretic effect kicks in.

Skin care

Pilots are often exposed to a number of different skin irritants. Ethylene glycol, used as a deicing agent, can cause contact dermatitis and exposure to bare skin should be avoided. (Because of its low vapor pressure, inhalation is less of a problem, but service personnel should wear respirators.) The hydraulic fluid in wing flaps and other parts of the aircraft is also a strong skin and eye irritant, and you should wear rubber gloves and goggles while inspecting these areas. The same is true of jet fuel (Jet A or Jet B); you should be careful when visually inspecting tanks.

After sitting for hours in a cramped cockpit, many pilots are bothered by rectal itching. The problem is much worse for those who have hemorrhoids, and is aggravated by poor hygiene or using rough toilet paper. Rectal itching might seem like a trivial problem, but those who have had it know that the condition can be highly distracting, difficult to cure, and truly miserable. Not all physicians are very sympathetic. This is one case where you may just have to treat yourself. You should begin by taking extra care to ensure cleanliness and minimize sweating by frequent showers, changes of fresh underwear, and the use of drying powders. Avoid rough toilet paper or vigorous wiping. Many pilots swear by the use of Tucks, a brand name moisture-absorbent pad, inside the underwear and against the anus. Chronic rectal itching is still something of a medical mystery and has no specific cure, but with good care the condition will eventually go away.

Stress

Stress is the spice of life. The reason most pilots are attracted to flying is precisely because of the demands and thrill of operating in an extreme environment, where decisions have to be made quickly and precisely. Too much stress, however, can be overwhelming and is almost always a major factor in an accident.

"Stress is the price paid to be a race horse instead of a plow horse."

Managing stress is one of the greatest challenges for a pilot, and the first step is recognition of the common stress symptoms:

- Anxiety
- Irritability
- Insomnia
- Depression
- Trembling or weakness
- Fixated attention
- Speech difficulties
- Forgetfulness
- Nightmares
- Impulsive behavior
- Increased smoking or overeating
- Inability to concentrate
- Indigestion
- Loss of appetite
- Sweating
- Emotional tension
- Headache
- Confusion
- Neck pain
- Chronically tense muscles
- Increased self-doubt
- Susceptibility to accidents

The greatest source of stress is not the physical demand of flying, but in getting along with others. Crew Resource Management (CRM, initially developed as Cockpit Resource Management) was designed when the military and commercial airlines realized the vital role that interpersonal relations have in flight safety. There are countless stories of accidents that occurred because of miscommunication or personal problems among the crew.

Dead right

The first officer had just been hired by a commuter airline and was still in his probationary period. He had been warned that the captain was a domineering old man who was also the senior manager of the company. On the final approach after a long day, the first officer called out the checks but got no response from the captain. Afraid to question or challenge him, the first officer said nothing and let the captain retain control. A few minutes later, the aircraft flew into the ground short of the runway. It turned out that the captain did not respond because he had died during the approach.

CRM applies to solo pilots as well, when you consider that every pilot needs to deal with air traffic control, other aircraft, ground and fuel management personnel, etc.

How to reduce stress if you are a member of a crew

- Don't compete, get angry, shout, sulk, or let your bad mood show. Do what you can to make a good working atmosphere even if you don't like the others.

- Don't delay sharing your uncertainty or anxiety because you are worried about looking foolish or weak. Others may feel the same and will welcome your openness.

> "Pilots tend to want to fix what they can't tolerate, which may not work very well with family problems where they cannot 'fix' other people."

- When your opinion is sought, give it clearly without worrying about what others want to hear—but in a considerate way, without being overly critical ("Any fool can see that ...").

- Avoid arguing to push your own judgment.

- Approach the task on the basis of logic.

- Don't change your mind just to reach agreement and avoid conflict.

- Support only those solutions that you agree with, at least partially.

- Don't let others get into trouble just to look clever in comparison.

- View differences of opinion as helpful rather than a hindrance in making a decision.

- Try to avoid using majority vote, trading favors, averaging, or splitting the difference as a way to reduce conflict in reaching your decision. A compromise decision usually satisfies no one.

- If a group decision has been made, accept it unless you feel that it contains some hazard not appreciated by the other members of the group.

How to reduce stress if you are the leader of a crew

- Don't state your own opinion at the outset—otherwise, subordinate crew will be reluctant to give their opinions if they contradict you.

- Specifically ask for ideas and opinions of your crew, and encourage them to express doubts or objections. Make sure that potential problems are not ignored.

- When you have made a decision, explain your reasons to the crew. If you don't, the others may feel that their own ideas have not been considered or even heard.

Vaccines

Vaccinations are the greatest success of modern medicine. They are also perhaps the most unappreciated, to the point where a large segment of the population does not even bother with this quick, simple, and painless way to prevent disease. As a pilot, you should take every precaution against getting sick, and appropriate vaccinations are one of the best ways to do this. You should consider the following:

- *Influenza*: The flu changes every year and for that reason there is a new vaccine distributed every fall for that year's two or three most common virus strains. You should definitely get this. It is available in October or November.

- *Tuberculosis*: Because of circulated air, pilots are at high risk of exposure to tuberculosis and should have a skin test every year. If you test positive, you will be treated. This test is not a vaccine. (There is a vaccine, BCG, but it is not very effective and is not recommended in the United States.)

- *Tetanus and diphtheria*: These vaccines are usually given together. Get a booster every 10 years.

- *Pneumonia*: The pneumococcal vaccine is a single lifetime vaccination, usually given to elderly people or those with lung problems. But why take the risk? The vaccine is a simple shot, and vastly preferable to getting pneumonia.

- *Measles, mumps, and rubella (German measles)*: If you were born before 1957, you were probably exposed to these viruses and got natural immunity. After 1957, you should have been vaccinated for these and, more recently, for chicken pox (varicella). Any of these are usually mild diseases in childhood but can be quite nasty to get when you are an adult. Shingles, a painful skin rash, is a recurrence of the chicken pox virus. If, for some reason, you have not developed immunity, it is worth getting the vaccine.

- *Hepatitis A and B*: Hepatitis A is extremely common, especially in third-world countries, and a vaccine for this liver disease has only recently become available. Hepatitis B is a more dangerous infection, with a vaccine previously offered to health care workers and firefighters. It is now recommended that everyone get both of these vaccines. It requires more than one shot, and may be a bit expensive, but well worth the protection.

- *Other vaccines and preventive medications*: If you are traveling in tropical countries or places with unusual diseases, you should consult a travel medicine physician to consider appropriate precautions. Some of the vaccinations may be required, such as those for yellow fever. Others are optional, but highly recommended, such as those for malaria or typhoid, and some offer dubious protection, such as those for cholera. It depends not only on where you are going, but also on your activities and your mode of travel. If you will be working with animals, for example, you might consider vaccination against rabies and plague. Be sure to inform your travel medicine physician that you are a pilot. Some prophylactic medications are incompatible with flying. For example, mefloquine, the most popular anti-malarial, is not recommended for use by pilots because of side-effects that include dizziness, disturbed balance, and mood changes. For pilots, chloroquine is a better choice, unless you will be traveling to a chloroquine-resistant area.

Vaccinations are rarely harmful, and usually the worst side-effect is soreness at the site of injection, and occasionally headache, mild fever, or fatigue. The symptoms usually go away in a day or two and are alleviated by taking an aspirin or Tylenol. Immunizations are not disqualifying, and do not need to be reported on your medical application as a medication.

Weight and balance

Since the first humans walked the earth, the greatest fear of most people was starving to death. It is still the major worry for about half of the world's population. The other half now faces the opposite problem: they are simply too fat. It is estimated that about two-thirds of Americans are overweight, and every year the statistics seem to get worse. In just the few years from 1991 to 1998, the percent of those who are seriously obese went up 50 percent—from about 12% to 18%—and obesity now causes an estimated 300,000 deaths per year, more than lung, breast, colon, and prostate cancers combined.

Being overweight is not just a health problem for a pilot. It can also make it difficult to fly, or at least more expensive. If you are a big person and have ever tried to fit into a Cessna 152 or Piper Tomahawk, you know what I mean. When you add a large instructor, these aircraft will very likely exceed their load capacity. The FAA has always figured that the average pilot weighs 170 lbs (77 kg), but the true average has increased to an estimated 187 lb (85 kg), and this needs to be taken into consideration in light aircraft performance.

Ultimately, just as in aircraft, a good level of fitness is not only a matter of weight but also balance. Some people are naturally large. Others may be within the normal weight range, but so poorly conditioned that they run all the risks of obesity. The ideal weight for a person should not be determined by a number on a scale, but by an overall sense of vitality and well-being.

Diets

The worst way to try to lose weight is to go on a diet. Despite this fact, Americans spend almost as much money on diet books and food substitutes as they do on high-calorie fast foods. Diets don't work, and the reason is simple: If you try to starve yourself, your body will compensate by hoarding food. This makes a lot of sense on an evolutionary level. Your ancestors were the people who avoiding starving by developing a taste for fatty foods. As for the slimmer people, they didn't have as many children and did not survive the hard times. A fat person can starve for about six months and still survive, while a pleasingly slender person would expire after about a month. In most of the world, throughout history, fat was good. Being heavy meant hanging on through the drought, the winter, or the famine, and living to enjoy the return of good times. We are hard-wired to crave high-calorie and high-protein foods. For a million years, the smell of that sizzling char-broiled steak was the smell of survival.

The word starve comes from the German *sterb,* meaning "to die." If you try to starve (by going on a diet), your body will protect itself—by getting fatter!

Now, in the industrial world, the problem is more likely to be over-eating and people find themselves trying to lose the extra weight. There are countless diets, and not one of them has been medically proven to work. Even the famed Dr. Atkin's diet does not get rid of fat—the weight loss occurs by the loss of body water, which causes dehydration and makes you even worse off.

Just SuperSize it!

	Calories per portion				*Increase*
Cappucino	Naples, Italy	50	New York	140	180 %
Taco	Morelia, Mexico	180	New York	260	44 %
Soda	London	172	New York	410	138 %
Croissant	Paris	215	New York	430	100 %
French fries	London	486	New York	610	44 %
Steak	London	545	New York	1360	149 %
Fettucine alfredo	Rome	825	New York	1500	81 %

The best way to lose weight is to eat well. A good breakfast will increase your energy level and metabolic rate throughout the day, burning up extra calories every minute. A light, nutritious lunch will provide just enough to keep you going without feeling heavy and fatigued. Eat a very light dinner, or nothing at all—most of this food will just be stored. Nowadays, the purpose of dinner is mostly as a social occasion or as "comfort food" rather than an actual need to eat. It is best to just skip dinner entirely and go for a long walk or an exercise class instead. If you are not used to doing this, you will feel hungry for the first couple of weeks since your appetite is largely due to the programmed expectation of food rather than your body needing more nourishment. Once you get used to the new eating schedule, you won't feel hungry in the evenings and your increased sense of vitality will be astonishing.

I once worked with a crew from Saudi Arabia. It was the month of Ramadan. They explained that during this time, their religious observance required them to fast during the day. They then had a special meal after sunset to break their fast. I replied that I, too, fast regularly, but at night. And each morning I also break my fast with a special meal, which I call "break fast."

Overall, avoid foods that are high in sugar or fat, which means just about all processed food. When you discover a taste for fresh and wholesome foods, you will be able to keep your natural and healthy body weight without needing to diet.

To get rid of extra weight, it is necessary to increase your fuel burn, not limit consumption. The way to do this is by exercise.

Exercise

Surveys show that 65 percent of Americans get too little exercise, and 25 percent get none at all. Most pilots, unfortunately, are in this last group. As an absolute minimum, people should engage in aerobic activity at least three days a week, at least 20 minutes at a time. For really good fitness, the American College of Sports Medicine recommends exercising three to five days a week for about an hour at 50 to 85 percent of the training heart rate.

The Karvonen formula to estimate the training heart rate (THR) is:

$$THR = [\%Hr_{max} (Hr_{max} - Hr_{rest})] + Hr_{rest}$$

where: $\%Hr_{max}$ = the desired training intensity
Hr_{max} = maximal heart rate = 220 - age
Hr_{rest} = resting heart rate measured in the standing position

For example, let's say you are 30 years old and want to train at 70 percent of your maximal capacity. If you simply take 70% of your estimated maximal heart rate (220-30 = 190 bpm), you would train at a THR of 133 bpm. But you are more sophisticated than that. So you measure your standing resting heart rate, which is 70 bpm, and apply the Karvonen formula. Your THR would be calculated to be [0.7(190-70)] + 70 = 154 bpm. You set your heart-rate monitor to keep you between, say, 150 and 165, and away you go, training at maximum efficiency.

The problem with exercise is that most people consider it to be a disagreeable chore. It is the last thing added to the schedule, and the first to get bumped when you are busy or under stress.

First, let's get rid of some misconceptions:

- "No pain, no gain" is not only false but will lead to injury, if you haven't already quit by then. Exercise should feel pleasant. If it hurts, you are pushing too hard or doing it wrong.

- Aerobic exercise is any activity that raises your heart rate, especially those that leave you breathing hard, in a light sweat, and feeling pleasantly spent afterward. Nearly any activity will do—including the one you're thinking of—so long as you can keep doing it for at least about 20 minutes. A faster pulse means the heart is working to supply more oxygen to the tissues, which benefits the entire cardiovascular system.

- Exercise should be fun. If you don't like to run, don't run. Do something you do like—the only requirement is that it gets your heart rate up. Golf may be fun, as is shooting pool or playing darts. All of these may be official sports, but they do not qualify as exercise. If you want to make sure you are getting the exercise you need, use a heart rate monitor. Professional athletes and Olympians use one to train at optimal efficiency. Your heart rate will tell you if you are really getting exercise, and a leisurely stroll around a golf course probably won't do it. A heart rate monitor is helpful to keep you focused and honest.

- Weight lifting is good for you beyond just sculpting the body. It builds and tones the muscles, increasing metabolic rate, and enhances overall physical and psychological well-being. Just 15 minutes a day is plenty, two or three times a week, and doing one set to your maximum burn-out is actually better than doing three or four sets. In other words, a few minutes of weight-lifting is good, but more is not necessarily better. Focus on lifting slowly and with concentration and control.

- Stretching is vital to fitness, but do your really deep stretching after you have been exercising, not before. Warm up with some easy jogging, slow lap swimming, etc., then do your main game or routine, and follow it at the end by a variety of stretches, which can also serve as a cooling down period. If you try to stretch too vigorously at first, you may well injure yourself. Yoga, developed over thousands of years, provides a superb stretching program and will benefit everyone.

What is the absolute best way to exercise?

Extensive and very sophisticated research has been carried out to answer this question and the answer is … a dog. A dog encourages people to get out more often, have more fun, and do things they haven't done since childhood. Even just patting the dog has been shown to reduce blood pressure.

Cholesterol

Elevated cholesterol is linked to obesity and lack of exercise, but even quite fit people suffer from this condition. The solution is to get tested early and often, beginning at age 20 and every five years thereafter (for optimal values, see *Chapter 2: Heart or vascular trouble*). If your values are slightly elevated, you can bring them down into the healthy range by increasing physical activity and changing your diet. If this is not enough, you should consider one of the newer cholesterol-lowering medications. Several products are being marketed to replace the fat in processed foods. These products, such as Olestra, are meant to carry the taste of fat without the extra calories. However, they also tend to cause abdominal gas, intestinal cramps and frequent bowel movements or even diarrhea. This is clearly no good for a pilot, and these products are best avoided.

Vitamins and supplements

Do you need vitamins? Many people believe that vitamins and other nutritional supplements are necessary for optimal wellness. Most popular health advisors seem to agree (it must be just coincidence that they are often connected with companies that sell the vitamins). On the other hand, it doesn't seem logical that humans evolved to be vitamin deficient. People around the world seem to do just fine without them. Vitamins are not necessarily harmless, either. Vitamin E, for example, is an anticoagulant and may cause internal bleeding if taken in large amounts or with aspirin.

At the present, food supplements are not recommended by the American Heart Association or the American Cancer Society, if you lead a normal life and have a balanced diet. Those are big ifs. It is difficult for many harried pilots to maintain a healthy diet when they work odd hours and eat in airports and hotels. In this case, it might be helpful to add a daily supplement of:

A multivitamin
Vitamin C 500 mg
Vitamin E 400 IU
Calcium 1,000-1,500 mg

Other supplements need to be looked at carefully. Some expensive "stress formulas," for example, contain a multitude of obscure substances that probably do no harm. Any "energy increasing" mixture is likely to contain substances that are banned by the FAA, including ephedrine or ephedra, Ma Huang, or epitonin. Read the labels carefully, and ask your AME if you have a question about the contents.

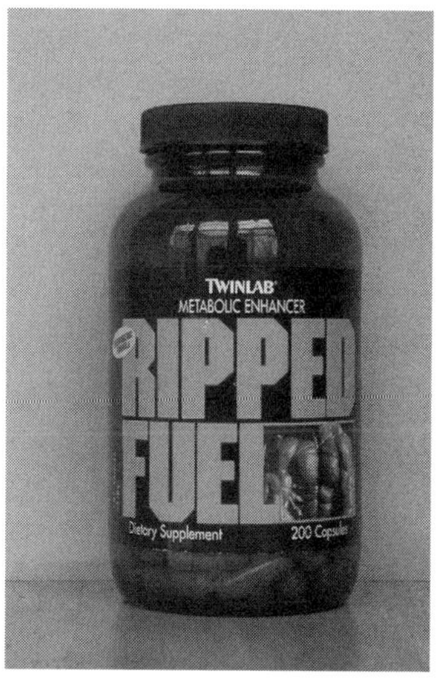

This product contains Ma Huang, prohibited by the FAA

Hearing loss

Airplanes and airports, especially the apron, are some of the noisiest places on earth. Hearing loss is a bothersome problem for pilots, and especially affects those who are older and have spent a lot of time in and around large airplanes. It begins to be noticeable when the pilot has trouble understanding people. Unfortunately, speaking louder doesn't help, and even makes things worse. The typical noise-induced hearing loss is at the higher frequencies, with the low frequencies affected only slightly or not at all. Speech recognition becomes a problem because consonants use higher frequencies, so that "ninety nine" sounds like "aye ee aye." Talking louder doesn't help (it sounds like "AYE EE AYE") and in fact, it can be even worse because people tend to emphasis the vowels when they speak louder.

A Life Flight pilot was talking to a nurse after her first trip in the helicopter. He noticed that she was speaking louder than necessary, and then tried to start her car although it was already running. When he asked if she had worn the earplugs he gave her, she said that she had taken them out because they were uncomfortable. She admitted to having trouble hearing and a buzzing noise in her ears.

Sound intensity, noticed as loudness, is measured in decibels (dB) on a logarithmic scale so that each unit is 10 times more intense. For example, a whisper is about 10 dB and a departing jet is about 100 dB, or 10 billion times louder. Long-term noise exposure should not be greater than 80 dB to avoid hearing loss. Sound greater than 120 dB is painful, and 140 dB can rupture the eardrums.

Exposure to loud sound will eventually damage the ear. At first this occurs for a short time, and the ear can recover. The feeling is often noticed as a sense of pressure, buzzing, or high-pitched ringing in the ears that goes away after a few hours. This is known as a temporary threshold shift (TTS). Eventually, the damage is permanent—causing a permanent threshold shift (PTS).

What's the difference between sound and noise? Is noise worse for hearing?

Noise is simply unwanted sound—in other words, it depends on whether you want to hear it. All sound can cause hearing damage if it is loud enough, whether it is great music or an aircraft engine (and to some pilots, they are the same). But because noise is annoying, it can cause fatigue and irritability and therefore interfere with performance. Even noise while off-duty can have a bad effect on health by disrupting rest and sleep.

There are many causes of hearing loss, both temporary and permanent. The best way to look at these is to consider the path of sound as it begins with vibrations in the air and continues through the ear and eventually is sensed by the brain.

The ear is designed to catch and amplify sound—which is why some animals have huge ears, and you can magnify sound by cupping your hand to your ear. The sound wave then travels through the ear canal to the eardrum. Earwax is produced to protect this canal by trapping dust, insects, and other intrusions. It slowly flows out and is washed away with normal cleaning of the outside ear. Some people have a build-up of wax, which can dry out into a hard plug and cause a hearing problem. The best way to get rid of this wax is to flush it out with warm water, using a soft rubber bulb syringe. Don't try to dig it out with a Q-tip, toothpick, key, or any other pointy object that people love to stick in their ears. At best, all this does is push the wax further into the ear; at worst it can puncture the eardrum (see *Chapter 2: Earwax*).

The eardrum separates the outer ear from the empty chamber of the middle ear. This thin membrane is truly a drum, and makes incoming sound waves 30 times louder. The eardrum can be stiff from being scarred by old injury or infection, or may be ruptured or torn.

The middle ear contains three small bones, linking the eardrum to the inner ear. The middle ear space is connected to the back of the throat by the auditory (Eustachian) tube. When this tube is blocked, the middle ear pressure cannot equalize, pulling on the eardrum (if the pressure is too low),

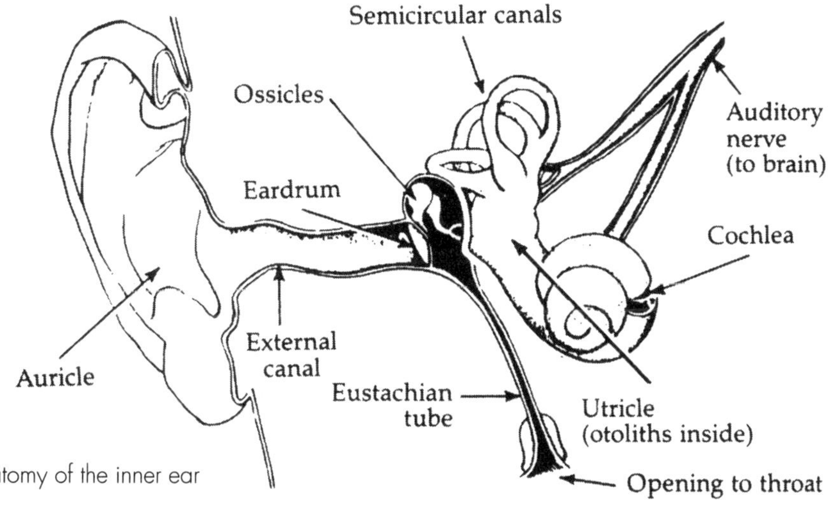

Anatomy of the inner ear

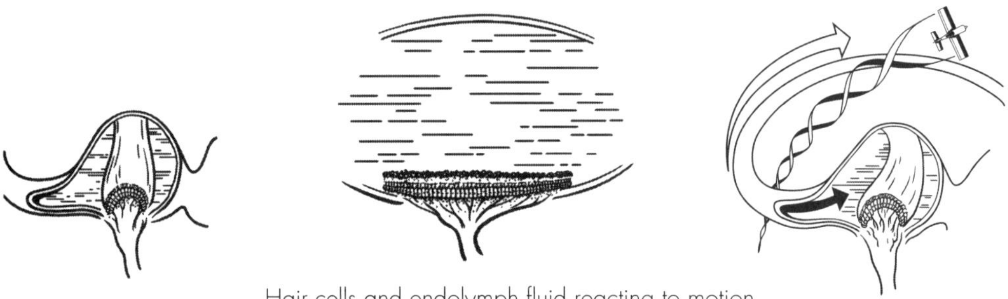

Hair cells and endolymph fluid reacting to motion

or pushing on it (if the pressure is too high). Either way, the result is a blocked ear that can be quite painful or even lead to the rupture of the drum. Typically, the pressure is worse on descending. During ascent, the middle ear has a higher pressure than the outside, and the extra pressure can usually leak out. During descent, when the middle ear pressure is too low, the tube tends to collapse and the only way to equalize pressure is to hold your nose and blow into it, pushing air back up the tube into the middle ear and popping the eardrum back to its normal position. With infections, such as a cold or flu, the middle ear can become filled with fluid, and you should not fly until it is relieved. Many pilots carry a decongestant nasal spray (such as Afrin) in their flight case, just to avoid this potential problem.

With age and noise exposure, the little bones that conduct sound from the eardrum to the inner ear tend to become stiff and calcified. Surgery can correct this problem, if it is bad enough, and will restore some hearing ability. This surgery is not disqualifying, but will require deferral to the FAA for review before you can be medically certified.

The inner ear is a fluid-filled chamber where fine membranes with microscopic hairs convert sound waves to vibrations in liquid and ultimately a nerve signal that goes to the brain.

Exposure to very loud sound can send a shock through this system, tearing out the hairs like a tornado in a wheat field. Another problem with the inner ear is the growth of tumors that can block off the nerve. A common symptom of inner ear damage is tinnitus—a constant ringing in the ears. A small amount of tinnitus may be normal, and almost everyone is aware of it in a very quiet space. If it is extreme, it can be masked with other noise or music. Unfortunately, there is no cure other than finding ways to ignore it. In the past ten years, a number of special clinics have opened to treat tinnitus, using Tinnitus Retraining Therapy (TRT). The program, developed at Emory University, helps patients adapt to the condition and claims an

80 percent improvement rate. Other therapies include vigorous massage of the base of the skull, acupuncture and acupressure, and daily doses of ginkgo biloba and zinc. All tinnitus sufferers should minimize use of caffeine and aspirin, and find alternatives to aggravating medications.

Other causes of hearing loss

- Alcohol
- Allergy
- Arthritis
- Aspirin
- Burns
- Cancer
- Chicken pox
- Cholesteatoma
- Colds
- Diabetes
- Ear infection
- Head injury
- Hypertension
- Hypothyroidism
- Influenza
- Measles
- Meniere's disease
- Meningitis
- Mononucleosis
- Mumps
- Otosclerosis
- Pneumonia
- Polyps
- Quinine
- Thrombosis
- Toxins
- Tumors

Hearing requirements

The normal hearing range is from about 20 to 20,000 Hz (cycles per second), from the lowest rumble to the highest pitch. Within this span of frequencies, the sound of the average human voice has a much smaller range of about 500 to 2,000 Hz. Human hearing is also most sensitive in this range, and this is the range tested by the FAA.

The aviation medical examination requires you to be able to hear an average conversational voice six feet away in a quiet room, using both ears and with your back turned to the speaker. If your hearing is worse than that, you can still be certified if you pass a more sophisticated audiometric test. In fact, you can get your certificate even if you are completely deaf, although there will be some restrictions. There are two audiometric tests; you can get your medical certificate if you pass either one:

1. *Audiometric speech discrimination test*
   You will need a score of at least 70 percent reception in one ear, and an intensity no greater than 65 dB.

2. *Pure tone unaided audiometric test*
   You will need a threshold no worse than:

	500 Hz	1000 Hz	2000 Hz	3000 Hz
Better ear	35 dB	30 dB	30 dB	40 dB
Worse ear	35 dB	50 dB	50 dB	60 dB

Note that you need only to have adequate hearing in one ear.

If you cannot meet the hearing requirement by any of these tests, but still think your hearing is satisfactory for safe flight, you can get your medical certificate by applying for a SODA (see *Chapter 3*). This will require a flight test, during which you will need to show your ability to:

- Hear radio and voice communications, and detect signals such as the marker beacon or Morse code identifiers.
- Understand a normal, conversational voice (without lip reading) with the engine off, with the engine running at different power settings, while on the ground and while airborne.
- Estimate a glide by sound in relation to speed.
- Recognize an approaching stall by change in sound related to a change in speed.

If you have severe hearing loss, or deafness, you will need to show that you can recognize:

- Engine power loss or engine failure by a change in vibration and by instrument scan.
- Approaching stall by aerodynamic buffet and visual cues.
- Retractable gear emergencies (if you fly an aircraft with retractable gear) by observing gear warning lights.

Deaf pilots

Deaf pilots have been common from the beginning of aviation, including Cal Rogers, who made the first cross-country flight from east to west, in 1911. There are now deaf flying instructors and a deaf aviation dealership. Currently, the International Deaf Pilots Association (IDPA), founded by Clyde Smith, has about 235 members.

Hearing protection

Working in and around aircraft used to be a common cause of hearing loss. Not long ago, most general aviation pilots used a hand-held microphone and no hearing protection. Now, a quality headset is one of the first purchases of a person learning to fly—and perhaps the most important investment.

How do you know if you need hearing protection? If you can't communicate comfortably, without shouting, you should be using a headset.

There are two types of hearing protection: noise attenuating and active noise reduction (ANR). Noise attenuating protection includes earplugs and ordinary headsets. Good quality, foam-moldable earplugs can reduce sound intensity by 15 to 20 dB, and are particularly effective at shielding high-frequency noise. The remarkable quality of earplugs is that they let lower frequency sounds through, so that you can understand speech even while being protected from the worst noise. Modern headsets, especially those with liquid-filled ear cups, are even better at sound reduction, shielding 20 to 25 dB, with more low frequency reduction. For this reason, some people in very high noise environments choose to use both earplugs and a headset to get both good high- and low-frequency noise protection.

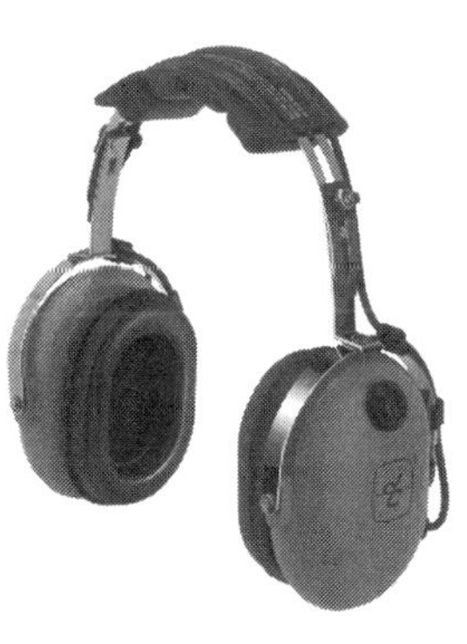

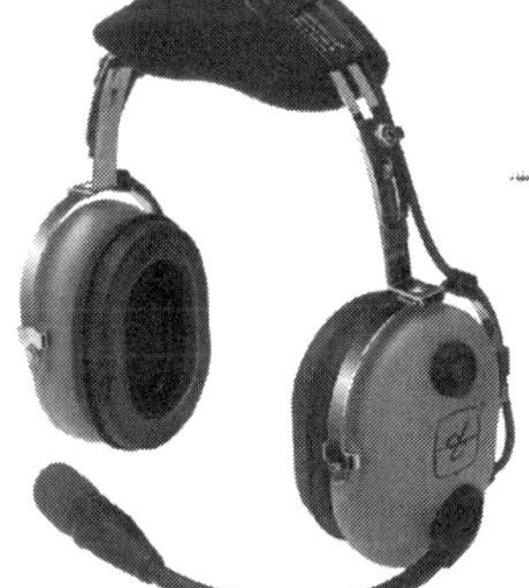

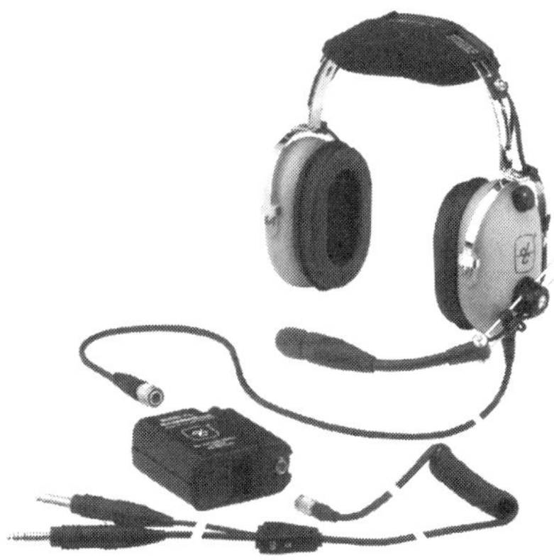

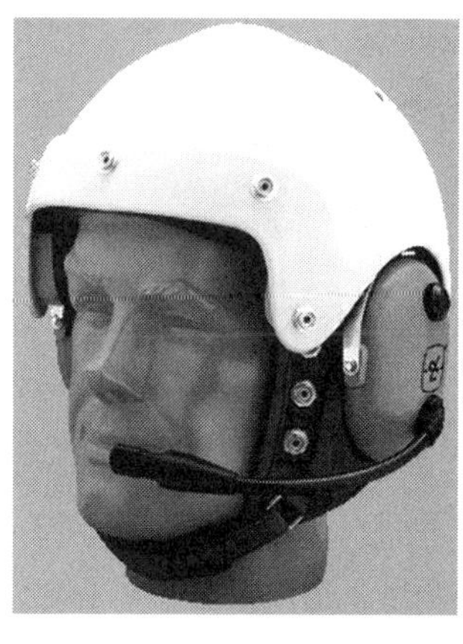

From left to right: Noise attenuating headset without microphone; NA headset with microphone; Active noise reduction headset; helmet headset

ANR is the latest, greatest achievement in noise protection. It works not by physically blocking sound, but by electronically generating the opposite sound wave and therefore canceling out the noise. The theory had been around for a long time, but sufficiently small and effective (and inexpensive) units have only recently become available. In order for ANR to work, the unit must first detect the sound, analyze it, and then generate its opposite. The lower the frequency, the easier this is to do. ANR therefore works primarily with low frequency protection and is typically embedded into a conventional noise-blocking headset that takes care of the higher frequencies. As technology becomes more sophisticated, it is likely that the future headset will be no larger than a hearing aid, and the bulky headsets will join leather helmets and flying scarves as relics of an earlier era.

Hearing aids

Can I use hearing aids during the medical exam? Do I then have to use them during flight?

Hearing aids are acceptable for a medical certificate at any class. If you choose to use them to pass the medical examination, your AME will add the limitation on your certificate: VALID ONLY WITH USE OF HEARING AMPLIFICATION. How you actually amplify your hearing is your decision. Some pilots who normally use hearing aids take them out while flying and turn up the volume on the headset instead. This practice is approved by the FAA, but you will need a medical flight test and a SODA. You should always have the hearing aids with you in case of headset failure.

Ear block

Ear block occurs when the air space in the middle ear is closed off to the outside, such that the inside air pressure becomes unequal to the outside pressure and causes a pushing or pulling on the eardrum. The result is pain that can be very severe. If the middle ear pressure differential is large enough, it will rupture the eardrum—not a pleasant feeling, but it does bring instant relief (and loss of hearing in that ear). Luckily, ruptured eardrums tend to heal well. You should not fly until healing is complete, which may take several weeks.

Ear block usually occurs on descent, when the outside air is pressing in, and clears on ascent. If you catch it early, you can do a Valsalva maneuver to equalize the pressure (hold your nose and blow).

The best way to handle ear block is

1. Stay ahead of your ears—perform Valsalva maneuvers often, before and during descent as needed, to relieve pressure.

2. Use a nasal decongestant, such as oxymetazoline (Afrin), if you are having problems.

I fly an air taxi service in an unpressurized aircraft, and show my passengers how to equalize their ears. But what can I do about infants?

Infants usually tolerate flying surprisingly well, especially if they are given a little sedative like a spoonful of Benadryl elixir beforehand. If the flight is long or you are worried about noise exposure, you can offer foam earplugs that may be trimmed to fit. A pacifier or bottle is useful to distract the baby and help it continually adjust ear pressure by swallowing. You should discourage parents from taking infants aboard if they are sick or have sinus problems.

Ear block is much more common if you are breathing supplemental oxygen. The reason for this is that the oxygen is absorbed from the inner ear, dropping the pressure even more than would occur just with altitude. Furthermore, the effect can continue for hours as the oxygen is slowly absorbed—even after the pilot has landed. You might go to bed after an evening flight and then wake up a couple of hours later with a splitting earache. The solution, of course, is to do the Valsalva maneuver after you get on the ground and as needed over the next few hours.

A pilot returned from a night flight in an old, unpressurized Beech twin. He had been on 100% oxygen at 15,000 feet while trying to get above some bad weather. The next morning, he felt pain in both ears and had difficulty hearing. When he managed to pop his ears, the pain was relieved.

Sinus block

Sinuses are air spaces in the head, with very small openings into the nasal cavity. If these openings get plugged, you can get a sinus block just like an ear block. The pain can be even worse than an earache and is said to feel like a knife in the face, making you close your eyes and wince in pain. If the maxillary sinus is affected, the pain can radiate to your back upper teeth, making it feel as if you have a toothache.

Sinus blocks usually occur in the frontal sinuses, above the eyes, and are noticeable in both ascent and descent. They are especially common in people with nasal polyps, which can plug the sinus openings. If you have polyps, you should have these taken care of by an ear, nose, and throat specialist and be very careful flying in unpressurized aircraft.

TEETH PRESSURE (BARODONTALGIA)

Teeth with cavities, abscesses, and improper fillings can have tiny air spaces trapped inside the tooth. These can cause pressure differential problems that have even resulted in an exploding tooth. More likely, there is tooth pain that increases with altitude and is relieved by descent. If you have these symptoms, the only cure is a dreaded visit to the dentist. Explain what you experienced, and the dentist should take care of the problem.

If you feel as if a whole row of top teeth are hurting, or if the pain is mainly on descent, you may have a maxillary sinus block.

VIBRATION EXPOSURE

Very low frequency sound waves are not heard, but felt as vibrations. When strong and persistent, the vibrations can cause fatigue and blurring of vision, as the eyes cannot continue to keep focus with the rapid disturbance.

With frequencies below about 10 Hz, the whole body begins to resonate with the vibration. The result is often back pain, frequently experienced by helicopter pilots.

> An older military pilot complained that his fingertips were turning white after a flight—a problem that had started years earlier as tingling and numbness after a mission. Now his fingers felt swollen, painful, and weak. A medical work-up revealed that he had developed hand-arm vibration syndrome.

Higher frequencies (between about 30 Hz to about 200 Hz, and again at 480 Hz) cause damage to the small blood vessels in the body part that is affected. This condition, sometimes called "vibration white finger," eventually results in injury to the nerves and bone as they are starved of blood. It is often seen in people who use vibrating hand tools, and in pilots gripping a vibrating control wheel. If you have these symptoms, you should discuss it with your AME and mechanic to arrive at an appropriate solution that can range from extra padding on the control handle to structural modifications of the aircraft.

Smoking

About 23 percent of American adults smoke (down from over 40 percent a couple of decades ago), and it is a sad fact that many pilots are among them. Smoking is bad not only for the smoker—it is distracting, irritating if you wear contact lens, and disruptive of cockpit operations, to say nothing of the pilot's health problems—but also bad for the airplane itself. Smoke is composed of microscopic liquid droplets (which is why smoke feels moist) that get into and ruin delicate instruments such as gyros and other avionics, and forms filmy deposits on windshields, visors, and glasses.

Passenger smoking is also a fire hazard when oxygen is being used or during maneuvers when someone might drop a cigarette on the carpet. During a seven-year period studied by the National Transport Safety Board, careless smoking was found to be the cause of six percent of all in-flight fires.

The real poison—carbon monoxide

Smoking has many bad effects on a pilot, and by far the greatest of these is the inhalation of carbon monoxide. When any carbon-containing material is burned, oxygen combines with carbon to produce the gas carbon dioxide, with the remaining material left as ash. This process is seldom 100 percent complete, and the result is only a partial combination of oxygen and carbon, producing carbon monoxide. Each cigarette replaces about 1 to 1.5 percent of the blood oxygen with carbon monoxide, and a typical smoker will have 5 to 10 percent of their blood hemoglobin bound with carbon monoxide. One accident investigation found a heavily smoking crewmember with a blood carbon monoxide level of 17 percent, which would be fatal for most

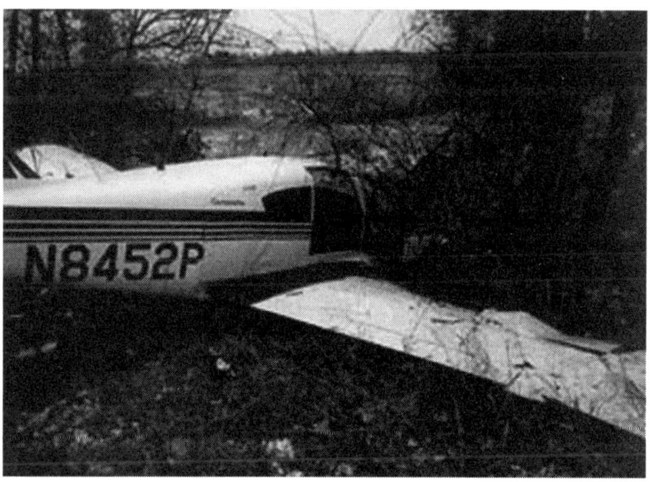

In December 1997, family physician Dr. Robert Frayser fired up his Piper Comanche 400 and took off from Hoisington, Kansas. Shortly after departure, he set his autopilot to cruise at 5,500 feet. That is the last thing he remembered. When he awoke some time later, he felt confused and disoriented, thinking he was still in the air. It took the groggy but uninjured pilot a few moments to realize that the engine was silent, and that he was on the ground, in a bean field—near Cairo, Missouri.

With the aircraft in stable flight, the pilot had lost consciousness. He later discovered the cause: a crack in the engine's exhaust system had allowed carbon monoxide to enter the aircraft cabin. The aircraft flew on autopilot until it ran out of gas and glided to a remarkably smooth landing.

people. This colorless, odorless, toxic gas binds hemoglobin 200 to 300 times more tightly than oxygen, displacing oxygen from the body and causing hypoxia. In fact, smoking just three cigarettes creates the same amount of hypoxia as ascending 5,000 to 8,000 feet in altitude. Night vision is normally lost with hypoxia, and carbon monoxide in smokers greatly increases this loss. It is estimated that a typical smoker has 20 percent less night vision, even at sea level. Unfortunately, it is not only smokers that are at risk, but also everyone breathing second-hand smoke.

Carbon monoxide exposure is insidious and can lead to hypoxia or loss of consciousness before it is noticed. Unless you have an open cockpit, it is highly recommended that you have a carbon monoxide detector in your airplane.

How to quit

OK, I know I need to quit smoking! Does the FAA allow any medication for this purpose?

Nicotine is believed to be the most addictive drug ever discovered—more addictive than heroin, cocaine, amphetamines, or alcohol. Since an average cigarette has about 15 to 25 mg of nicotine, it seems sensible to help smokers quit by giving them nicotine in some other form until they can break the habit. The FAA approves smoking cessation with nicotine replacement. A variety of products are available, including skin patches (Nicoderm, Habitrol, Nicotrol, or Prostep), chewing gums (Nicorette, Nicotine polacrilex), tablets (Nicolar), elixir (Nicotinex), and a nasal spray (Nicotrol).

Anti-depressant medications to help you quit, such as Zyban (bupropion), are not permitted during flight. However, you may obtain permission from your AME to use the medication for smoking cessation if you do not take it for at least 72 hours before flight.

Using oxygen

Over 2,000 years ago, Aristotle noticed that people walking up Mt. Olympus became more breathless than would be expected just from the exercise. Over the following centuries, speculation increased about the effects of altitude. In 1643, Evangelista Torricelli invented the barometer to study the effects of atmospheric pressure on living creatures. He discovered that the seemingly endless atmosphere was really quite a thin layer of air that drops off quickly as one goes higher.

From sea level to outer space

From the ground or in the air, the atmosphere that allows flight to take place can seem like a vast region, far greater than the two-dimensional surface of land and water. In fact, viewed from outer space, the atmosphere is just a wispy covering of the planet. If the earth were the size of a basketball, the majority of the atmosphere would be the thickness of Saran wrap.

Looked at more closely, this thin layer can be divided into four zones:

- *Physiologic zone*, from sea level to about 10,000 feet. Humans are generally well adapted to this zone and require no special equipment for ascent or descent.

- *Physiologically deficient zone*, from 10,000 feet to about 50,000 feet. Adaptation gradually fails here because of the decrease in air pressure and available oxygen. Some individuals have a remarkable tolerance for high-altitude environments, as demonstrated by those who have climbed Mt. Everest without oxygen. At an altitude of about 40,000 feet, supplemental oxygen is not only necessary but must be given in a pressurized form to be effective.

- *Space-equivalent zone*, from about 50,000 feet to about 50 miles. A pressurized suit or cabin becomes necessary. At 63,000 feet, atmospheric pressure is so low that blood will boil and fluids quickly evaporate out of an unprotected body.

- *Space*, arbitrarily defined to begin at 50 miles above sea level. If you can reach this altitude, you qualify for astronaut status. Only a tiny percentage of the atmosphere remains, and it continues its decline to essentially disappear at about 120 miles, but this small amount is enough to support some types of flight. On July 17, 1962, USAF Major Robert M. White flew an X-15 to an altitude of 95 km and became the first winged pilot-astronaut.

Altitude and air pressure

	Altitude		*Pressure*			
	M	ft	mb	in Hg	mm Hg	PSIA
Sea level	0	0	1013	29.9	760	14.7
	20	655	989	29.2	742	14.4
	50	1,640	955	28.2	716	13.8
	1000	3,280	899	26.6	674	13.0
	2000	6,560	795	23.5	596	11.5
	5000	16,400	540	15.9	405	7.8
	10,000	32,800	265	7.8	199	3.8
	15,000	49,200	121	3.6	91	1.8
	20,000	65,600	55	1.0	41	0.8

Altitude and hypoxia

The amount of oxygen in the atmosphere is constant, at 20.93 percent, up to about 70,000 feet. With increasing altitude, however, the pressure of this oxygen decreases along with the air pressure, so that although the *percentage* is the same, the *quantity* of oxygen available to the body is much less. At first, the body can compensate by breathing faster and deeper. After spending time at high altitude, the body can also adapt in further ways by producing more red blood cells, thickening the blood and allowing it to carry more oxygen. For example, people living in Leadville, Colorado (elevation about 10,000 ft) have a much easier time handling high altitude than those at sea level. When these people come down to sea level, they have an advantage in endurance sports because of the extra oxygen-carrying capacity of their blood. This is why many athletes train at Colorado Springs.

Adapting to altitude is one way to get the body to handle more oxygen. There are also artificial ways to do this: getting a blood transfusion of extra red blood cells, or taking EPO (erythropoietin; a hormone that increases production of red blood cells). Both methods have been illegally used by Olympic athletes.

As the amount of oxygen decreases, the pilot responds by first taking deeper breaths, and then more frequent breaths. This can be noticed at as little as 4,000 feet. By about 8,000 feet, the increased breathing rate will have the effect of blowing off the carbon dioxide in the blood, making it more alkaline. This causes the small blood vessels to constrict, decreasing blood flow to the brain and to the eyes, resulting in poorer thinking and vision. The heart rate and blood pressure increase to try to catch up to send more blood to the brain. The racing heart contributes to the feeling of anxiety that many people experience.

Some symptoms of hypoxia

Air hunger, gasping, faster and deeper breathing
Feelings of anxiety, irritability, or euphoria and false sense of well-being
Fatigue, weakness, or drowsiness
Difficulty speaking clearly
Poor coordination, slowed reaction time
Nausea
Headache
Dizziness
Hot and cold flashes
Blurred vision, tunnel vision, or trouble switching from near to far vision
Numbness or tingling
Poor judgment

"The flyer who is suffering from want of oxygen is far from normal. He may be exhilarated, he may be simply dull and sleepy, or, if he is in a position of danger he may fail to take the measures necessary for the safety of himself and those with him, even when he is well aware of the danger."
—*United States War Department, 1919*

Pilots are affected in different ways by hypoxia, and each person not only has an individual response, but the response may change depending on other factors such as illness, obesity, smoking, fatigue, and age. Most people experience a change in personality, becoming anxious, aggressive, or euphoric with a loss of inhibitions or self-criticism. Short-term memory is affected, so that the pilot is easily distracted, forgetful, and absent-minded. Vision is affected very early, with difficulty reading fine print. Color vision also deteriorates. Muscular control is affected, especially the performance of finely coordinated movements. With increasing hypoxia, the fingers and lips may turn blue and the person begins to hyperventilate in a futile effort to try to get more air. Eventually, the level of consciousness drops into confusion, unconsciousness, and finally death. All of this can occur within minutes in cases of rapid hypoxia.

Susceptibility to hypoxia is increased by:

Exercise—increases need for oxygen
Cold—increases need for oxygen
Illness—lowers tolerance for hypoxia
Fatigue—lowers tolerance for hypoxia
Smoking—produces carbon monoxide; smoking a pack a day is the same as an extra 7,000 ft of altitude
Drugs or alcohol—an ounce of alcohol has the same effect as an extra 2,000 ft of altitude

Although the effects of hypoxia are the same, there are actually different types of hypoxia and the pilot may experience more than one type.

- *Hypoxic hypoxia*, such as that caused by altitude, is the most common kind of hypoxia, beginning at about 5,000 feet.

- *Anemic hypoxia* is due to a decrease in the ability of the blood to carry oxygen, either by a reduced number of red blood cells or by a problem with these cells or their hemoglobin. Carbon monoxide causes this type of hypoxia. Other causes include various drugs and certain blood conditions such as sickle cell anemia.

- *Stagnant hypoxia* is due to a decrease in blood flow. Even though there is plenty of oxygen and the blood is healthy, it may not do much good if the blood cannot get to where it is needed. This type of hypoxia is experienced in aerobatic maneuvers while "pulling Gs" and to a lesser extent in pilots with varicose veins or poor circulation, causing the blood to pool in the legs.

- *Histotoxic hypox*ia is experienced when the cells cannot use oxygen, no matter how much is available from the blood. This occurs with exposure to alcohol, narcotics, cyanide, and other poisons.

Stages of hypoxia

Hypoxia is dangerous because it is so sneaky. At the mild levels, in particular, there is no discomfort, pain, change in appearance, or obvious loss of functioning. There may be only a slight increase in breathing, beyond the normal range of 12 to 16 breaths per minute. But this is likely to go unnoticed, since few people pay much attention to their breath rate and it naturally increases with stress or exercise. The effect of mild hypoxia is more pronounced at night, when visual sensitivity is decreased by 10 percent at 5,000 ft, and by 28 percent at 10,000 ft. It is not just a matter of altitude, but also of time at altitude: spending a few hours at 8,000 ft has the same effect as a half hour at 16,000 ft.

With the decrease in oxygen, the person progresses through the following stages:

1. *Indifferent stage:* Altitude 0-10,000 ft breathing ambient air, or 34,000-39,000 ft unpressurized oxygen

   Blood oxygen approx. 90 to 98 percent

So-called because the pilot is usually unaware of the effects, and indifferent to the slight changes that take place: an increase in heart rate and breathing, along with a gradual decrease in overall performance and night vision.

2. *Compensatory stage:* Altitude 10,000-15,000 ft breathing ambient air, or 39,000-42,500 ft unpressurized oxygen

   Blood oxygen approx. 80 to 90 percent

Also called the zone of adaptation, the body tries to compensate for the decreased oxygen with a further increase in heart rate and breathing. Because the brain is getting less oxygen, there is poor judgment, concentration, and coordination. Along with the impaired overall performance, there may be feelings of well-being or euphoria.

3. *Disturbance stage:* Altitude 15,000-20,000 ft breathing ambient air, or 42,500-44,800 ft unpressurized oxygen

Blood oxygen approx. 70 to 80 percent

At this stage, the body can no longer compensate and is markedly impaired. The pilot may have difficulty with flight controls, speaking and writing. Many people suffer headaches and the loss of peripheral vision. Hyperventilation is common, along with drowsiness, fatigue, or euphoria.

4. *Critical stage*: Altitude 20,000-23,000 ft breathing ambient air, or 44,800-45,500 ft unpressurized oxygen

Blood oxygen approx. 60 to 70 percent

At this stage, the body's compensation for lack of oxygen breaks down entirely. There may be convulsions, heart failure, and death. The usual progression is dizziness, followed by loss of consciousness.

Normal blood oxygen saturation levels at sea level are 96 to 100 percent. Ninety-five percent is considered minimal. This decreases to 93 to 95 percent at 5,000 feet, 90 to 93 percent at 7,500 feet, 88 to 92 percent at 10,000 feet, 83 to 87 percent at 12,500 feet, and 77 to 83 percent at 14,000 feet. Below 90 percent, most people begin to experience signs of hypoxia.

To avoid the subtle onset of hypoxia, an increasing number of pilots are using a portable oxygen monitor. Just a few years ago, these would have been too cumbersome and expensive to consider for use in general aviation, but new products are appearing

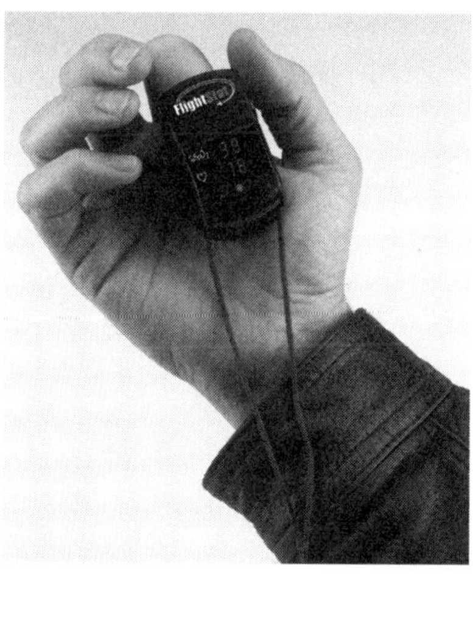

FlightStat Pulse Oximeter

which are small, inexpensive, and very convenient. They will probably become a standard item in future cockpits. One such product, the Nonin FlightStat, slips on to your fingertip and measures saturation by shining red and infrared light through the tissue. It displays pulse rate and oxygen saturation with an accuracy within two percent.

On a January evening in 1980, a Cessna 441 left Shreveport, Louisiana on a flight to Baton Rouge. A short time later, the pilot reported bad weather and requested a climb to 21,000 ft. Air traffic controllers lost radio contact and noticed the aircraft continuing to climb. The Air Force was alerted and sent out two aircraft to intercept the Cessna. They found it near Raleigh, North Carolina at 40,000 ft, continuing out over the Atlantic. Offshore, the Cessna nosed over into a spiraling descent and struck the water. The final investigation showed that the pilot and passenger had lost consciousness from hypoxia, leaving the plane on autopilot until it ran out of fuel.

Rapid decompression

The danger from hypoxia is greatest when cabin pressurization is suddenly lost. Instead of a slow and insidious progression of symptoms, the pilot may lose consciousness within minutes, or even seconds. There may be a warning sign of sudden decompression:

- Noise—ranging from a swishing sound to an explosion.
- Air blast—as air rushes out.
- Cold—the sudden decrease in pressure will lower the temperature, even to the point of freezing.
- Fogging—the lower temperature may cause condensation.
- Body air pressure—as the outside pressure is suddenly decreased, there may be a gasp as air escapes from the lungs. Pressure in the ears and sinuses will also be noticeable and perhaps painful. The abrupt loss of air pressure can even cause decompression sickness if it occurs at an altitude of 25,000 feet or more.

Explosive decompression—defined as loss of pressure in less than 0.5 seconds—is more likely in occur in smaller aircraft. Since human lungs usually require about 0.2 seconds to release their air, this type of decompression can result in rupture of the airways. More common is rapid decompression (0.5 seconds to 10 seconds). With subtle decompression, pressure is lost gradually and often insidiously.

> *"Explosive decompression and emergency descent drills are practiced at least once a year by all jet pilots during recurrent training and I am often amazed at the casual attitude shown towards these emergency situations. The actuality will not bear any resemblance to the neat and orderly drill accomplished in training."—Linda Pendleton, Citation instructor*

The Effective Performance Time (EPT) is the amount of time available to effectively function before the pilot is incapacitated by the lack of oxygen. At 43,000 feet, this will shrink to about 10 seconds—just enough time for the oxygen-starved blood to move from the lungs to the brain.

Effective performance time

Altitude (feet)	*Time*
15,000 to 18,000	about 30 minutes
22,000	5-10 minutes
25,000	3-5 minutes
30,000	2-3 minutes
35,000	30 to 60 seconds
40,000	15 to 20 seconds
45,000	9 to 15 seconds

Another indicator of the critical time left after sudden decompression is the Time of Useful Consciousness (TUC). This is the interval between the beginning of oxygen deprivation and unconsciousness.

Time of useful consciousness

Altitude (feet)	*Time*
20,000	10 minutes
22,000	6 minutes
24,000	3 minutes
25,000	2 minutes
30,000	30 seconds
35,000	20 seconds
40,000	15 seconds

Altitude chamber

Because of the danger of hypoxia, it is recommended that all pilots—especially those who fly pressurized aircraft—experience oxygen deprivation first-hand. It is one thing to study hypoxia and be aware of it. It

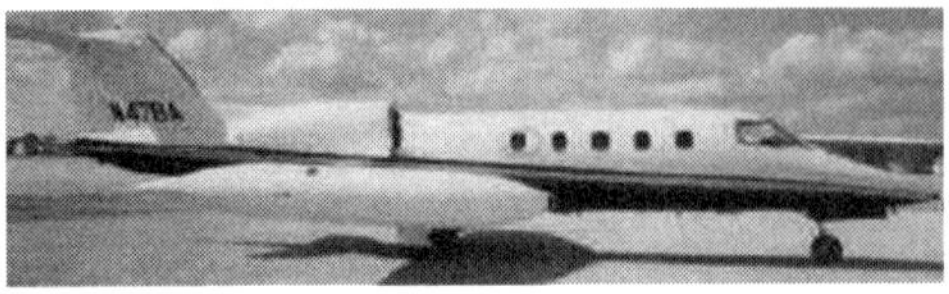

A dramatic, recent case of rapid decompression took place on October 25, 1999, with the death of golfer Payne Stewart. As his Lear 35A climbed past the assigned altitude of 39,000ft, air traffic control lost communication. The Air Force dispatched tracking aircraft, which came close enough to see that the windshields were heavily frosted. National news media tracked the jet for four hours, as millions watched in horror and fascination, until it dropped in a near-vertical dive into a farm field near Mina, South Dakota. The passengers and both pilots had almost certainly expired from hypoxia before the fatal impact.

Why did this happen? There may have been a flaw in the aircraft's oxygen system, or perhaps (as required by FAR 135.89) there was not at least one pilot wearing a mask above 35,000 feet—a common infraction in small, privately operated jets.

is quite another to observe yourself becoming incapacitated even while you are convinced that you are just fine. Learning how you react to hypoxia in the safety of an altitude chamber will prepare you for the real thing, should you ever encounter it, and may well save your life.

> *"There is no doubt that the altitude chamber experience literally saved my neck."—Mark Patiky*

Altitude chambers can be found at a number of Air Force bases, and at the Civilian Aerospace Medical Institute in Oklahoma City. To locate the nearest one, call AOPA or your Regional Flight Surgeon (see *Appendix* for phone numbers or websites).

The usual altitude chamber flight takes place as follows:

1. A briefing describes the program, with a warning that you should not participate if you have certain medical conditions such as ear or sinus problems.

2. You will learn how to don an oxygen mask and ensure a good fit. You will also learn how to use the intercom system, and how to signal the attendants. Participants are usually assigned in pairs, and you will be asked to keep an eye on your partner to observe anything unusual.

3. Once seated in the altitude chamber, the pressure will be lowered to a simulated altitude of 5,000 or 6,000 feet, at a rate of about 3,000 ft/min, and then returned to local ground pressure. This allows you to

practice clearing your ears and get accustomed to the chamber—and discontinue the test if you have any problems.

4. While you have your mask on, the simulated altitude is brought to 8,000 feet, followed by a rapid decompression to 18,000 feet. There may be a sudden noise or fog and cooling of the air as this occurs.

5. The simulated altitude is brought to 25,000 feet. At this point, you will be asked to remove your mask to experience hypoxia. You may also be given small tasks, such as adding a column of numbers, answering questions, or completing a puzzle. You can put on your mask at any time, or signal to the attendant for help. After five minutes (the EPT at this altitude), everyone will put their masks back on (see if you have problems doing this!), and the pressure is returned to ground level.

6. The overall experience is discussed by the group and instructors.

> My own experience in the CAMI altitude chamber was quite an eye-opener. After I took off my mask at 25,000 feet, I was not aware of any problems other than noticing it was a bit hard to do simple arithmetic problems, which I attributed to being distracted by the others. In fact, I was sure that I was completely unaffected, and even suspected that they hadn't really done anything. I looked over at my partner and watched as he went into convulsions, thinking "now why is he acting silly?"—It didn't occur to me that he was having a problem. After the five minutes, I only reluctantly put the mask back on, convinced that I was not only fine, but actually feeling great. In fact, I was dangerously incapacitated—something I would never have realized in an actual flight.
>
> As for my partner, he recovered as soon as the attendant put the mask back on him. He not only remembered nothing of what happened to him, he wouldn't believe us when we told him!

Sickle cell anemia

Sickle cell is an inherited condition of the blood, which makes the person more sensitive to hypoxia. There are two forms: sickle cell anemia, which can be a crippling disease, and sickle cell trait, which may be so mild as to go unnoticed but still predispose individuals to hypoxia. Both forms are found mainly in those of African or Mediterranean ancestry.

A person with sickle cell anemia will probably not be certified to fly because of the high risk of experiencing hypoxia. A person with sickle cell trait, however, may tolerate altitude quite well, although some experience problems with exertion. In 1981, the US Air Force began to accept candidates with sickle cell trait for flight training.

Other blood traits with risk of hypoxia are less common, and include Hemoglobin S and the various forms of thalassemia (formerly called Cooley's anemia). For someone with any of these conditions, the decision whether to fly is based on their ability and tolerance.

Hyperventilation

Breathing too fast and deep is a common response to hypoxia (and to excitement, fear, certain drugs and poisons, and other conditions), but actually decreases the delivery of oxygen to the brain. Breathing fast lowers the amount of the carbon dioxide in the blood, which causes a constriction of the blood vessels, decreasing blood flow not only to the brain but everywhere else in the body. This produces the hyperventilation symptoms of tingling, muscle spasms, cold clammy skin, numbness, and dizziness. Many of these symptoms are the same as those experienced with hypoxia, encouraging you to breathe even faster.

The best way to manage hyperventilation is to breathe slowly at a steady, even rate. If a person is hyperventilating because of panic, it is useful to breathe into a bag, which will collect the carbon dioxide and help reverse the process. Neither of these is easy to do when you are disoriented at night in poor weather, when you switch fuel tanks and the engine quits, or when you are following a heavy transport in clear blue skies—and suddenly get flipped sideways from the vortex. In these cases, there are two simple ways to control breathing:

1. Breathe through your nose, not your mouth.
2. Exhale twice as long as inhale.

It is a good idea to breathe like this *all the time*—slow, deep, steady—and you won't have a problem when things get tense.

Using oxygen

When is oxygen needed? The FAA has regulations as to when oxygen is required, but pilots should consider using oxygen more extensively if available. Studies by the FAA have shown that pilots flying unpressurized aircraft at 8,000 to 12,000 feet without supplemental oxygen make more procedural errors than pilots who use oxygen. Night vision is helped with oxygen and many pilots use it over 5,000 feet. The military requires night combat pilots to use oxygen from the ground up; this is a good policy, since it removes one more task to carry out while aloft. Smokers and others at higher risk of hypoxia should also consider using oxygen at lower altitudes.

> "Regardless of the numbers, if at anytime you do not feel right at altitude, turn on the oxygen supply. If your symptoms improve, remain on oxygen. If they don't, land as soon as possible. You may be suffering from carbon monoxide poisoning, which even high oxygen flows won't eliminate." —*Fred Furgang, MD*

Some people are concerned that overuse of oxygen is dangerous. It is true that continuous use of 100 percent oxygen for a long time can be toxic. However, this applies to periods much longer than a flight, and pilots should not be concerned about oxygen toxicity.

The FAR require oxygen use for:
Pilots at or above 12,500 ft for more than 30 minutes
Pilots at or above 14,000 ft any time
All occupants at or above 15,000 ft any time

If the aircraft is pressurized, with cabin oxygen:
Above 25,000 ft one pilot must wear a mask, unless quick-donning masks are available
Above 35,000 ft one pilot must be wearing a mask at all times

Oxygen systems come in three basic types:

- *Continuous flow*. Useful up to 30,000 feet, this type of system simply provides a flow of 100 percent oxygen until the valve is turned off or the tank is empty. Different masks are available, including the Hudson mask and Scott Sky mask (hospital-type masks with a rebreather bag attached), Scott Duo-Seal mask (with microphone), and Scott Executive Mark III (with altitude-compensating flow).

- *Diluter demand*. Useful up to 34,000 feet, these systems allow a mixture of outside air with the oxygen to last longer.

- *Pressure demand*. Designed for use up to about 45,000 feet and with extreme maneuvers, this type of system can add positive pressure from the regulator. Because of the pressurized gas, the facemask is large and tight-fitting to ensure a good fit.

Nasal cannulas are a popular alternative to face masks at lower altitudes.

They are much more comfortable and allow you to eat and drink and talk through a regular microphone instead of the muffled microphones built into facemasks. They are also useful for men with beards and mustaches that interfere with mask fitting. Cannulas can be used only up to 18,000 feet, and you must carry a normal facemask for use in case the cannula does not provide enough oxygen.

The oxygen used for flying is not the same as other types of oxygen. Aviation oxygen is classified as Grade A, Type I. Medical oxygen is not suitable because it contains moisture, which could freeze at high altitudes. Some pilots argue that this doesn't really matter, and that the moisture actually comes from the medical oxygen equipment and not the oxygen itself. If you want to experiment with the cheaper medical oxygen, you should make sure that you use it only in situations that are not critical.

All oxygen is extremely flammable. You should not use sunblock, lip balms, lipstick, or other petroleum-based skin products while using oxygen, since these can burn.

SCUBA diving

Depressurization and the bends

Decompression sickness occurs when there is a great decrease in the pressure around the body. As the diver descends in the water, gases dissolve in the blood and body fluids under the increased pressure. When the diver ascends, these gases come back out of solution. If the ascent occurs too quickly, bubbles form in the blood and body fluids, in the same way that fizz occurs when the top is taken off a carbonated drink. The bubbles can have a number of effects, depending on their size and location. Even very small bubbles can be trapped in fine blood vessels, blocking blood flow and causing pain or injury to the tissue. In the skin, this can feel like tingling, itching, numbness, or cold or warm sensations, and create a mottled appearance. In the joints, bubbles are more likely to cause a deep, gnawing pain, often severe enough to make the victim double over (the bends). A further effect is due to the chemical make-up of the bubble surface, which causes blood platelets to clump up and release hormones that constrict blood vessels. (Since air is not normally present in the blood, the body reacts to air as if it was a cut, and constricts blood vessels.) Bubbles in the blood vessels around the lungs can cause a burning sensation in the chest that can worsen to a stabbing pain with deep breathing, somewhat like a stitch after exercising without warming up. There may be a dry, irritable cough and feeling of suffocation. In the brain, bubbles cause headache, disorientation, paralysis, inability to speak or hear, and visual symptoms such as flashing lights.

Decompression sickness is classified as Type I, with pain in the joints and skin effects, or as the more serious Type II, in which the bubbles affect the internal organs of the body and can lead to heart failure or stroke. Type I usually resolves without treatment, but Type II requires immediate transfer to a recompression (hyperbaric) chamber.

Susceptibility to decompression sickness increases with age, obesity, and strenuous activity. The effect of age is not well understood, although it may relate to the generally poorer circulation of people as they get older. Obesity is more obviously a risk factor for the bends. Blood is considered a fast-phase tissue, releasing its nitrogen quickly, while fat is a slow-phase tissue, absorbing up to six times more nitrogen than blood and releasing it much more slowly. Exercise just works more compressed nitrogen into the tissues. The treatment for localized decompression sickness is therefore relaxation and immobilization of the affected joint.

> Altitude decompression sickness is rare, but struck a 51-year-old Air Force pilot on March 13, 1987. The pilot had become very obese, weighing over 300 pounds. He took a surplus military jet to 28,000 feet, lost pressurization, and noticed he was having trouble breathing. After landing, he felt better and refused medical care, although the line crew noted that he looked pale and short of breath. The base flight surgeon was contacted, and ordered the pilot to be treated with oxygen and transferred by emergency helicopter to a recompression chamber. In the chamber, the pilot initially improved, but then took a turn for the worse and died.

Pilots exposed to sudden decompression, especially at altitudes above 25,000 feet, are at risk of the bends, but by far the most common cause of flight-related decompression sickness is flying after SCUBA diving.

Flying after diving

SCUBA diving dramatically increases the amount of nitrogen absorbed into the body. An hour at a depth of 60 feet will double the body nitrogen content. The compressed nitrogen will gradually come out of the blood after surfacing—studies have shown the persistence of tiny bubbles in divers as long as 13 hours after a dive to just 32 feet. Flying after diving greatly increases the pressure differential and the rate of bubble formation. Standard recommendations have been developed to prevent this, and are repeated in the Airman's Information Manual (AIM).

Undersea and Hyperbaric Medical Society recommendations

1. *No-decompression dive*
   a. less than 2 hours' accumulated dive time in the 48 hours before final dive
      Minimum surface interval = 12 hours
   b. multi-day unlimited diving
      Minimum surface interval = 24 hours

2. *Decompression dive*
   Minimum surface interval = 24 to 48 hours

3. *Saturation dive*
   May require weeks of decompression.

Bends after no-decompression dives
A young woman made two dives, each to a depth of about 30 feet for about 45 minutes. She flew home about five hours later, and developed the bends.

A scuba-diving pilot dove to 80 feet, with a bottom time of 35 minutes. He flew home four hours later in his unpressurized aircraft, but was careful to stay at 5,000. Despite this precaution, he experienced numbness and pain in one hand—a severe enough condition of the bends to require treatment in a recompression chamber.

If you have to fly before the recommended wait, you can decrease the risk of decompression sickness by breathing 100 percent oxygen for 30 minutes before flight.

"There have been cases of divers getting the bends while attempting a drive home over a mountain pass after making SCUBA dives."—*Divers Alert Network*

High altitude and Nitrox diving

The extraordinary popularity of SCUBA diving is due in large part to the emphasis on safety. In the early years of the sport, even divers with little training or experience would dive to great depths, and injuries were common. To prevent such mishaps, the PADI Dive Manual gives a maximum depth of 60 feet for the novice and 100 feet for the advanced sports diver. At these depths, decompression is usually not necessary. However, if the dive takes place at a high altitude, such as Lake Tahoe where the surface is at 6,200 feet, decompression tables are altered, and both decompression rates and the risk of flying after diving are increased.

Another trend of the last few years is Nitrox diving, using 36 percent oxygen and 64 percent nitrogen. Although the body theoretically has less nitrogen, using this mixture does not change the flying-after-diving recommendations.

Recompression chambers

With symptoms of decompression sickness, it is better to be prudent and call for help rather than wait to see if the situation improves. The Divers Alert Network (DAN) is a civilian organization developed to promote diving safety. Its headquarters at Duke University Medical Center, in Durham, North Carolina, keeps track of recompression chambers around the world. The DAN emergency number is 800-446-2671 or 919-684-8111.

DAN will also give non-emergency information at 919-684-2948, but because they do not want you to have old and possibly incorrect information, they will only give you the address of a recompression chamber if you actually need it for a dive emergency.

If you require air transport to a recompression chamber, consider the choice of aircraft carefully. Most airliners maintain cabin pressure at 7,000 to 8,000 feet, and can increase pressure if necessary. The Super King Air B200 can provide sea level cabin pressure to 17,000 feet, but smaller aircraft are generally inadequate.

After treatment in a recompression chamber, a person should not fly until at least 72 hours after the disappearance of all symptoms.

Women's health

Women were involved in aviation from the very beginning. One of the first people to take to the air was Madame Thible of France, who flew in one of the Montgolfier balloons in the eighteenth century. The first woman officially licensed as a pilot was Elise Deroche, in 1910. Harriet Quimby was the first licensed female pilot in the United States. Dozens of altitude and distance records were set by Ruth Law Oliver and Ruth Nichols, who encouraged other aviation pioneers such as Beryl Markham, Jacqueline Cochran, and Amelia Earhart.

Women were clearly at no disadvantage in flight, and many trained the male pilots during the First and Second World Wars. The restrictions against women in various piloting roles gradually disappeared. Women now hold virtually every type of crew status in both military and commercial aviation operations, including about three dozen US Air Force combat fighter pilots.

Oral contraceptives

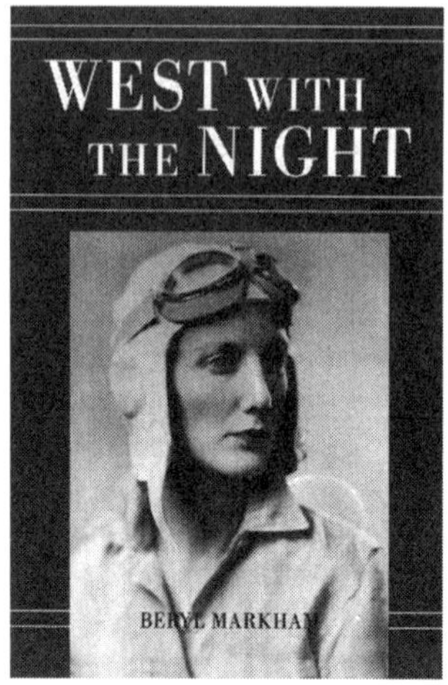

An AME is likely to approve any oral contraceptive once you are familiar and comfortable with it. The problem is that it can take a least a month and sometimes longer to adjust to taking these hormonal supplements. In the meantime, you can experience bloating, depression, and any of a large number of other complaints. The military policy is to ground women starting birth control pills for 30 days to detect significant side-effects. The FAA leaves it open, treating contraceptives the same as any other medication that may have side-effects.

Despite all this concern, there have been no significant reports of adverse reactions to oral contraceptives in the female flying population. This may be because female pilots tend to be healthy, and those using contraceptives have already done so for some time before their aviation medical exam. If you smoke, have a tendency to blood disorders or other chemical imbalances, or have had trouble with depression, you should be more cautious about beginning use of oral contraceptives and perhaps consider other methods of birth control.

Menstrual discomfort

Many women have noticed irregular menstrual cycles or increased menstrual discomfort after beginning work as a flight crewmember. This probably has to do with the general stress of a new job and tends to go away with time and experience. Research on female flight attendants shows that many of them have increased menstrual discomfort, but this is due to jet-lag rather than flying itself, and is made worse by the long sessions of sitting or standing.

> "There is no solid evidence that menses causes performance decrement or increased absenteeism among female pilots."
> —*Fundamentals of Aerospace Medicine*

There are two types of menstrual problem: primary and secondary. The primary type is most common, and can be treated with birth control pills or over-the-counter medication such as ibuprofen (Motrin, Advil, etc). It usually does not interfere with flight. The secondary type is due to some underlying disease, which should be treated appropriately.

Pregnancy

Flight in itself is not hazardous to the fetus, even at altitudes where some amount of hypoxia is present. FAA studies on baboons have shown that the fetus is also well protected from sudden deceleration. If the mother can tolerate it, the baby can too. The major concerns with pregnancy are nausea, the discomfort of lap and shoulder belts, and the possibility that delivery might occur. Although flying is theoretically safe right up to the time of delivery, all of these concerns tend to increase as pregnancy advances. Pregnant women experience nausea and vomiting, fatigue, emotional swings, and other distractions that can impair their performance. Most aviation operations have an arbitrary cut-off time for working on a flight crew. Pilots are usually taken off the flight line as soon as they know they are pregnant. Flight attendants may work longer, usually until about 20 to 27 weeks of gestation. There is some concern that long flights might expose the unborn child to high amounts of radiation. If this is indeed a hazard, it would be most injurious to the fetus during the first eight weeks after conception, when women often do not even realize they are pregnant.

During pregnancy, seat restraints become increasingly uncomfortable. If a lap belt only is used, it should be worn low, under the fetus, rather than high, although the higher position may feel more natural.

By 1935, U.S. airlines were carrying a million passengers per year, still far behind trains, which carried five hundred times as many. Most travelers considered flying too risky. To encourage people to fly, the airlines needed to change this attitude—and especially that of men, who did the most traveling.

A woman, Ellen Church, found the solution. She went to United Airlines and suggested that they put young nurses on board their planes to care for their frightened and airsick passengers. Men would be reluctant to admit their anxiety when they saw the women handling flight with poise and assurance. The stewardess program was a resounding success and led commercial aviation to become the dominant mode of travel (to the detriment of the passenger railways). Women now work in all areas of aviation, as mechanics, air traffic controllers and they account for about 10 percent of pilots, while an increasing number of flight attendants are male.

Sleep and fatigue

A study by the National Transport Safety Board of airline accidents found that half of the captains had been awake for more than 12 hours before the accident, and fatigue was the most common cause of pilot error. This will come as no surprise to any pilot who is well-acquainted with the effects of fatigue: decreases in alertness, performance, judgment, situation awareness, memory, reaction time, concentration, motivation, and mood. Laboratory studies show that these effects begin after just two hours less sleep than usual.

Lack of enough restful sleep is the curse of the modern world. We now sleep, on average, about 6.5 hours a day—20 percent less than a century ago. It is not just a matter of fewer hours of sleep, but a lower quality of those hours. Noise is perhaps the worst offender, but caffeine, nicotine, alcohol, and stimulation all contribute to a restless night. Most adults need about eight hours of good sleep, with some requiring as little as six hours and others up to ten hours. With aging, sleep is generally less deep, night-time awakenings are more frequent, and therefore the overall period of sleep needs to be longer. When sleep is missed, it builds up a deficit that can take two or more days to completely resolve.

Sleepiness is not the same as fatigue. For most people with a normal daily cycle, sleepiness peaks at about 3:00 to 5:00 AM and again in the afternoon at about 3:00 to 5:00 PM. Oddly, humans do not have a natural 24-hour cycle, but rather a 25- or 26-hour cycle. This means that you naturally want to stay awake a little later each day and get up a bit later. This is why people typically stay up later on the weekend, and then face Monday morning with a sleep deficit. Daylight helps to reset the biological clock each day.

Although you can become accustomed to working for long periods without sleep, it is a myth that you can train yourself to function on less sleep overall. Sleep is a physiological requirement, and the deficit will result in diminished performance. Eventually, there are involuntary "microsleep" lapses from a few seconds to a few minutes, in which you may not be aware that you have been asleep. Like hypoxia, symptoms of inadequate sleep are subtle and insidious.

Stages of sleep

Sleep is separated into dreaming and non-dreaming sleep. Dreaming sleep is usually referred to as REM (rapid eye movement) sleep since the eyes tend to flicker while the rest of the body is relaxed—in fact, the dreamer may even feel paralyzed. The function of dreams is still controversial and not well understood. It is likely a sort of reset of the brain. What is known is that dreaming sleep is essential, and anything that interferes with it—such as alcohol, drugs, stress, noise, or being frequently interrupted—will result in non-productive sleep. Everyone has periods of dreaming about every 90 minutes during sleep, even though most people remember few, if any, of their dreams.

There are four basic stages of non-dreaming sleep, which typically repeat in a 90-minute cycle and alternate with REM sleep:

1. In the first stage, you are still awake but drowsy. Brain waves slow down and temperature, breathing and heart rate decrease. There may be an occasional jerk of a muscle as the body relaxes.

2. During the second stage, brain activity slightly increases with short bursts of thoughts and memories. Your muscles are more relaxed and breathing becomes deep and steady. You might still think you are awake at this point, and insist that you weren't sleeping if you are awakened.

3. The third stage is a deeper sleep during which you are harder to awaken. If you are interrupted at this point, you may feel irritable and even more tired.

4. The fourth stage is the deepest part of sleep. If you are awakened, you may feel disoriented and take a few minutes to fully wake up. This is also the most restful stage of sleep. As people get older, they spend less time in this stage and sleep is no longer as restful.

Snoring

Most people snore occasionally, making a sound that ranges from a gentle purr to a loud roar that can be heard through walls. As muscles relax during sleep, the soft tissues of the nose, palate, tongue, tonsil, and uvula (that little dangly piece of flesh at the back of your mouth) all relax as well. When they constrict the airflow, you will begin to snore. When they completely cut off the airflow, you stop breathing momentarily until your body is pulled out of deep sleep to begin breathing again—a condition called sleep apnea.

Mild snoring is mainly a problem for others, while the snorers themselves are blissfully unaware of the disturbance. This is one reason why you should never be without earplugs. Most pilots I know would rather fly through a squall line than spend a night in a hotel room with a "heroic" snorer.

You can relieve snoring by:

- Losing weight: the bigger you are, the more likely you are to snore.

- Exercise regularly to firm up muscle tone.
- Avoid alcohol: it disturbs sleep and further relaxes the tongue and throat muscles.
- Avoid sleeping pills, tranquilizers, and antihistamines.
- Don't eat a heavy meal within three hours of bedtime.
- Don't sleep on your back: gravity will help collapse your airway.
- Elevate the head of the bed, or use extra pillows, to keep the head more upright.
- Treat any nasal congestion to breathe freely through the nose.
- Consider using breathing strips to keep the nose open.

And if that doesn't work, consider using:

- A CPAP or BIPAP machine.
- A dental device that supports the soft palate.
- Laser therapy or radio-wave treatment (somnoplasty) to shrink tissue.
- Surgery to cut away extra tissue.

What, me snore?
I once had a layover at a remote airstrip in the Canadian Northwest Territories, sharing a small Quonset hut with a couple of other pilots. Their combined snoring rattled the aluminum roof to such a deafening racket that I seriously considered taking my sleeping bag outside to a snow bank. The next morning, they both gave *me* dirty looks and said, "That's it, man! You kept us awake with your [deleted] snoring. You're outta here." The next night, I was out on the snow bank, under the stars, sleeping peacefully.

Sleep apnea

While mild snoring is harmless, more severe snoring indicates a potentially serious health problem. Sleep apnea, from the Greek "without breath," is defined as an interruption of breathing for more than 10 seconds. Obstructive apnea occurs when the airway is blocked—usually by the tongue or tissue at the back of the throat that is too relaxed or too thick. The typical pattern is deeper and louder snoring, building up to a complete block of breathing and ending with a choking gasp as breathing is resumed. It is very difficult to get restful sleep with this condition, as sleep might be interrupted hundreds of times during the night. Sleep apnea affects more than 12 million Americans. It is most common in middle age, affecting about four percent of men and two percent of women.

The major therapies for sleep apnea are surgery to remove the excess tissue at the back of the throat, or breathing-support machines (CPAP or BIPAP). Both of these are well tolerated and are allowed by the FAA (see *Chapter 2: Sleep disorders*).

Fatigue

Fatigue is not the same as drowsiness, and can be a significant problem even when a person is getting enough sleep. Like hypoxia or alcohol, fatigue is dangerous because the main symptom is a lack of awareness of its effects. There are three types of fatigue:

- *Physical fatigue*—resulting from exertion, muscle soreness, and illness. It is also caused by sleep deprivation.
- *Mental fatigue*—resulting from boredom or prolonged mental strain. Research has shown that monotonous vigilance tasks decreased alertness by 80 percent in one hour.
- *Emotional fatigue*— resulting from personal strains, such as family, co-worker, or authority conflicts. This type of fatigue is often called burnout.

Causes of fatigue

Lack of restful sleep	Hypoxia
Dehydration	Impaired vision
Caffeine	Temperature too hot or too cold
Noise and vibration	Movement restriction
Illness	Boredom
Medications	Jet lag
Hypoglycemia	Stress

Symptoms of fatigue
Delayed reaction time
Insensitive to signals
Poor timing
Lower accuracy
Poor awareness
Easily distracted
Neglect minor tasks
Inattention to detail
Cannot multitask (can think only of one thing at a time)
Fixate (stare at a single item or instrument)
Short-term memory loss (quickly forget ATC's last clearance)
Poor judgment and decision making
Decreased visual perception
Loss of initiative
Don't care attitude
Personality change, gloomy outlook on life

FAA REGULATIONS FOR FLIGHT TIME AND REST SCHEDULES

When the Airline Pilots Association (ALPA) was formed in 1931, one of its first concerns was fatigue. Until then, pilots had been required to fly up to 150 hours a month. The organization convinced the FAA to set limits for domestic carrier crews at 1,000 hours in a calendar year, 100 hours in a calendar month, and 30 hours in seven consecutive days. Under Part 135, the limit was slightly higher at 120 hours per month, and 1,200 annually. Individual air carriers and union contracts set maximal flight times at lower amounts.

On final approach to its home base, a DC-8 cargo aircraft was caught in a wind shear microburst and crashed with the loss of life of everyone aboard. Later analysis showed that the crew was experienced and the captain was a simulator instructor who taught how to handle this exact situation. The first officer began the corrective action but was over-ruled by the captain, who performed the wrong operation and did not recognize his error until it was too late. In the previous two days, the captain had had 14 hours of flight time and two hours of ground preparation, along with jet lag resulting from a transfer from Europe. Despite his extensive knowledge, his probable fatigue caused his misjudgment of the situation.

Current FAA regulations (Part 121.471) for flight time and rest periods for scheduled domestic commercial carriers limit crewmembers to a maximum total flying time of:

- 30 hours in 7 consecutive days
- 8 hours between required rest periods

During the 24 hours before a scheduled flight, there must be at least:

- 9 hours rest for less than 8 hours scheduled flight time.
- 10 hours rest for 8 to 9 hours scheduled flight time.
- 11 hours rest for 9 hours or more scheduled flight time.

Jet Lag

Jet lag is defined as "a syndrome of general malaise frequently experienced after transmeridian jet travel across multiple time zones." When a person travels eastward, the day becomes shorter, and with travel westward, the day becomes longer. Either way, the normal daily sleep-wake cycle is disturbed and the traveler has to adjust to a new one. It is not only sleep that is disturbed, because the entire body functions on an internal clock. Hormonal levels vary during the day, as do sensations of hunger and physical alertness. These are known as circadian rhythms, daily cycles that are established by zeitgebers (from the German for "time givers") such as daylight hours, regular meals, work and rest schedules.

The usual formula for recovery from jet lag is about one day for each hour of time zone difference. It is a bit easier to adjust to east-west flight, since the day is naturally longer, fitting the body's tendency to stay awake longer. But with major time changes such as 10 to 12 hours, it no longer makes much difference and it can take over a week to readjust.

Ways to minimize jet lag:

- Before the flight, reset your watch to the time at the destination.
- Try to do activities you would normally do at the new time.
- Drink plenty of fluids, but not alcohol.
- Get into the sun as soon as possible on arrival at the destination.

> The US Army studied the "Argonne jet lag diet"—a program of eating specific foods at specific times three days before flight—and found that it actually made jet lag worse.

If you are going to your new destination for less than three days, it is better to remain on home time rather than try to adapt to the new time zone and then re-adapt on your return. This is done by keeping your watch on home time and taking your meals and sleep to your home schedule, as much as possible.

Sleep hygiene

One of the greatest causes of sleepiness and fatigue is lack of good sleep and insomnia. To improve the quality of sleep, the following sleep hygiene techniques are recommended:

- Aerobic exercise for 20-30 minutes improves general fitness and will encourage restful sleep, but should be avoided three to four hours before bedtime.

- Allow an hour or two to "wind down" and prepare for sleep, doing relaxing activities.

- Avoid caffeine or stimulants at least four hours before bedtime.

- Certain foods make you more or less drowsy. Carbohydrates increase sleepiness and are good for dinner, but you should avoid a heavy carbohydrate meal at lunchtime unless you want to fall asleep in the afternoon. Protein and fat makes you more alert. Sugar gives a quick energy burst but will lead to drowsiness as it wears off.

- Do not use alcohol as a sedative. Although it may make you relaxed or sleepy, it disrupts the sleep cycle and interferes with deep sleep.

- Make the bedroom a relaxing place, associated with sleep. Do not use your bedroom for work activities, exercise, or entertainment.

- Your bedroom should be dark and quiet. Windows can be blocked, or you can use a sleep mask over your eyes. Earplugs are helpful to block noise, and some people like the white noise of fans or air conditioners to mask outside noise.

- Anxiety about missing a wake-up call can be alleviated by setting two alarm clocks.

- Many relaxation recordings and techniques are available to guide you into a calm and pleasant state.

Is it helpful to take a nap when sleepy in the daytime?

There are really two types of naps. A short nap (less than 40 minutes) can be very helpful to take a break. It is designed to be a restorative rest period, but without going into deep sleep. It is sometimes called a "power nap." Research has shown that a short nap can provide an extra two to four hours of physical and mental activity. This can be done for several days, until your sleep deficit builds up.

Long naps are about three to four hours and go into deep sleep. They can keep you going for four to five days before sleep deficit is overwhelming.

You should decide what type of nap you want to take—either short or long, but not in between. If you are awakened after an hour or two, you may feel groggy and irritable.

Sleeping pills

Sleeping pills can be useful for people suffering from short-term anxiety, jet lag, or other sleep disturbance. All of these medications have a depressing effect on the nervous system and should not be used unless they are really necessary. Most sleeping pills are either antihistamines (over-the-counter, such as Sleep-Eze) or benzodiazepines (prescription, such as Halcion). None of these is permitted for use before or while acting as a flight crew.

What about melatonin?

Melatonin came under investigation as a natural sleeping aid since the brain produces melatonin and it is linked to the sleep-wake cycle. However, research did not show that taking melatonin reliably improves sleep. Some people swear by it anyway. Like other herbal medications, melatonin may be used if it does not affect flight performance. In other words, it may be used only if it does not make you sleepy!

... and if you can't sleep, some facts to ponder

- A duck's quack doesn't echo, and no one knows why.
- An ostrich's eye is bigger than its brain.
- Opossums playing possum aren't "playing." They have passed out from sheer fright.
- The longest recorded flight of a chicken is 13 seconds.
- More people are killed by donkeys annually than in plane crashes.

6

Military Pilots

COL. CHRISTOPHER R. KLEINSMITH D.O., M.P.H.
DIRECTOR OF INTERNATIONAL MEDICAL TRAINING, UNITED STATES AIR FORCE

Flying is a fascinating, dangerous activity that is both loved and feared: loved because of its grace and beauty, feared because of the chance of catastrophe. Thus, the issues involved may be summarized as "flying and dying".
—*USAF Flight Surgeon's Guide*

Military medical requirements

Each of the four branches of the US Armed Forces has its own aviation medical system and pilot medical requirements. In general, these are quite similar to the civilian requirements, but are somewhat less tolerant of illness and disabilities.

The medical management of all military air crew is the duty of flight surgeons. A flight surgeon is assigned to every flying unit, and must fly with them at least four hours per month. The flight surgeon acts as a general medical officer to the flying squadron and deploys with them. In this manner, the flight surgeon has intimate knowledge of the crew.

In no other field of medicine do physicians end up identifying so strongly with their patients, often changing their outward personality, so that they begin thinking of themselves more as fliers than as doctors.
—*USAF Aerospace Medicine Program*

Like the FAA system, there is a program by which the aviator who does not meet the medical requirement may apply for a waiver. Ultimately, the decision whether to grant a waiver is made by a delegated USAF Surgeon General authority. This decision may be carried out at different levels (e.g., base, major command) depending upon the medical condition.

Air force

In 1994, all USAF medical facilities were reorganized into objective medical groups. In all but the smallest facilities, the medical group is organized into four squadrons: the Dental Squadron, the Medical Support Squadron, the Medical Operations Squadron, and the Aerospace Medicine Squadron. For USAF aviators, there are three medical classes that qualify for flying duties:

- Flying Class I (FC-I) for entry into pilot training.
- Flying Class II (FC-II) for individuals who are in pilot training, rated officers, and physicians who are Flight Surgeons.
- Flying Class III (FC-III) for non-rated individuals whose duties involve flying (e.g., boom operators, crew chiefs, load masters).

AF regulation AFI 40-502 requires that body weight be maintained within a prescribed range depending on height (given in AFVA 40-503, USAF Maximum Allowable Weight Table), or determined by the percentage of body fat. If it is beyond the weight limit, the aviator will be removed from flying status until a satisfactory weight is achieved.

Army

The Army flying duty medical examination classification is not the same as that of the Air Force. Army flight surgeons perform the following examinations:

Class 1 and 1A: Flying duty medical examinations for initial entry warrant (1) and commissioned (1A) officers.

Class 2: Flying duty medical examinations for initial entry flight surgeons, aeromedical physician assistants, air traffic controllers, Department of the Army or contract civilian pilots, and special civilian pilot-to-army flight school candidates; and annual examinations for all aviation officers, flight surgeons, air traffic controllers, and Department of the Army or contract civilian pilots.

Class 3: Initial entry and annual flying duty medical examinations for crew chiefs, flight medics, aerial observers, aerial gunners, and non-crewmember personnel on flight status; and annual examinations of aeromedical physician assistants.

HALO: Initial entry and routine airborne physical examinations for special forces operations High-Altitude, Low-Opening parachutists.

DIVING: Initial entry and routine diving physical examinations for Army divers.

Disqualifications for flying duties are stated in Army Regulation 40-501, Standards of Medical Fitness.

Mental health

Few question the motivation of civilian pilot candidates—if the applicant has the time and the money, and passes a medical examination, no further questions are usually asked. Flight training is like any other service that is purchased, and buyers generally have the right to buy what they want. If people want to learn how to fly a jet purely for ego reasons, not only are they allowed to do so, but flight schools are happy to get the business.

In contrast, military flight training has a completely different mission. In this case, the military, and ultimately the taxpayer, pays for flight training. The tremendous investment to fully train a pilot calls for careful selection of applicants. A major concern is their reason for wanting to fly. For example, some want to fly so that they can live out a parent's fantasy, or become more powerful than a parent (usually the father), or prove to themselves or to others that they are not afraid. Some just love risk-taking and are in search of new thrills. There is no way to completely screen out pilot applicants who want to fly for the wrong reasons. Studies show that jet pilots tend to be independent (narcissistic), controlling (stubborn, obsessive), active (high stimulus threshold), and goal-directed (competitive). Some are counterphobic, meaning that they deliberately seek exposure to situations that they fear consciously or unconsciously. Divorce rates are very high among military pilots. The typical aviator going through a divorce is a 35-year-old captain with 1700 hours. The preceding marital discord extended over 2.5 years. The wife initiated divorce proceedings in 90 percent of the cases, citing poor communication with an authoritarian, over-controlled husband/pilot, conflicts between marital goals and career goals, and too-frequent TDYs.

"Remember that flying is not a recognized form of psychotherapy. Any flier who says 'Flying is the only thing I enjoy any more!' should probably be grounded."—*USAF Flight Surgeon's Guide*

To assess motivation and personality that is best suited for pilot training, the Adaptability Rating for Military Aviation (ARMA) is used. The adaptability rating (AR) is not a formal psychiatric interview, but takes the form of an interested conversation between the flight surgeon and the aviator applicant. Only "ARMA-SAT" (satisfactory) and "ARMA-UNSAT" (unsatisfactory) are used in the decision to permit flight training.

Critical Incident Stress Management (CISM)

Varieties of combat fatigue have been known since the beginning of human warfare. It has been referred to by countless names ("shell shock" seems so much simpler and more direct than the current favorite, Post-Traumatic Stress Disorder). During the World Wars, it became evident that soldiers given immediate psychological support in the field recovered more quickly than those who were managed later in hospital settings.

CISM is a comprehensive, organized approach for the reduction and control of harmful symptoms due to stressful events. The technique was developed in the 1980s to prevent post-traumatic stress among those responding to emergencies. In the Air Force, it is carried out by a Critical Incident Stress Team (CIST), typically composed of medical and mental health professionals, chaplain, and trained emergency responders, and appointed at each station by the wing commander.

The key components of CISM are:

- *Critical Incident Stress Debriefing (CISD)*: a group meeting, lasting 1.5 to 3 hours, in which the event is reviewed in a systematic manner:
    - *Introduction*: everyone is introduced and process is described.
    - *Facts*: each participant describes the incident from his or her own perspective.
    - *Thoughts*: participants describe their reactions to the incident.
    - *Emotional responses*: participants describe their most traumatic reaction, and emotional responses.
    - *Symptoms*: participants identify their personal symptoms of distress.

- *Teaching*: team members educate the group about normal reactions to stress and coping mechanisms.
- *Re-entry*: opportunities to clarify ambiguities and prepare for termination.

- *Defusing*: a shortened version of CISD, lasting 20 to 60 minutes, provided within 8 hours of the incident. This is used for smaller groups and consists of:
  - Introduction
  - Exploration of facts
  - Informal teaching.
- *Demobilization*: a group meeting lasting 1.5 to 3 hours, usually in response to a large-scale event, for groups of 100 or more. This involves a 10-minute information talk from a CISD member, followed by 20 minutes of food and rest for the participants.

Substance abuse

Alcohol and drug abuse has been a persistent problem in the armed forces for thousands of years, from the very beginning of organized conflict. The reasons, of course, are quite obvious. The tremendous stress, loneliness, isolation, foreign environments—and soldier's youth—predispose them to use recreational drugs. Since the time of the Roman Empire, the western favorite has been alcohol. Not until 1968 did the British Royal Navy finally stop the tradition of giving sailors rations of rum.

In a study made of military aviators with psychiatric hospitalization, 57 percent were for alcohol-related problems. More U.S. military members exceed five drinks per week (32 percent) than does the general population (14 percent). The cultural role of alcohol was firmly established in long-standing traditions concerning O-clubs (for example, having to "buy the bar" as a penalty for placing one's flight cap on the bar, or being paged by one's spouse), various party traditions (e.g., chug-a-lug contests) and squadron functions (e.g., keg parties and Friday evening commanders' calls at the bar).

In the Air Force, if an alcohol problem is suspected, the situation becomes a matter of official USAF policy. The flight surgeon must inform the aviator's commander. The commander must then request an Alcohol and Drug Abuse Prevention and Treatment (ADAPT) evaluation and counsel the aviator about the situation. The ADAPT team will then perform an evaluation within seven days. The diagnosis of alcohol abuse or dependence results in immediate DNIF (Duties Not to Include Flying) as well as Medical Disqualification (DQ) for flying duties. Disqualification continues until full remission, but lasts not less than six months. Diagnosed patients are also placed on S4T profile (ordinarily a six-month ineligibility for deployment or mobility). The flier may be considered for a waiver when treatment and aftercare is complete, and has been sober and off Antabuse or naltrexone for six months.

Allowable medications

The following medications may be used without consultation or waiver action:

Skin antiseptics, topical antifungals, one percent hydrocortisone cream, or benzoyl peroxide for either minor wounds or acute skin diseases which do not interfere with the performance of flying duties or wear of personnel equipment.

Single doses of aspirin, acetaminophen, or ibuprofen to provide pain relief for minor self-limiting conditions.

Antacids for mild, isolated episodes of upset stomach.

Hemorrhoidal suppositories.

Bismuth subsalicylate for mild cases of diarrhea without fever.

Oxymetazoline or phenylephrine nasal sprays may be used by aircrew as "get me downs" should unexpected ear or sinus block occur during flight. These should not be used to treat symptoms of congestion existing prior to flight.

The following medications may be used without consultation or waiver once the potential for individual reactions has been excluded:

Isoniazid for prophylactic therapy for aviators reacting to tuberculin, who do not have active tuberculosis. A minimum of seven days ground trial needed.

Oral contraceptives, implantable timed release progestin, estrogen alone or with progestin as replacement therapy. A minimum of 28 days ground trial is needed. Changes in dosage or brand require an additional 28-day observation period.

Chloroquine phosphate, primaquine phosphate, or doxycycline for antimalarial prophylaxis. A single dose ground trial is advised.

Pyridostigmine for chemical warfare prophylaxis. A single dose ground trial is needed.

Anti-motion sickness medications may be used by students in flying training programs provided certain requirements are met. Usually, non-medical interventions (such as dietary modifications, keeping the eyes looking inside or outside the cockpit, keeping the cockpit as cool as possible, or using 100 percent oxygen) are tried first. If these are not successful, anti-motion sickness medications may be used if ground-testing is performed before use, the pilot-in-command is aware of the student's medication use, and medication use is restricted for a brief period. Scopalamine alone or in combination with dextroamphetamine or ephedrine are the medications used. Failure to adapt to flying after a brief course of such therapy will usually result in elimination from the flying training program.

Doxycycline (100 mg) administered twice a day for five days may be used to treat mild diarrhea. Doxycycline may also be used for prophylaxis against diarrhea in deployed personnel, with the total period of use not to exceed two weeks.

Topical antibiotics for control of acne.

Topical tretinoin for control of acne, so long as local irritation does not interfere with wearing life-support equipment.

Topical acyclovir.

Completion of a course of oral penicillin, oxacillin, dicloxacillin, erythromicin, sulfamethoxazole-trimethoprim, tetracycline, ampicillin, doxycycline, or cephalexin, once an infection is no longer symptomatic.

Vaginal creams or suppositories for treatment of vaginitis once the condition is no longer symptomatic.

Temazepam, if such use is essential for the safe execution of an operational mission and only after MAJCOM coordination and approval. A single dose ground trial is required.

Vaccines, but these should be given on non-flying days.

Nicorette or transdermal nicotine. A minimum of 72 hours' ground trial required.

Resin binding agents such as cholestyramine for control of high blood cholesterol.

The following list of medications for conditions may be waived by the MAJCOM surgeon:

Chlorothiazide or hydrochlorothiazide for control of hypertension.

Triamterene for control of hypertension.

Probenecid for treatment of gout or hyperuricemia.

Allopurinol for treatment of gout or hyperuricemia.

Combination therapy of thiazide with triamterine, probenecid, allopurinol, or oral potassium supplements.

Epinephrine derivatives without added action agents, or beta blockers (timolol), both for topical use only, for control of glaucoma.

Synthroid or dessicated thyroid for treatment of thyroid hypofunction or for thyroid suppression.

Tetracycline, erythromicin, doxycycline in standard doses for acne management.

Folic acid in the treatment of sprue.

Sucralfate for prevention of recurrent, uncomplicated duodenal ulcers. A minimum of seven days' observation is required.

Topical flunisolide or beclomethasone or cromolyn nasal spray for control of mild to moderate allergic rhinitis, nonallergic rhinitis, or vasomotor rhinitis. Observation for control of rhinitis (usually 7 to 14 days) is required.

Ranitidine may be considered for a categorical IIA waiver.

Griseofulvin for treatment of fungal infections may be granted a one-year non-renewable waiver after a four-week ground trial.

Clomiphene citrate for treatment of infertility.

Lovastatin and gemfibrozil may be considered for a categorical IIA waiver.

The use of other medications singly or in combination requires a review by HQ AFMOA/SGPA, Bolling AFB DC 20332-6188.

Any medication effect that may affect flying safety, such as nervousness, mental performance decrement, or nausea, is cause for immediate grounding and reassessment of the therapy.

These are some actual maintenance work orders submitted by US Air Force pilots and the replies from the maintenance crews.

Problem: Left inside main tire almost needs replacement.
Solution: Almost replaced left inside main tire.

Problem: Test flight OK, except autoland very rough.
Solution: Autoland not installed on this aircraft.

Problem: #2 Propeller seeping prop fluid.
Solution: #2 Propeller seepage normal—#1 #3 and #4 propellers lack normal seepage.

Problem: Something loose in cockpit.
Solution: Something tightened in cockpit.

Problem: Evidence of leak on right main landing gear.
Solution: Evidence removed.

Problem: DME volume unbelievably loud.
Solution: Volume set to more believable level.

Problem: Dead bugs on windshield.
Solution: Live bugs on order.

Problem: Autopilot in altitude hold mode produces a 200 fpm descent.
Solution: Cannot reproduce problem on ground.

Problem: IFF inoperative.
Solution: IFF always inoperative in OFF mode.

Problem: Friction locks cause throttle levers to stick.
Solution: That's what they're there for.

Problem: Number three engine missing.
Solution: Engine found on right wing after brief search.

Problem: Target Radar hums.
Solution: Reprogrammed Target Radar with the words.

Problem: Aircraft handles funny.
Solution: Aircraft warned to straighten up, "fly right" and be serious.

Appendix I

Further Information

FAA addresses

The FAA is a large organization, and they are not immune to error or misplacing documents. Always keep copies of everything you send. It is also helpful to send important documents as certified mail with a return receipt request.

FAA Aerospace Medical Certification Division

For most purposes, such as submitting or requesting information by regular mail, the address is:

FAA Aerospace Medical Certification Division
PO Box 26080
Oklahoma City OK 73126

For express mail service, use:

FAA Aerospace Medical Certification Division
CAMI Building Room B59
6700 S. MacArthur Blvd.
Oklahoma City, OK 73169
Telephone: 405-954-4821 or 800-350-5286

Since phone volume is very high at the beginning of the week, it is best to call Wednesday to Friday.

Motor vehicle actions

You are legally required to report each motor vehicle action to the FAA within 60 days of its occurrence. A letter must be sent to:

FAA Civil Security Division
AMC-700
PO Box 25810
Oklahoma City, OK 73125

To get a copy of your National Driver Registry (NDR) file, you must submit a notarized request to:

DOT
NHTSA
NTS-24
400 7th Street, SW
Washington, D.C. 20590-0001

ALTITUDE CHAMBERS

The FAA's Civil Aerospace Medical Institute (CAMI) operates a hypobaric pressure chamber at its facility in Oklahoma City. Other chambers are located around the country, mostly at military bases. A list of them is given in www.cami.jccbi.gov/aam-400/asemphys.html. Currently, all scheduling for civil aviation pilots is by the CAMI Airman Education Program Branch in Oklahoma City. To schedule a course, call CAMI at 405-954-4837. They will mail you an application form and notification letter, and assign a training date. The application must be completed and mailed to the address provided within 30 days of the scheduled training, along with a $50 nonrefundable fee made payable to the FAA. You should take the notification letter, along with your current medical certificate, to the training location on the day of your scheduled course. After you complete it, you will receive a certificate noting that you have completed the FAA's physiological training course. There is no annotation in your logbook.

Pilot resources

AOPA

The Aircraft Owners and Pilots Association is the oldest and largest such organization in the world. If you are (or planning to be) a pilot it is well worth joining. For the current annual dues of $39 per year you get an enormous variety of benefits, including the monthly AOPA Pilot magazine. An online tool, TurboMedical, provides help filling out Form 8500-8.

AOPA also provides support for pilots having trouble with medical certification. The first step is the inexpensive publication: *A Pilot's Guide to Medical Certification.* Further information is available online at:

www.aopa.org/members/files/medical/medcert.html
and by telephone at 800-USA-AOPA (872-2672)

If you need help right away, you can call the AOPA Pilot Assistance Hotline (800-872-2376).

For medico-legal advice, you can subscribe to the AOPA Legal Services Plan for an additional fee.

PILOT MEDICAL SOLUTIONS, INC.

This is a relatively new service to help general aviation pilots get their medical certificate. Their website (www.leftseat.com) provides a good amount of useful information, including a list of supportive AMEs, and promises more specialized help for a fee. They may also be reached at 800-699-4457.

The disadvantage of this type of service is the cost involved. On the other hand, it may be well worth the expense to save mountains of paperwork and months of delays.

Pilot Medical Solutions is located right in Oklahoma City and seems to have a pretty good pipeline to the FAA head offices. Given that the FAA resources are stretched to the limit, and unlikely to improve any time soon, it might be cost-effective to have a professional service handle the paperwork for you.

Virtual Flight Surgeons, Inc.

VFS is a group of board-certified aerospace medicine specialists who personally answer questions and help prepare and file paperwork, for a fee. The group has been providing this sort of service for airline pilots since the 1970s through the Airline Pilots Association (ALPA). With the new website (www.AviationMedicine.com) they are broadening their market beyond professional pilots to general aviation.

Like other such services, their help might be expensive, but well worth it if you can save months (or even years) of frustration and endless paperwork.

International Wheelchair Aviators

Information on all types of handicaps, including paraplegic certification and hand control suppliers, can be obtained at www.wheelchairaviators.org/info.html, or by contacting:

International Wheelchair Aviators
Mike Smith, Secretary
PO Box 2799
Big Bear City, CA 92314
Ph 909-585-9663
Fax 909-585-7156

For helicopter information, contact:

- Mike Higgins, Bellevue, WA; 206-462-7320
- Joris Naiman, Waltham, MA; 781-642-6842, joris@naiman.net
- Alto Puerto FBO, PO Box 810, Patagonia, AZ 85624

For amputee information, contact:

- Sheri Coin Marshall, ATP and Flight Instructor; 662-893-0044, doufly@earthlink.net
- Bryant Gains, who flies an A-36 Bonanza, Ft. Worth, TX, bwgaines@flash.net
- Dave Thompson, Scappose, OR; 503-543-2910, beavis@dsinw.com

For hearing impaired, contact:

- Clyde Smith, IDPA President, 1 Galena Dr., Apt. D, Jacksonville, FL 62650; 217-243-0065

Regional flight surgeons

Alaska Region
Robert W. Rigg, M.D.
Phone 907-271-5431
Fax 907-271-3769

Great Lakes Region
Illinois, Indiana, Minnesota, Michigan, Ohio, Wisconsin, North Dakota, South Dakota
Paul L. Brattain, M.D.
Phone 847-294-7491
Fax 847-294-7808

Western Pacific Region
Arizona, California, Hawaii, Nevada, American Samoa, Guam, Marshall Islands, Wake Island
Stephen H. Goodman, M.D.
Phone 310-725-3750, or 800-471-6736
Fax 310-536-8650

Northwest Mountain Region
Colorado, Idaho, Montana, Oregon, Utah, Washington, Wyoming
Michael D. Jones, M.D.
Phone 800-233-5811, or 425-227-2300
Fax 425-227-1300

Southwest Region
Arkansas, Louisiana, New Mexico, Oklahoma, Texas
G.J. Salazar, M.D.
Phone 817-222-5300
Fax 817-222-5965

Central Region
Iowa, Kansas, Missouri, Nebraska
Joel Dickman, M.D.
Phone 800-832-6421, or 816-329-3251
Fax 816-426-5685

Eastern Region
Delaware, District of Columbia, Maryland, New Jersey, New York, Pennsylvania, Virginia, West Virginia
Nicholas M. Lomangino, M.D.
Phone 800-322-2180, or 718-553-3304
Fax 718-995-5698

New England Region
Connecticut, Maine, Massachusetts, New Hampshire, Rhode Island, Vermont
Paul H. Clark, M.D.
Phone 781-238-7300
Fax 781-238-7306

Southern Region
Alabama, Florida, Georgia, Kentucky, Mississippi, North Carolina, South Carolina, Tennessee, Puerto Rico, Virgin Islands
David P. Millett, M.D.
Phone 404-305-6150
Fax 404-305-6161

Appendix II

Code of Federal Regulations Title 14 Part 67
Federal Aviation Regulations: Medical Standards and Certification

Outline

Subpart A—General
- 67.1 Applicability.
- 67.3 Issue.
- 67.7 Access to the National Driver Register.

Subpart B—First-Class Airman Medical Certificate
- 67.101 Eligibility.
- 67.103 Eye.
- 67.105 Ear, nose, throat, and equilibrium.
- 67.107 Mental.
- 67.109 Neurologic.
- 67.111 Cardiovascular.
- 67.113 General medical condition.
- 67.115 Discretionary issuance.

Subpart C—Second-Class Airman Medical Certificate
- 67.201 Eligibility.
- 67.203 Eye.
- 67.205 Ear, nose, throat, and equilibrium.
- 67.207 Mental.
- 67.209 Neurologic.
- 67.211 Cardiovascular.
- 67.213 General medical condition.
- 67.215 Discretionary issuance.

Subpart D—Third-Class Airman Medical Certificate
- 67.301 Eligibility.
- 67.303 Eye.
- 67.305 Ear, nose, throat, and equilibrium.
- 67.307 Mental.
- 67.309 Neurologic.
- 67.311 Cardiovascular.
- 67.313 General medical condition.
- 67.315 Discretionary issuance.

Subpart E—Certification Procedures
- 67.401 Special issuance of medical certificates.
- 67.403 Applications, certificates, logbooks, reports, and records: falsification, reproduction, or alteration; incorrect statements.
- 67.405 Medical examinations: Who may give.

67.407 Delegation of authority.
67.409 Denial of medical certificate.
67.411 Medical certificates by flight surgeons of Armed Forces.
67.413 Medical records.
67.415 Return of medical certificate after suspension or revocation.

Medical standards and certification

Subpart A—General

Sec. 67.1 Applicability.
This part prescribes the medical standards and certification procedures for issuing medical certificates for airmen and for remaining eligible for a medical certificate.

Sec. 67.3 Issue.
Except as provided in Sec. 67.5, a person who meets the medical standards prescribed in this part, based on medical examination and evaluation of the person's history and condition, is entitled to an appropriate medical certificate.

Sec. 67.7 Access to the National Driver Register.
At the time of application for a certificate issued under this part, each person who applies for a medical certificate shall execute an express consent form authorizing the Administrator to request the chief driver licensing official of any state designated by the Administrator to transmit information contained in the National Driver Register about the person to the Administrator. The Administrator shall make information received from the National Driver Register, if any, available on request to the person for review and written comment.

Subpart B—First-Class Airman Medical Certificate

Sec. 67.101 Eligibility.
To be eligible for a first-class airman medical certificate, and to remain eligible for a first-class airman medical certificate, a person must meet the requirements of this subpart.

Sec. 67.103 Eye.
Eye standards for a first-class airman medical certificate are:

(a) Distant visual acuity of 20/20 or better in each eye separately, with or without corrective lenses. If corrective lenses (spectacles or contact lenses) are necessary for 20/20 vision, the person may be eligible only on the condition that corrective lenses are worn while exercising the privileges of an airman certificate.
(b) Near vision of 20/40 or better, Snellen equivalent, at 16 inches in each eye separately, with or without corrective lenses. If age 50 or older, near vision of 20/40 or better, Snellen equivalent, at both 16 inches and 32 inches in each eye separately, with or without corrective lenses.
(c) Ability to perceive those colors necessary for the safe performance of airman duties.
(d) Normal fields of vision.
(e) No acute or chronic pathological condition of either eye or adnexa that interferes with the proper function of an eye, that may reasonably be expected to progress to that degree, or that may reasonably be expected to be aggravated by flying.
(f) Bifoveal fixation and vergence-phoria relationship sufficient to prevent a break in fusion under conditions that may reasonably be expected to occur in performing airman duties. Tests for the factors named in this paragraph are not required except for persons found to have more than 1 prism diopter of hyperphoria, 6

prism diopters of esophoria, or 6 prism diopters of exophoria. If any of these values are exceeded, the Federal Air Surgeon may require the person to be examined by a qualified eye specialist to determine if there is bifoveal fixation and an adequate vergence-phoria relationship. However, if otherwise eligible, the person is issued a medical certificate pending the results of the examination.

Sec. 67.105 Ear, nose, throat, and equilibrium.

Ear, nose, throat, and equilibrium standards for a first-class airman medical certificate are:

(a) The person shall demonstrate acceptable hearing by at least one of the following tests:

(1) Demonstrate an ability to hear an average conversational voice in a quiet room, using both ears, at a distance of 6 feet from the examiner, with the back turned to the examiner.

(2) Demonstrate an acceptable understanding of speech as determined by audiometric speech discrimination testing to a score of at least 70 percent obtained in one ear or in a sound field environment.

(3) Provide acceptable results of pure tone audiometric testing of unaided hearing acuity according to the following table of worst acceptable thresholds, using the calibration standards of the American National Standards Institute, 1969 (11 West 42d Street, New York, NY 10036):

Frequency (Hz)	500	1000	2000	3000
Better ear (dB)	35	30	30	40
Poorer ear (dB)	35	50	50	60

(b) No disease or condition of the middle or internal ear, nose, oral cavity, pharynx, or larynx that:

(1) Interferes with, or is aggravated by, flying or may reasonably be expected to do so; or

(2) Interferes with, or may reasonably be expected to interfere with, clear and effective speech communication.

(c) No disease or condition manifested by, or that may reasonably be expected to be manifested by, vertigo or a disturbance of equilibrium.

Sec. 67.107 Mental.

Mental standards for a first-class airman medical certificate are:

(a) No established medical history or clinical diagnosis of any of the following:

(1) A personality disorder that is severe enough to have repeatedly manifested itself by overt acts.

(2) A psychosis. As used in this section, "psychosis" refers to a mental disorder in which:

(i) The individual has manifested delusions, hallucinations, grossly bizarre or disorganized behavior, or other commonly accepted symptoms of this condition; or

(ii) The individual may reasonably be expected to manifest delusions, hallucinations, grossly bizarre or disorganized behavior, or other commonly accepted symptoms of this condition.

(3) A bipolar disorder.

(4) Substance dependence, except where there is established clinical evidence, satisfactory to the Federal Air Surgeon, of recovery, including sustained total abstinence from the substance(s) for not less than the preceding 2 years. As used in this section—

(i) "Substance" includes: alcohol; other sedatives and hypnotics; anxiolytics; opioids; central nervous system stimulants such as cocaine, amphetamines, and similarly acting sympathomimetics; hallucinogens; phencyclidine or similarly acting arylcyclohexylamines; cannabis; inhalants; and other psychoactive drugs and chemicals; and

(ii) "Substance dependence" means a condition in which a person is dependent on a substance, other

than tobacco or ordinary xanthine-containing (e.g., caffeine) beverages, as evidenced by—
(A) Increased tolerance;
(B) Manifestation of withdrawal symptoms;
(C) Impaired control of use; or
(D) Continued use despite damage to physical health or impairment of social, personal, or occupational functioning.

(b) No substance abuse within the preceding 2 years defined as:
(1) Use of a substance in a situation in which that use was physically hazardous, if there has been at any other time an instance of the use of a substance also in a situation in which that use was physically hazardous;
(2) A verified positive drug test result acquired under an anti-drug program or internal program of the U.S. Department of Transportation or any other Administration within the U.S. Department of Transportation; or
(3) Misuse of a substance that the Federal Air Surgeon, based on case history and appropriate, qualified medical judgment relating to the substance involved, finds—
(i) Makes the person unable to safely perform the duties or exercise the privileges of the airman certificate applied for or held; or
(ii) May reasonably be expected, for the maximum duration of the airman medical certificate applied for or held, to make the person unable to perform those duties or exercise those privileges.

(c) No other personality disorder, neurosis, or other mental condition that the Federal Air Surgeon, based on the case history and appropriate, qualified medical judgment relating to the condition involved, finds—
(1) Makes the person unable to safely perform the duties or exercise the privileges of the airman certificate applied for or held; or
(2) May reasonably be expected, for the maximum duration of the airman medical certificate applied for or held, to make the person unable to perform those duties or exercise those privileges.

Sec. 67.109 Neurologic.
Neurologic standards for a first-class airman medical certificate are:

(a) No established medical history or clinical diagnosis of any of the following:
(1) Epilepsy;
(2) A disturbance of consciousness without satisfactory medical explanation of the cause; or
(3) A transient loss of control of nervous system function(s) without satisfactory medical explanation of the cause.

(b) No other seizure disorder, disturbance of consciousness, or neurologic condition that the Federal Air Surgeon, based on the case history and appropriate, qualified medical judgment relating to the condition involved, finds—
(1) Makes the person unable to safely perform the duties or exercise the privileges of the airman certificate applied for or held; or
(2) May reasonably be expected, for the maximum duration of the airman medical certificate applied for or held, to make the person unable to perform those duties or exercise those privileges.

Sec. 67.111 Cardiovascular.
Cardiovascular standards for a first-class airman medical certificate are:

(a) No established medical history or clinical diagnosis of any of the following:
(1) Myocardial infarction;
(2) Angina pectoris;
(3) Coronary heart disease that has required treatment or, if untreated, that has been symptomatic or clinically significant;

(4) Cardiac valve replacement;
(5) Permanent cardiac pacemaker implantation; or
(6) Heart replacement;

(b) A person applying for first-class medical certification must demonstrate an absence of myocardial infarction and other clinically significant abnormality on electrocardiographic examination:
  (1) At the first application after reaching the 35th birthday; and
  (2) On an annual basis after reaching the 40th birthday.
(c) An electrocardiogram will satisfy a requirement of paragraph (b) of this section if it is dated no earlier than 60 days before the date of the application it is to accompany and was performed and transmitted according to acceptable standards and techniques.

Sec. 67.113 General medical condition.
The general medical standards for a first-class airman medical certificate are:
(a) No established medical history or clinical diagnosis of diabetes mellitus that requires insulin or any other hypoglycemic drug for control.
(b) No other organic, functional, or structural disease, defect, or limitation that the Federal Air Surgeon, based on the case history and appropriate, qualified medical judgment relating to the condition involved, finds—
  (1) Makes the person unable to safely perform the duties or exercise the privileges of the airman certificate applied for or held; or
  (2) May reasonably be expected, for the maximum duration of the airman medical certificate applied for or held, to make the person unable to perform those duties or exercise those privileges.
(c) No medication or other treatment that the Federal Air Surgeon, based on the case history and appropriate, qualified medical judgment relating to the medication or other treatment involved, finds—
  (1) Makes the person unable to safely perform the duties or exercise the privileges of the airman certificate applied for or held; or
  (2) May reasonably be expected, for the maximum duration of the airman medical certificate applied for or held, to make the person unable to perform those duties or exercise those privileges.

Sec. 67.115 Discretionary issuance.
A person who does not meet the provisions of Secs. 67.103 through 67.113 may apply for the discretionary issuance of a certificate under Sec. 67.401.

Subpart C—Second-Class Airman Medical Certificate

Sec. 67.201 Eligibility.
To be eligible for a second-class airman medical certificate, and to remain eligible for a second-class airman medical certificate, a person must meet the requirements of this subpart.

Sec. 67.203 Eye.
Eye standards for a second-class airman medical certificate are:
(a) Distant visual acuity of 20/20 or better in each eye separately, with or without corrective lenses. If corrective lenses (spectacles or contact lenses) are necessary for 20/20 vision, the person may be eligible only on the condition that corrective lenses are worn while exercising the privileges of an airman certificate.
(b) Near vision of 20/40 or better, Snellen equivalent, at 16 inches in each eye separately, with or without corrective lenses. If age 50 or older, near vision of 20/40 or better, Snellen equivalent, at both 16 inches and 32 inches in each eye separately, with or without corrective lenses.

(c) Ability to perceive those colors necessary for the safe performance of airman duties.
(d) Normal fields of vision.
(e) No acute or chronic pathological condition of either eye or adnexa that interferes with the proper function of an eye, that may reasonably be expected to progress to that degree, or that may reasonably be expected to be aggravated by flying.
(f) Bifoveal fixation and vergence-phoria relationship sufficient to prevent a break in fusion under conditions that may reasonably be expected to occur in performing airman duties. Tests for the factors named in this paragraph are not required except for persons found to have more than 1 prism diopter of hyperphoria, 6 prism diopters of esophoria, or 6 prism diopters of exophoria. If any of these values are exceeded, the Federal Air Surgeon may require the person to be examined by a qualified eye specialist to determine if there is bifoveal fixation and an adequate vergence-phoria relationship. However, if otherwise eligible, the person is issued a medical certificate pending the results of the examination.

Sec. 67.205 Ear, nose, throat, and equilibrium.
Ear, nose, throat, and equilibrium standards for a second-class airman medical certificate are:
(a) The person shall demonstrate acceptable hearing by at least one of the following tests:
   (1) Demonstrate an ability to hear an average conversational voice in a quiet room, using both ears, at a distance of 6 feet from the examiner, with the back turned to the examiner.
   (2) Demonstrate an acceptable understanding of speech as determined by audiometric speech discrimination testing to a score of at least 70 percent obtained in one ear or in a sound field environment.
   (3) Provide acceptable results of pure tone audiometric testing of unaided hearing acuity according to the following table of worst acceptable thresholds, using the calibration standards of the American National Standards Institute, 1969:

Frequency (Hz)	500	1000	2000	3000
Better ear (dB)	35	30	30	40
Poorer ear (dB)	35	50	50	60

(b) No disease or condition of the middle or internal ear, nose, oral cavity, pharynx, or larynx that—
   (1) Interferes with, or is aggravated by, flying or may reasonably be expected to do so; or
   (2) Interferes with, or may reasonably be expected to interfere with, clear and effective speech communication.
(c) No disease or condition manifested by, or that may reasonably be expected to be manifested by, vertigo or a disturbance of equilibrium.

Sec. 67.207 Mental.
Mental standards for a second-class airman medical certificate are:
(a) No established medical history or clinical diagnosis of any of the following:
   (1) A personality disorder that is severe enough to have repeatedly manifested itself by overt acts.
   (2) A psychosis. As used in this section, "psychosis" refers to a mental disorder in which:
      (i) The individual has manifested delusions, hallucinations, grossly bizarre or disorganized behavior, or other commonly accepted symptoms of this condition; or
      (ii) The individual may reasonably be expected to manifest delusions, hallucinations, grossly bizarre or disorganized behavior, or other commonly accepted symptoms of this condition.
   (3) A bipolar disorder.

(4) Substance dependence, except where there is established clinical evidence, satisfactory to the Federal Air Surgeon, of recovery, including sustained total abstinence from the substance(s) for not less than the preceding 2 years. As used in this section—
   (i) "Substance" includes: alcohol; other sedatives and hypnotics; anxiolytics; opioids; central nervous system stimulants such as cocaine, amphetamines, and similarly acting sympathomimetics; hallucinogens; phencyclidine or similarly acting arylcyclohexylamines; cannabis; inhalants and other psychoactive drugs and chemicals; and
   (ii) "Substance dependence" means a condition in which a person is dependent on a substance, other than tobacco or ordinary xanthine-containing (e.g., caffeine) beverages, as evidenced by—
      (A) Increased tolerance;
      (B) Manifestation of withdrawal symptoms;
      (C) Impaired control of use; or
      (D) Continued use despite damage to physical health or impairment of social, personal, or occupational functioning.

(b) No substance abuse within the preceding 2 years defined as:
   (1) Use of a substance in a situation in which that use was physically hazardous, if there has been at any other time an instance of the use of a substance also in a situation in which that use was physically hazardous;
   (2) A verified positive drug test result acquired under an anti-drug program or internal program of the U.S. Department of Transportation or any other Administration within the U.S. Department of Transportation; or
   (3) Misuse of a substance that the Federal Air Surgeon, based on case history and appropriate, qualified medical judgment relating to the substance involved, finds—
      (i) Makes the person unable to safely perform the duties or exercise the privileges of the airman certificate applied for or held; or
      (ii) May reasonably be expected, for the maximum duration of the airman medical certificate applied for or held, to make the person unable to perform those duties or exercise those privileges.

(c) No other personality disorder, neurosis, or other mental condition that the Federal Air Surgeon, based on the case history and appropriate, qualified medical judgment relating to the condition involved, finds—
   (1) Makes the person unable to safely perform the duties or exercise the privileges of the airman certificate applied for or held; or
   (2) May reasonably be expected, for the maximum duration of the airman medical certificate applied for or held, to make the person unable to perform those duties or exercise those privileges.

67.209 Neurologic.

Neurologic standards for a second-class airman medical certificate are:

(a) No established medical history or clinical diagnosis of any of the following:
   (1) Epilepsy;
   (2) A disturbance of consciousness without satisfactory medical explanation of the cause; or
   (3) A transient loss of control of nervous system function(s) without satisfactory medical explanation of the cause;

(b) No other seizure disorder, disturbance of consciousness, or neurologic condition that the Federal Air Surgeon, based on the case history and appropriate, qualified medical judgment relating to the condition involved, finds—
   (1) Makes the person unable to safely perform the duties or exercise the privileges of the airman certificate applied for or held; or
   (2) May reasonably be expected, for the maximum duration of the airman medical certificate applied for or held, to make the person unable to perform those duties or exercise those privileges.

67.211 Cardiovascular.
Cardiovascular standards for a second-class medical certificate are no established medical history or clinical diagnosis of any of the following:
(a) Myocardial infarction;
(b) Angina pectoris;
(c) Coronary heart disease that has required treatment or, if untreated, that has been symptomatic or clinically significant;
(d) Cardiac valve replacement;
(e) Permanent cardiac pacemaker implantation; or
(f) Heart replacement.

67.213 General medical condition.
The general medical standards for a second-class airman medical certificate are:
(a) No established medical history or clinical diagnosis of diabetes mellitus that requires insulin or any other hypoglycemic drug for control.
(b) No other organic, functional, or structural disease, defect, or limitation that the Federal Air Surgeon, based on the case history and appropriate, qualified medical judgment relating to the condition involved, finds—
  (1) Makes the person unable to safely perform the duties or exercise the privileges of the airman certificate applied for or held; or
  (2) May reasonably be expected, for the maximum duration of the airman medical certificate applied for or held, to make the person unable to perform those duties or exercise those privileges.
(c) No medication or other treatment that the Federal Air Surgeon, based on the case history and appropriate, qualified medical judgment relating to the medication or other treatment involved, finds—
  (1) Makes the person unable to safely perform the duties or exercise the privileges of the airman certificate applied for or held; or
  (2) May reasonably be expected, for the maximum duration of the airman medical certificate applied for or held, to make the person unable to perform those duties or exercise those privileges.

Sec. 67.215 Discretionary issuance.
A person who does not meet the provisions of Secs. 67.203 through 67.213 may apply for the discretionary issuance of a certificate under Sec. 67.401.

Subpart D—Third-Class Airman Medical Certificate

Sec. 67.301 Eligibility.
To be eligible for a third-class airman medical certificate, or to remain eligible for a third-class airman medical certificate, a person must meet the requirements of this subpart.

Sec. 67.303 Eye.
Eye standards for a third-class airman medical certificate are:
(a) Distant visual acuity of 20/40 or better in each eye separately, with or without corrective lenses. If corrective lenses (spectacles or contact lenses) are necessary for 20/40 vision, the person may be eligible only on the condition that corrective lenses are worn while exercising the privileges of an airman certificate.
(b) Near vision of 20/40 or better, Snellen equivalent, at 16 inches in each eye separately, with or without corrective lenses.
(c) Ability to perceive those colors necessary for the safe performance of airman duties.

(d) No acute or chronic pathological condition of either eye or adnexa that interferes with the proper function of an eye, that may reasonably be expected to progress to that degree, or that may reasonably be expected to be aggravated by flying.

Sec. 67.305 Ear, nose, throat, and equilibrium.

Ear, nose, throat, and equilibrium standards for a third-class airman medical certificate are:

(a) The person shall demonstrate acceptable hearing by at least one of the following tests:

(1) Demonstrate an ability to hear an average conversational voice in a quiet room, using both ears, at a distance of 6 feet from the examiner, with the back turned to the examiner.

(2) Demonstrate an acceptable understanding of speech as determined by audiometric speech discrimination testing to a score of at least 70 percent obtained in one ear or in a sound field environment.

(3) Provide acceptable results of pure tone audiometric testing of unaided hearing acuity according to the following table of worst acceptable thresholds, using the calibration standards of the American National Standards Institute, 1969:

Frequency (Hz)	500	1000	2000	3000
Better ear (dB)	35	30	30	40
Poorer ear (dB)	35	50	50	60

(b) No disease or condition of the middle or internal ear, nose, oral cavity, pharynx, or larynx that—

(1) Interferes with, or is aggravated by, flying or may reasonably be expected to do so; or

(2) Interferes with clear and effective speech communication.

(c) No disease or condition manifested by, or that may reasonably be expected to be manifested by, vertigo or a disturbance of equilibrium.

Sec. 67.307 Mental.

Mental standards for a third-class airman medical certificate are:

(a) No established medical history or clinical diagnosis of any of the following:

(1) A personality disorder that is severe enough to have repeatedly manifested itself by overt acts.

(2) A psychosis. As used in this section, "psychosis" refers to a mental disorder in which—

(i) The individual has manifested delusions, hallucinations, grossly bizarre or disorganized behavior, or other commonly accepted symptoms of this condition; or

(ii) The individual may reasonably be expected to manifest delusions, hallucinations, grossly bizarre or disorganized behavior, or other commonly accepted symptoms of this condition.

(3) A bipolar disorder.

(4) Substance dependence, except where there is established clinical evidence, satisfactory to the Federal Air Surgeon, of recovery, including sustained total abstinence from the substance(s) for not less than the preceding 2 years. As used in this section—

(i) "Substance" includes: alcohol; other sedatives and hypnotics; anxiolytics; opioids; central nervous system stimulants such as cocaine, amphetamines, and similarly acting sympathomimetics; hallucinogens; phencyclidine or similarly acting arylcyclohexylamines; cannabis; inhalants; and other psychoactive drugs and chemicals; and

(ii) "Substance dependence" means a condition in which a person is dependent on a substance, other than tobacco or ordinary xanthine-containing (e.g., caffeine) beverages, as evidenced by—

(A) Increased tolerance;

(B) Manifestation of withdrawal symptoms;

(C) Impaired control of use; or
(D) Continued use despite damage to physical health or impairment of social, personal, or occupational functioning.

(b) No substance abuse within the preceding 2 years defined as:
(1) Use of a substance in a situation in which that use was physically hazardous, if there has been at any other time an instance of the use of a substance also in a situation in which that use was physically hazardous;
(2) A verified positive drug test result conducted under an anti-drug rule or internal program of the U.S. Department of Transportation or any other Administration within the U.S. Department of Transportation; or
(3) Misuse of a substance that the Federal Air Surgeon, based on case history and appropriate, qualified medical judgment relating to the substance involved, finds—
(i) Makes the person unable to safely perform the duties or exercise the privileges of the airman certificate applied for or held; or
(ii) May reasonably be expected, for the maximum duration of the airman medical certificate applied for or held, to make the person unable to perform those duties or exercise those privileges.

(c) No other personality disorder, neurosis, or other mental condition that the Federal Air Surgeon, based on the case history and appropriate, qualified medical judgment relating to the condition involved, finds—
(1) Makes the person unable to safely perform the duties or exercise the privileges of the airman certificate applied for or held; or
(2) May reasonably be expected, for the maximum duration of the airman medical certificate applied for or held, to make the person unable to perform those duties or exercise those privileges.

Sec. 67.309 Neurologic.

Neurologic standards for a third-class airman medical certificate are:

(a) No established medical history or clinical diagnosis of any of the following:
(1) Epilepsy;
(2) A disturbance of consciousness without satisfactory medical explanation of the cause; or
(3) A transient loss of control of nervous system function(s) without satisfactory medical explanation of the cause.

(b) No other seizure disorder, disturbance of consciousness, or neurologic condition that the Federal Air Surgeon, based on the case history and appropriate, qualified medical judgment relating to the condition involved, finds—
(1) Makes the person unable to safely perform the duties or exercise the privileges of the airman certificate applied for or held; or
(2) May reasonably be expected, for the maximum duration of the airman medical certificate applied for or held, to make the person unable to perform those duties or exercise those privileges.

Sec. 67.311 Cardiovascular.

Cardiovascular standards for a third-class airman medical certificate are no established medical history or clinical diagnosis of any of the following:

(a) Myocardial infarction;
(b) Angina pectoris;
(c) Coronary heart disease that has required treatment or, if untreated, that has been symptomatic or clinically significant;
(d) Cardiac valve replacement;
(e) Permanent cardiac pacemaker implantation; or
(f) Heart replacement.

Sec. 67.313 General medical condition.

The general medical standards for a third-class airman medical certificate are:

(a) No established medical history or clinical diagnosis of diabetes mellitus that requires insulin or any other hypoglycemic drug for control.

(b) No other organic, functional, or structural disease, defect, or limitation that the Federal Air Surgeon, based on the case history and appropriate, qualified medical judgment relating to the condition involved, finds—

(1) Makes the person unable to safely perform the duties or exercise the privileges of the airman certificate applied for or held; or

(2) May reasonably be expected, for the maximum duration of the airman medical certificate applied for or held, to make the person unable to perform those duties or exercise those privileges.

(c) No medication or other treatment that the Federal Air Surgeon, based on the case history and appropriate, qualified medical judgment relating to the medication or other treatment involved, finds—

(1) Makes the person unable to safely perform the duties or exercise the privileges of the airman certificate applied for or held; or

(2) May reasonably be expected, for the maximum duration of the airman medical certificate applied for or held, to make the person unable to perform those duties or exercise those privileges.

Sec. 67.315 Discretionary issuance.

A person who does not meet the provisions of Secs. 67.303 through 67.313 may apply for the discretionary issuance of a certificate under Sec. 67.401.

Subpart E—Certification Procedures

Sec. 67.401 Special issuance of medical certificates.

(a) At the discretion of the Federal Air Surgeon, an Authorization for Special Issuance of a Medical Certificate (Authorization), valid for a specified period, may be granted to a person who does not meet the provisions of subparts B, C, or D of this part if the person shows to the satisfaction of the Federal Air Surgeon that the duties authorized by the class of medical certificate applied for can be performed without endangering public safety during the period in which the Authorization would be in force. The Federal Air Surgeon may authorize a special medical flight test, practical test, or medical evaluation for this purpose. A medical certificate of the appropriate class may be issued to a person who does not meet the provisions of subparts B, C, or D of this part if that person possesses a valid Authorization and is otherwise eligible. An airman medical certificate issued in accordance with this section shall expire no later than the end of the validity period or upon the withdrawal of the Authorization upon which it is based. At the end of its specified validity period, for grant of a new Authorization, the person must again show to the satisfaction of the Federal Air Surgeon that the duties authorized by the class of medical certificate applied for can be performed without endangering public safety during the period in which the Authorization would be in force.

(b) At the discretion of the Federal Air Surgeon, a Statement of Demonstrated Ability (SODA) may be granted, instead of an Authorization, to a person whose disqualifying condition is static or nonprogressive and who has been found capable of performing airman duties without endangering public safety. A SODA does not expire and authorizes a designated aviation medical examiner to issue a medical certificate of a specified class if the examiner finds that the condition described on its face has not adversely changed.

(c) In granting an Authorization or SODA, the Federal Air Surgeon may consider the person's operational experience and any medical facts that may affect the ability of the person to perform airman duties including—

(1) The combined effect on the person of failure to meet more than one requirement of this part; and
(2) The prognosis derived from professional consideration of all available information regarding the person.

(d) In granting an Authorization or SODA under this section, the Federal Air Surgeon specifies the class of medical certificate authorized to be issued and may do any or all of the following:
(1) Limit the duration of an Authorization;
(2) Condition the granting of a new Authorization on the results of subsequent medical tests, examinations, or evaluations;
(3) State on the Authorization or SODA, and any medical certificate based upon it, any operational limitation needed for safety; or
(4) Condition the continued effect of an Authorization or SODA, and any second- or third-class medical certificate based upon it, on compliance with a statement of functional limitations issued to the person in coordination with the Director of Flight Standards or the Director's designee.

(e) In determining whether an Authorization or SODA should be granted to an applicant for a third-class medical certificate, the Federal Air Surgeon considers the freedom of an airman, exercising the privileges of a private pilot certificate, to accept reasonable risks to his or her person and property that are not acceptable in the exercise of commercial or airline transport pilot privileges, and, at the same time, considers the need to protect the safety of persons and property in other aircraft and on the ground.

(f) An Authorization or SODA granted under the provisions of this section to a person who does not meet the applicable provisions of subparts B, C, or D of this part may be withdrawn, at the discretion of the Federal Air Surgeon, at any time if—
(1) There is adverse change in the holder's medical condition;
(2) The holder fails to comply with a statement of functional limitations or operational limitations issued as a condition of certification under this section;
(3) Public safety would be endangered by the holder's exercise of airman privileges;
(4) The holder fails to provide medical information reasonably needed by the Federal Air Surgeon for certification under this section; or
(5) The holder makes or causes to be made a statement or entry that is the basis for withdrawal of an Authorization or SODA under Sec. 67.403.

(g) A person who has been granted an Authorization or SODA under this section based on a special medical flight or practical test need not take the test again during later physical examinations unless the Federal Air Surgeon determines or has reason to believe that the physical deficiency has or may have degraded to a degree to require another special medical flight test or practical test.

(h) The authority of the Federal Air Surgeon under this section is also exercised by the Manager, Aeromedical Certification Division, and each Regional Flight Surgeon.

(i) If an Authorization or SODA is withdrawn under paragraph (f) of this section the following procedures apply:
(1) The holder of the Authorization or SODA will be served a letter of withdrawal, stating the reason for the action;
(2) By not later than 60 days after the service of the letter of withdrawal, the holder of the Authorization or SODA may request, in writing, that the Federal Air Surgeon provide for review of the decision to withdraw. The request for review may be accompanied by supporting medical evidence;
(3) Within 60 days of receipt of a request for review, a written final decision either affirming or reversing the decision to withdraw will be issued; and
(4) A medical certificate rendered invalid pursuant to a withdrawal, in accordance with paragraph (a) of this section, shall be surrendered to the Administrator upon request.

(j) No grant of a special issuance made prior to September 16, 1996, may be used to obtain a medical certificate after the earlier of the following dates:

(1) September 16, 1997; or
(2) The date on which the holder of such special issuance is required to provide additional information to the FAA as a condition for continued medical certification.

Sec. 67.403 Applications, certificates, logbooks, reports, and records:
Falsification, reproduction, or alteration; incorrect statements.

(a) No person may make or cause to be made—
(1) A fraudulent or intentionally false statement on any application for a medical certificate or on a request for any Authorization for Special Issuance of a Medical Certificate (Authorization) or Statement of Demonstrated Ability (SODA) under this part;
(2) A fraudulent or intentionally false entry in any logbook, record, or report that is kept, made, or used, to show compliance with any requirement for any medical certificate or for any Authorization or SODA under this part;
(3) A reproduction, for fraudulent purposes, of any medical certificate under this part; or
(4) An alteration of any medical certificate under this part.

(b) The commission by any person of an act prohibited under paragraph (a) of this section is a basis for—
(1) Suspending or revoking all airman, ground instructor, and medical certificates and ratings held by that person;
(2) Withdrawing all Authorizations or SODAs held by that person; and
(3) Denying all applications for medical certification and requests for Authorizations or SODAs.

(c) The following may serve as a basis for suspending or revoking a medical certificate; withdrawing an Authorization or SODA; or denying an application for a medical certificate or request for an authorization or SODA:
(1) An incorrect statement, upon which the FAA relied, made in support of an application for a medical certificate or request for an Authorization or SODA.
(2) An incorrect entry, upon which the FAA relied, made in any logbook, record, or report that is kept, made, or used to show compliance with any requirement for a medical certificate or an Authorization or SODA.

Sec. 67.405 Medical examinations: Who may give.

(a) First-class. Any aviation medical examiner who is specifically designated for the purpose may give the examination for the first-class medical certificate. Any interested person may obtain a list of these aviation medical examiners, in any area, from the FAA Regional Flight Surgeon of the region in which the area is located.

(b) Second- and third-class. Any aviation medical examiner may give the examination for the second- or third-class medical certificate. Any interested person may obtain a list of aviation medical examiners, in any area, from the FAA Regional Flight Surgeon of the region in which the area is located.

Sec. 67.407 Delegation of authority.

(a) The authority of the Administrator under 49 U.S.C. 44703 to issue or deny medical certificates is delegated to the Federal Air Surgeon to the extent necessary to—
(1) Examine applicants for and holders of medical certificates to determine whether they meet applicable medical standards; and
(2) Issue, renew, and deny medical certificates, and issue, renew, deny, and withdraw Authorizations for Special Issuance of a Medical Certificate and Statements of Demonstrated Ability to a person based upon meeting or failing to meet applicable medical standards.

(b) Subject to limitations in this chapter, the delegated functions of the Federal Air Surgeon to examine applicants for and holders of medical certificates for compliance with applicable medical standards and to issue, renew, and deny medical certificates are also delegated to aviation medical examiners and to authorized representatives of the Federal Air Surgeon within the FAA.

(c) The authority of the Administrator under 49 U.S.C. 44702, to reconsider the action of an aviation medical examiner is delegated to the Federal Air Surgeon; the Manager, Aeromedical Certification Division; and each Regional Flight Surgeon. Where the person does not meet the standards of Secs. 67.107(b)(3) and (c), 67.109(b), 67.113(b) and (c), 67.207(b)(3) and (c), 67.209(b), 67.213(b) and (c), 67.307(b)(3) and (c), 67.309(b), or 67.313(b) and (c), any action taken under this paragraph other than by the Federal Air Surgeon is subject to reconsideration by the Federal Air Surgeon. A certificate issued by an aviation medical examiner is considered to be affirmed as issued unless an FAA official named in this paragraph (authorized official) reverses that issuance within 60 days after the date of issuance. However, if within 60 days after the date of issuance an authorized official requests the certificate holder to submit additional medical information, an authorized official may reverse the issuance within 60 days after receipt of the requested information.

(d) The authority of the Administrator under 49 U.S.C. 44709 to re-examine any civil airman to the extent necessary to determine an airman's qualification to continue to hold an airman medical certificate, is delegated to the Federal Air Surgeon and his or her authorized representatives within the FAA.

Sec. 67.409 Denial of medical certificate.

(a) Any person who is denied a medical certificate by an aviation medical examiner may, within 30 days after the date of the denial, apply in writing and in duplicate to the

Federal Air Surgeon
Attention: Manager
Aeromedical Certification Division, AAM-300
Federal Aviation Administration
P.O. Box 26080
Oklahoma City, Oklahoma 73126

for reconsideration of that denial. If the person does not ask for reconsideration during the 30-day period after the date of the denial, he or she is considered to have withdrawn the application for a medical certificate.

(b) The denial of a medical certificate—-
(1) By an aviation medical examiner is not a denial by the Administrator under 49 U.S.C. 44703.
(2) By the Federal Air Surgeon is considered to be a denial by the Administrator under 49 U.S.C. 44703.
(3) By the Manager, Aeromedical Certification Division, or a Regional Flight Surgeon is considered to be a denial by the Administrator under 49 U.S.C. 44703 except where the person does not meet the standards of Secs. 67.107(b)(3) and (c), 67.109(b), or 67.113(b) and (c); 67.207(b)(3) and (c), 67.209(b), or 67.213(b) and (c); or 67.307(b)(3) and (c), 67.309(b), or 67.313(b) and (c).

(c) Any action taken under Sec. 67.407(c) that wholly or partly reverses the issue of a medical certificate by an aviation medical examiner is the denial of a medical certificate under paragraph (b) of this section.

(d) If the issue of a medical certificate is wholly or partly reversed by the Federal Air Surgeon; the Manager, Aeromedical Certification Division; or a Regional Flight Surgeon, the person holding that certificate shall surrender it, upon request of the FAA.

Sec. 67.411 Medical certificates by flight surgeons of Armed Forces.

(a) The FAA has designated flight surgeons of the Armed Forces on specified military posts, stations, and facilities, as aviation medical examiners.

(b) An aviation medical examiner described in paragraph (a) of this section may give physical examinations for the FAA medical certificates to persons who are on active duty or who are, under Department of Defense medical programs, eligible for FAA medical certification as civil airmen. In addition, such an examiner may issue or deny an appropriate FAA medical certificate in accordance with the regulations of this chapter and the policies of the FAA.

(c) Any interested person may obtain a list of the military posts, stations, and facilities at which a flight surgeon has been designated as an aviation medical examiner from the Surgeon General of the Armed Force concerned or from the

Manager
Aeromedical Education Division, AAM-400
Federal Aviation Administration
P.O. Box 26082
Oklahoma City, Oklahoma 73125

Sec. 67.413 Medical records.

(a) Whenever the Administrator finds that additional medical information or history is necessary to determine whether an applicant for or the holder of a medical certificate meets the medical standards for it, the Administrator requests that person to furnish that information or to authorize any clinic, hospital, physician, or other person to release to the Administrator all available information or records concerning that history. If the applicant or holder fails to provide the requested medical information or history or to authorize the release so requested, the Administrator may suspend, modify, or revoke all medical certificates the airman holds or may, in the case of an applicant, deny the application for an airman medical certificate.

(b) If an airman medical certificate is suspended or modified under paragraph (a) of this section, that suspension or modification remains in effect until the requested information, history, or authorization is provided to the FAA and until the Federal Air Surgeon determines whether the person meets the medical standards under this part.

Sec. 67.415 Return of medical certificate after suspension or revocation.

The holder of any medical certificate issued under this part that is suspended or revoked shall, upon the Administrator's request, return it to the Administrator.

Notes and References

Introduction: Fit for Flight

The story of von Richthofen is summarized from the article: Manfred Freiherr von Richthofen's medical record—was the "Red Baron" fit to fly? Allmers H. *Lancet* 1999; 354:502-04

The statistics for the aviation accident rate due to human factors are from DeHart R. *The historical perspective. Fundamentals of Aerospace Medicine*, 2nd ed. DeHart R, ed. Baltimore: William & Wilkins, 1996

Early understanding of health hazards of flight are described in Anderson HG. *The Medical and Surgical Aspects of Aviation*. London: Oxford University Press, 1919

Aviation accident statistics are taken from Lane JC, Brown TC. Probability of casualties in an airport disaster. *Aviat Space Environ Med* 1975; 46: 958

Fatal aviation accident investigations are described by Moher SR. Civil aviation medicine. IN: *Fundamentals of Aerospace Medicine*, 2nd ed. Chap 24. DeHart R, ed. Baltimore: William & Wilkins, 1996

"Your odds of dying from..." is based on: *Wired*, March 2002, p 59

Quote from: Lowery J. *Professional Pilot*. 2nd ed. Ames, IA: Iowa State University Press, 2001

Pilot health symptoms survey reported in Reinhart RO. *Fit for Flight: Flight Physiology and Human Factors for Aircrew.* 2nd ed. Ames, Iowa: Iowa State University Press, 1999.

"I'm Safe" checklist is from Trollip SR, Jensen RS. *Human Factors Manual for General Aviation.* Englewood, CO: Jeppesen Sanderson, 1991.

An excellent description of the early flights over the Western Sahara is provided by Schiff S. *Saint-Exupery: A Biography.* New York: Knopf, 1994.

Chapter 1: How Can I Pass the FAA Medical Exam?

The possibility that recreational pilots may be exempt from the FAA medical examination is discussed in Reinhart RO. *FAA Medical Certification: Guidelines for Pilots.* 3rd ed. Ames, Iowa: Iowa State University Press, 1997

Airline pilot age restrictions are discussed in Institute of Medicine. *Airline Pilot Age, Health, and Performance.* Washington, D.C.: National Academy Press, 1981; Broach D. Pilot age and accident rates: a re-analysis of the 1999 Chicago Tribune report and discussion of technical considerations for future analyses. *FAA Civil Aerospace Medical Institute AAM-00-A-HRR-520*; and *NTSB and FAA Stat Handbook*. Pilot Age and Accidents, 1982-1985. Washington, D.C.: US Govt Printing Office, 1982-1985.

Face of cod anecdote is from Machado R. *AOPA Pilot*, Sept 2001, p 46.

Dr. Reinhart quoted from: Reinhart RO. *FAA Medical Certification: Guidelines for Pilots*. 3rd ed. Ames, Iowa: Iowa State University Press, 1997

Dr. Jordan quoted from: *The Federal Air Surgeon's Bulletin*, Spring 2001, p 2

"Flyin' the ointment" This clever name was taken form the Australian internet column by Dr. Dougal Watson, http://members.ozemail.com.au/~dxw/Articles/ointment

The list of acceptable medications is based in part on: Silberman WS. What Is Acceptable and What Is Not. *Federal Air Surgeon's Bulletin*, Winter 1997, and one compiled by the AOPA Medical Certification Department and confirmed by the FAA Aerospace Medical Certification Division in Oklahoma City.

Viagra use is discussed in: Borrillo DJ. Dangers of Viagra use in pilots. *Federal Air Surgeon's Medical Bulletin*. Fall 1998

FAA categorization of drugs is described in: Moher SR. Civil aviation medicine. IN: *Fundamentals of Aerospace Medicine*, 2nd ed. Chap 24. DeHart R, ed. Baltimore: William & Wilkins, 1996

Chapter 2: Conditions That *May* Disqualify You

B. The cause of fainting spells is discussed in: Kappor WN, et al. A prospective evaluation and followup of patients with syncope. *N Engl J Med* 1983; 309:197.

C. Causes of sudden loss of consciousness are reviewed in: Jones DR, Katchen MS, Patterson JC, Rea M. Neuropsychiatry in aerospace medicine. IN: *Fundamentals of Aerospace Medicine*, RL DeHart, ed, 2nd ed. Chap 18. Baltimore: William & Wilkins, 1996

Head injury research showing subsequent epilepsy is reported in: Annegers J, Hauser WA, Coan SP, Rocca WA. A population-based study of seizures after traumatic brain injuries. *N Engl J Med* 1998; 338: 20-24.

FAA head-injury guidelines are taken from: Fiedler E, Orme D, Mills W, Patterson JC. Assessment of head-injured aircrew: comparison of FAA and USAF procedures. US DOT FAA document DOT/FAA/AM-01/11, Washington, DC: Office of Aerospace Medicine, July 2001.

D. The airline accident attributed to improper use of corrective lenses is described in: Reinhart RO. *Fit for Flight: Flight Physiology and Human Factors for Aircrew*. 2nd ed. Ames, Iowa: Iowa State University Press, 1999.

The use of blue-blocker sunglasses is questioned in: Clinical Aerospace Physiology Review for Aviation Medical Examiners, *CAMI Training Manual*, 1999.

The story of color vision loss resulting in missing a red warning light is adapted from: Reinhart RO. *FAA Medical Certification: Guidelines for Pilots*. 3rd ed. Ames, Iowa: Iowa State University Press, 1997.

The human-bird eyesight comparison is taken from http://magazine.audubon.org/ask/ask0007.html and http://www.stanfordalumni.org/birdsite/text/essays/Hawk-Eyed.html.

Alternative color vision tests are described in: Reinhart RO. *FAA Medical Certification: Guidelines for Pilots*. 3rd ed. Ames, Iowa: Iowa State University Press, 1997.

Corrective eye surgery is discussed in: Nakagawara VB, Wood KJ, Montgomery RW. LASIK refractive surgery: clinical considerations for the pilot. *Federal Air Surgeon's Medical Bulletin*. Winter 1998, and Wayda M. Considering LASIK eye surgery? Think again. *Federal Air Surgeon's Medical Bulletin*. Spring 2001

The option of surgery to correct one eye for near vision and the other for distance is described by: Baldwin G. Good news for older pilots (including me!). *Federal Air Surgeon's Medical Bulletin*. Fall 2000, p 5

One-eyed pilots are discussed in: Moher SR. Civil aviation medicine. IN: *Fundamentals of Aerospace Medicine*, 2nd ed. Chap 24. DeHart R, ed. Baltimore: William & Wilkins, 1996

E. Antihistamine effects are explained by Simons FER. *Clin Exp Allergy* 1999; 29 Suppl 3: 125. Second generation antihistamines are described in: Medical Letter On Drugs and Therapeutics. Newer antihistamines. *Med Letter* 2001; April 30: 35; Side-effects are discussed by Shamsi Z, Hindmarch I. *Hum Psychopharmacol Clin Exp* 2000; 15 suppl 1:S3

G. The unnecessary treadmill test story is derived from: Walker JS. Calm down! Don't feel pressured by a hypertension diagnosis. *AOPA Pilot* 1999; June: 22-23

The report of arrhythmia leading to loss of consciousness among airline pilots is from: Epstein AE, Miles WM, et al. Personal and public safety issues related to arrhythmias that may affect consciousness: implications for regulation and physician recommendations. *Circulation* 1996; 94: 1147-66

Bundle branch block is described in: Rowlands DJ. Left and right bundle branch block, left anterior and left posterior hemiblock. *European Heart Journal* 1985; 5 (Supplement): 99-105.

H. The blood pressure quote is taken from: Walker JS. Calm down! Don't feel pressured by a hypertension diagnosis. *AOPA Pilot* 1999; June: 22-23

M. The quotes on depression are from Stoutt GR. Depression: a recoverable stall. *Federal Air Surgeon's Medical Bulletin*, Summer 2000

Pilot use of lithium is discussed in: Fries, IB. Can I fly on lithium? *Flying* Jan, 1998: 49

The stress of flying quote is from: Jones DR, Katchen MS, Patterson JC, Rea M. Neuropschiatry in aerospace medicine. IN: *Fundamentals of Aerospace Medicine*, 2nd ed. Chap 18. DeHart R, ed. Baltimore: William & Wilkins, 1996

The gender dysphoria example is taken from: Feinberg M. Difficulties inherent in certifying people with gender dysphoria. *Federal Air Surgeon's Medical Bulletin*. Summer 1998

The case of the pilot with Alzheimer's disease is described by: Angelici A. Alzheimer's disease in an airman. *Federal Air Surgeon's Medical Bulletin*, Spring 2001

N. Transporting intoxicated passengers is discussed in: Yodice, J. Alcohol and drugs. *AOPA Pilot* 1999; July: 131-132

Impaired performance due to even very small amounts of alcohol are reported in: Aksnes EG. Effects of small dosages of alcohol upon performance in Link trainer. *J Aviat Med* 1954; 25: 680-683; and Billings CE, Wick RL, Gerke RJ. Chase RC, et al. Effects of alcohol on pilot performance during instrument flight. *Office of Aviation Medicine Report AM-72-4*. US Govt Printing Office, Washington, D.C.: Federal Aviation Administration, 1972; Yesaverge J, Leirer V. Hangover effects on aircraft pilots 145 hours after alcohol ingestion: A preliminary report. *Am J Psychol* 1986; 143: 1546-1550.

PAN is described in Money KE, et al. The mechanism of positional alcohol nystagmus. *Can J Otolaryngol* 3: 302-313; Ryback RS, Dowd PJ. Aftereffects of various alcoholic beverages on positional nystagmus and Coriolis acceleration. *Aerospace Med* 1970; 41: 429-435.

The effect of alcohol at high altitude is described in: Nelson TO, et al. Cognition and metacognition at extreme altitudes on Mount Everest. *J Exp Psychol Gen* 1990; 119: 367-374; and Freedman R, et al. Electrophysiological effects of low dose alcohol on human subjects at high altitude. *Alcohol Drug Res* 1985-86; 6:289-297

Alcohol abuse and alcoholism among pilots is documented in: Masters RL, Kohn GM. Aeromedical support to airline and civilian professional crew. IN: *Fundamentals of Aerospace Medicine*, 2nd ed. Chap 25. DeHart R, ed. Baltimore: William & Wilkins, 1996; data from FAA Aeromedical Certification Division, as of 1/1/2001. Alcohol-related aviation accidents are discussed in: Modell JG, Mountz JM. Drinking and flying—the problem of alcohol use by pilots. *N Engl J Med* 1990; 323: 455-461.

Q. Motion sickness among pilots described in: James M, Green R. Airline incapacitation survey. *Aviat Space Environ Med* 1991; 62:1068-1072; and when using flight simulators: Gillingham KK, Previc FH. Spatial orientation in flight. IN: DeHart et al. *Fundamentals of Aerospace Medicine*. 2nd ed. Baltimore: Lippincott Williams & Wilkins, 1996: 309-397

Airsickness and flicker vertigo anecdotes are modified from similar stories in Clinical Aerospace Physiology Review for Aviation Medical Examiners, CAMI Training Manual, 1999

The example of pilots in Florida who were allowed to fly despite having their driver's license revoked is provided by: Reinhart RO. *FAA Medical Certification: Guidelines for Pilots*. 3rd ed. Ames, Iowa: Iowa State University Press, 1997

Mark Sweeney's report of the effectiveness of the NDR program is stated in: FAA program probes pilot sobriety. *Federal Air Surgeon's Medical Bulletin*, Summer 2001. The sample DUI Report letter is derived from one suggested by *AOPA Aviation Services*. The most common loss of aviation certificates is failing to report a DUI, reported in: Yodice JS. Alcohol and drugs. *AOPA Pilot* 1999; July: 131-132

Richard Logan's quote is from: Armour K. No longer the exception: disabled pilots work to gain acceptance. *AOPA Pilot* 1999; Oct: 67-77

Chapter 3: Getting a SODA

The sample Authorization of Special Issuance letter is based on: Silberman WS. Managing the special issuance system. *Federal Air Surgeon's Medical Bulletin*. Fall, 1999.

Chapter 4: Flying High: Drug-Testing Programs

The long-distance truck driver statistic is from: Potter BA, Orfali J. *Drug Testing at Work: A Guide for Employers.* Berkeley, CA: Ronin, 1998

No commercial airline accident because of pilot drug use, reported in: American Civil Liberties Union. *In Brief: Privacy in America: Workplace Drug Testing*, 1996

Reagan's drug testing program: *Omnibus Transportation Employee Testing Act of 1991*. Public Law 102-143, 102nd Congress, October 28, 1991. DOT and USCG programs: Department of Health and Human Services. Mandatory guidelines for federal workplace drug testing programs. *Federal Register* 1988;53 (April 11): 11,970-89. NRC program: Nuclear Regulatory Commission. Fitness-for-duty programs. *Federal Register* 1989;54 (June 7):24,468-508

Drug use among pilots: 2000 NAL report: General Aviation Accident Trends and Factors for 1999. AOPA Air Safety Foundation, 2001, p 23. Drugs found on investigation of aircraft mishaps: McMeekin RR. Aircraft accident investigation. IN: *Fundamentals of Aerospace Medicine*, 2nd ed. Chap 28. DeHart R, ed. Baltimore: William & Wilkins, 1996

Case history of award-winning pilot dead after drug use: Gibbons HL, Snyder RG. Aircraft accidents: prevention, survival, and rescue. IN: *Fundamentals of Aerospace Medicine*, 2nd ed. Chap 32. DeHart R, ed. Baltimore: William & Wilkins, 1996

NIDA 5 drugs: Swotinsky R, Smith D. *The Medical Review Officer's Manual: MROCC's Guide to Drug Testing* Boca Raton, FL: OEM Press, 1999.—This is the standard text by the Medical Review Officer Certification Council, an excellent review of the issues involved in drug testing of the NIDA-5 drugs

The story of a pilot taking non-NIDA 5 drugs: Silberman W. Beyond drug screening. *Federal Air Surgeon's Medical Bulletin*. Winter, 2000, p 3

Definition of "mature minor" for drug screening programs: English A., Matthews M., Extravour K, et al. *State Minor Consent Statutes: A Summary*. San Francisco, CA: National Center for Youth Law for Continuing Education in Adolescent Health, April 1995

Job interview questions allowed by ADA, based on the very straightforward and helpful summary of this issue in: Potter BA, Orfali J. *Pass the Test: An Employee Guide to Drug Testing*. Berkeley, CA: Ronin, 1999

FAA policy on drug screening is specified in a memorandum from Jane Garvey: USDOT FAA: Agency Policy on Substance Abuse, Oct 14, 1999

Greater likelihood of dark-skinned people testing positive for drugs: Potter BA, Orfali J. *Pass the Test: An Employee Guide to Drug Testing*. Berkeley, CA: Ronin, 1999. For a review of hair testing, see: Cone EJ, Welch MJ, Babecki MG (eds.) *Hair Testing for Drugs of Abuse: International Research on Standards and Technology*. National Institute on Drug Abuse. NIH Publication No. 95-3727. Rockville, MD: Superintendent of Documents, U.S. Government Printing Office, 1995

Chain of custody is described in: Substance Abuse and Mental Health Services Administration. *Urine Specimen Collection Handbook for Federal Workplace Drug Testing Programs*. DHHS Publication No. (SMA)96-3114, 1996. Urine collection for drug screening is described in: Judson, BA, Himmelberger DU, Goldstein A. Measurement of urine temperature as an alternative to observed urination in narcotic treatment programs. *Am J Drug Alcohol Abuse* 1979; 6:197. Adulterated urine samples: Peron, NB, Ehrenkranz JRL. Fake urine samples for drug analysis: hot but not hot enough. *JAMA* 1988; 259: 841. Urine creatinine levels: Cone, EJ, Lange R, Darwin WD. In vivo adulteration: excess fluid ingestion causes false-negative marijuana and cocaine urine test results. *J Anal Toxicol* 1998;22:460-73

Urine adulterants are illegal in some states: Neb. Rev. Stat. Section 48-1909; Tex. Health and Safety Code Ann. Section 481.133

Passive marijuana exposure is discussed in: Perez-Reyes M., Diguiseppi S, Mason AP, Davis KH. Passive inhalation of marijuana smoke and urinary excretion of cannabinoids. *Clin Pharmacol Ther* 1983;34:36-41; Law B, Mason PA, Moffat AC, et al. Passive inhalation of cannabis smoke. *J Pharm Pharmacol* 1984;36:578-81; Cone, EJ, Johnson RE, Darwin M, et al. Passive inhalation of marijuana smoke: urinalysis and room air levels of delta THC. *J Anal Toxicol* 1987;11:89-96. Cocaine exposure: Siegel RK, ElSohly MA, Plowman T, et al. Cocaine in herbal tea. *JAMA* 1986;255:40

Chapter 5: Cleared for Flight

Percent of adults who have pain: The Arthritis Foundation.

Most degenerative disk disease is asymptomatic: Boden SD, et al. Abnormal magnetic resonance imaging scans of the lumbar spine in asymptomatic subjects: A prospective investigation. *Journal of Bone and Joint Surgery* 1990; 72A:403-408

Stress quote is taken from: Reinhart RO. *Fit for Flight: Flight Physiology and Human Factors for Aircrew*. 2nd ed. Ames, Iowa: Iowa State University Press, 1999. Quote of pilots not being able to fix everything is taken from: *Clinical Aerospace Physiology Review Manual for Aviation Medical Examiners*, 1999. Common stress symptoms are given in: Reinhart RO. *Ibid.*

"Dead Right" is modified from a story quoted in Green RG, Muir H, James M, Gradwell D, Green RL. *Human Factors for Pilots*. 2nd ed. Brookfield, VT: Ashgate Publishing, 1996

How to reduce stress is summarized from Green RG, Muir H, James M, Gradwell D, Green RL. *Human Factors for Pilots*. 2nd ed. Brookfield, VT: Ashgate Publishing, 1996

Immunizations are reviewed in: Borrillo DJ. Immunizations and flying. *Federal Air Surgeon's Medical Bulletin*. Winter, 2000, p 4

Obesity statistics are from: *JAMA*, Oct 1999. The obsolete estimate of the 170 lb pilot is discussed in: Borrillo DJ. Dispelling the 170-pound myth: unacknowledged obesity as a hazard to flight safety. *Federal Air Surgeon's Medical Bulletin*. Fall, 2000, p 4-5

Just SuperSize it! data are taken from *Readers Digest*, April 2002, from an article that earlier appeared in *Self* magazine.

Olestra problems are described in: Breuder AJ. Olestra, Precose, carboxyhemoglobin, and smoking. *Federal Air Surgeon's Medical Bulletin*. Fall 1998

Tinnitus advice is given in Avery P. *Stop Your Tinnitus*. Hygeia Pub, 1993.

The list of causes of hearing loss is taken in part from: Reinhart RO. *Fit for Flight: Flight Physiology and Human Factors for Aircrew*. 2nd ed. Ames, Iowa: Iowa State University Press, 1999.

Statistic of in-flight fires due to smoking provided by: Lowery J. *Professional Pilot*. 2nd ed. Ames, IA: Iowa State University Press, 2001. Carbon monoxide in aviation accidents described in: McMeekin RR. Aircraft accident investigation. IN: *Fundamentals of Aerospace Medicine*, 2nd ed. Chap 28. DeHart R, ed. Baltimore: William & Wilkins, 1996; and Reinhart RO. *Fit for Flight: Flight Physiology and Human Factors for Aircrew.* 2nd ed. Ames, Iowa: Iowa State University Press, 1999.

Symptoms of hypoxia described in: Reinhart RO. *Fit for Flight: Flight Physiology and Human Factors for Aircrew*. 2nd ed. Ames, Iowa: Iowa State University Press, 1999, and Green RG, Muir H, James M, Gradwell D, Green RL. *Human Factors for Pilots*. 2nd ed. Brookfield, VT: Ashgate Publishing, 1996. Susceptibility to hypoxia is outlined in: Reinhart RO. *Ibid.*

The fatal hypoxia story was reported in: Moher SR. Civil aviation medicine. IN: *Fundamentals of Aerospace Medicine*, 2nd ed. Chap 24. DeHart R, ed. Baltimore: William & Wilkins, 1996. Sudden decompression is described in: Sheffield PJ, Stork RL. Protection in the pressure environment: cabin pressurization and oxygen equipment. IN: *Fundamentals of Aerospace Medicine*, RL DeHart, ed, 2nd ed. Chap 6. Baltimore: William & Wilkins, 1996. Paticky's quote is from: Lowery J. *Professional Pilot*. 2nd ed. Ames, IA: Iowa State University Press, 2001.

Rapid decompression is reviewed in the excellent article by Pendleton L. When humans fly: what pilots should know about high-altitude physiology, hypoxia, and rapid decompression, available online www.avweb.com/articles/highalt/

Sickle cell in pilots is discussed in: Sears DA. The morbidity of sickle cell trait, a review of the literature. *Am J Med* 1978; 64: 1021-1036; and Moser R. Additional medical and surgical conditions of aeromedical concern. IN: *Fundamentals of Aerospace Medicine*, RL DeHart, ed, 2nd ed. Chap 19. Baltimore: William & Wilkins, 1996

The FAA's supplemental oxygen studies are reported in an article by F Furgang, Hypoxia, Oxygen, and Pulse Oximetry, available online at www.nonin.com

Susceptibility to decompression sickness is described in: Heimbach RD, Sheffield PJ. Decompression sickness and pulmonary overpressure accidents. IN: *Fundamentals of Aerospace Medicine*, RL DeHart, ed, 2nd ed. Chap 7. Baltimore: William & Wilkins, 1996. Anecdotes of bends when flying after diving are taken from: Lowery J. *Professional Pilot*. 2nd ed. Ames, IA: Iowa State University Press, 2001. Quote of diver getting the bends after driving over mountain pass, is from: Clinical Aerospace Physiology Review for Aviation Medical Examiners, *CAMI Training Manual*, 1999.

Oral contraceptive use by female pilots is discussed in *United States Air Force Surgeon's Guide*, see below, Military Pilots.

Menstrual discomfort is discussed in: Cameron RG. Effects of flying on the menstrual function of air hostesses. *Aerospace Med* 1969; 40:1020-1023; Preston FS, Baterman SC, Short RV, Wilkinson RT. Effects of flying and of time changes on menstrual cycle length and on performance in airline stewardesses. *Aerospace Med* 1973; 44:438-443; and Iglesias R, Terres A, Chavarria A. Disorders of the menstrual cycle in airline stewardesses. *Aviat Space Environ Med* 1980; 51:518-520. The quote is from: Rayman RB. Aircraft health crew maintenance. IN: *Fundamentals of Aerospace Medicine*, RL DeHart, ed, 2nd ed. Chap 14. Baltimore: William & Wilkins, 1996. Pregnant flight attendant work regulations are reviewed in: Scholter P. Pregnant stewardess—should she fly? *Aviat Space Environ Med* 1976; 47: 77-81; and Raymond RB. Genitourinary. IN: Rayman RB, ed. *Clinical Aviation Medicine*, 2nd ed. Philadelphia: Lea & Febiger, 1990.

The aviation stewardess story is derived from a report given in: http://www.pbs.org/kcet/chasingthesun/series/series_2.html

Sleep cycles are described in: Battelle Memorial Institute. *A Review of Issues Concerning Duty Period Limitations, Flight Time Limitations, and Rest Requirements*. Federal Aviation Administration (AAR-100): Washington, D.C., 1998.

Sleep apnea is described in: Alan M. Sleep apnea. *Federal Air Surgeon's Medical Bulletin*. Fall, 2000, p 6-11.

Fatigue is described in: Colquhoun P. Psychological and Psychophysiological Aspects of Work and Fatigue. *Activitas Nervosa Superior* 1976; 18: 257-263.

Jet lag definition is taken from: Jones DR, Katchen MS, Patterson JC, Rea M. Neuropsychiatry in aerospace medicine. IN: *Fundamentals of Aerospace Medicine*, RL DeHart, ed, 2nd ed. Chap 18. Baltimore: William & Wilkins, 1996

Chapter 6: Military Pilots

Much of this chapter is from the *United States Air Force Surgeon's Guide*, which may be downloaded from wwwsam.brooks.af.mil/af/files/fsguide.html

Quote is taken from: USAF Aerospace Medicine Program. IN: *Flight Surgeon's Check List.* San Antonio, Texas: Society of USAF Flight Surgeons, 1993: 1-5.

Flying as a loved and feared activity is from Bond DD. *The Love and Fear of Flying*. New York: International Universities Press, 1952

CISM was developed by Dr. Jeffrey Mitchell: Mitchell JT. When disaster strikes: the critical incident stress debriefing process. *J Emerg Med Svcs* 1983; 8: 36-39

Psychiatric hospitalization due to alcohol abuse is discussed in: Flynn CF, McGlohn S, Miles RE. Occupational outcomes in military aviators after psychiatric hospitalization. *Aviat Space Environ Med* 1996; 67(1):8-13

Appendix II: FAR

This document contains FAR Part 67 including Amendment 67-17 published in the Federal Register on 3/19/96, and Amendment 67-18 published in the Federal Register on 10/5/98. Authority: 49 U.S.C. 106(g), 40113, 44701-44703, 44707, 44709-44711, 45102-45103, 45301-45303.

Acknowledgments

When I began to float the idea of writing this book, I received unexpected enthusiasm from many people. I would especially like to thank Dr. Warren Silberman, Manager of the Civil Aerospace Medical Institute, for his very detailed corrections to the manuscript, and David Hale, of Pilot Medical Solutions, Inc., who pointed out much that I had missed in the morass of regulations. AOPA's Gary Crump, and FAA medical examiners Dr. Layne Kamalu and Dr. Letitia Archuleta gave helpful comments and advice. Dr. Hemming Allmers kindly provided a superb contribution to the history of flight with his research on the Baron von Richthofen and accompanying photos. Colonel Christopher Kleinsmith supplied valuable perspective on the medical requirements for military pilots. Sheri Coin Marshall provided great insight into the special problems of disabled pilots, and I was very fortunate when she agreed to write a section for the book.

Finally, I would like to thank editor Lesley Baxter for her tireless efforts to turn an almost impossibly cluttered manuscript into a readable document.

Photographic acknowledgments

Cover: Getty Images
Page 3, 4: USAF National Archives
Page 5: Dr. H. Allmers
Page 84: Mediven, Inc.
Page 127: Woodside Biomedical, Inc. and Travelband International
Page 137: ResMed, Corp.
Page 150, 151: Capt. Sheri Coin Marshall
Page 185, 186: Dr. A. J. Parmet
Page 189: David Clark, Inc.
Page 193: Dr. Robert Frayser
Page 199: Nonin Medical, Inc.
All other photos provided by Sagebrush Press.

Index

A

Abdominal gas 183
Abdominal surgery 94
Accident 2, 7
  aviation 6
  cause 7
  defined 7
  fatal 7
Acoustic neuroma 51
Active noise reduction (ANR) 189
Acupressure wrist bands 127
ADAPT 226
adaptability rating (AR) 224
Adaptability Rating for Military Aviation (ARMA) 224
Administrative action 34
Admission to hospital 130
Adulterated specimen 162
Adulteration products 164
Aerobatics 128
Aerospace Medical Certification Division 36, 62, 142
Aerospace Medicine Squadron 221
Afrin 186. *See* Oxymetazoline
Age 60 rule 17
Age requirements 16
AIDS 140
Air Commerce Act of 1926 4
Air force 222
Air traffic controller 13
Aircraft
  air carrier 6
  general aviation 6
  modified 18
Airline Pilots Association (ALPA) 28, 78, 216
Airline Transport Pilot (ATP) 15
Airports 6
Airsickness 123
Alcohol 55
  abuse 171
  dependence 117
Alcoholics Anonymous (AA) 121
Alcoholism 118
Allegra. *See* Fexofenadine
Allergies 68
Altitude chamber 201, 202
AME 24
  Senior 25
American Cancer Society 183
American College of Sports Medicine 181
American Heart Association 183
Americans with Disabilities Act (ADA) 157
Amiodarone 80
Amphetamine 40, 153
Amputation 23
Anger 108
Angina pectoris 20, 75
Annulus fibrosis 172
Anti-depressant medications 194
Anticoagulants 85
Anticonvulsants 104
Antihistamine 37, 69, 126
Anxiety 109, 110
AOPA Medical Certification Dept. 41
AOPA Pilot 24
Appeals 146
Argonne jet lag diet 216
Aristotle 194
ARMA-SAT 224
ARMA-UNSAT 224
Army 222
Army Air Corps 171
Arrhythmias
  atrial 78
  ventricular 78
Aspirin 40
Asthma 71
Astigmatism 55, 64
Atrial flutter 80
Atropine 94
Attention Deficit Disorder (ADD) 40, 110
Attention Deficit Hyperactivity Disorder (ADHD) 110

Auditory (Eustachian) tube 185
Automatic external defibrillators 86
Aviation Medical Examiners (AME) 11
Aviation Security Division 132
Avionics 193

B

Back pain 171
Bacterial meningitis 104
Barium swallow 92
Barodontalgia 192
Basal cell 138
BCG 177
Benadryl. *See* Diphenhydramine
Bends 206
BIPAP 215
Bipolar disorder 20, 109
Birthday 17
Black out 54
Blindness 63
Blood pressure 19
Blood testing 160
Blue-blockers 59
Boeing 7
Boelcke, Oswald 4
Bradyarrhythmia 78
Breguet mail planes 7
Buclizine 126
Bundle Branch Block (BBB) 80
Bupropion 194
Burnout 215

C

Caffeine 79, 173, 218
CAGE questions 119
Calcium 183
Carbamazepine 104
Carbon dioxide 193
Carbon monoxide 193, 197
Cardiac catheterization 81
Cardiomyopathy 78, 80
Cardiovascular evaluation 76
Carotid arteriogram 105
Cataract 60, 66
Cauda equina syndrome 172
Cerebrovascular accident (CVA) 104
Chain of custody 161
Chicken pox 177
Chiropractic 173
Chloroquine 178
Chlorpheniramine 69
Cholera 178
Cholesterol 73, 182
Chronic bronchitis 72
Chronic inflammatory bowel diseases 93
Chronic obstructive pulmonary disease (COPD) 72
Church, Ellen 210
Circadian rhythms 217
Citizenship 31
Civil Aerospace Medical Institute (CAMI) 26
Civil Aviation Medical Association (CAMA) 28
Claritin. *See* Loratidine
Clotting 84
Cocaine 154, 170
Cochran, Jacqueline 209
Cockpit humidity 173
Cockpit Resource Management. *See* Crew Resource Management
Coffee 173
Cognitive testing 140
COGSCREEN 139
Color blind 19, 60
Color deficiency 60
Color signal control 61
Color vision 197
Colorado Springs 196
Colostomy 93
Concussion 53
Conductive keratoplasty 64
Confirmation test 156, 163
Congenital heart disease 78
Contact lenses 57
Continuous flow mask 205
Control towers 6
Control zones 22
Conviction 34
Cooley's anemia. *See* Thalassemia
Coolidge, President Calvin 4
Coronary angiography 77
Coronary artery disease 75
Coronary heart disease (CHD) 20
Coumadin 80

CPAP 215
Crew Resource Management (CRM) 175
Critical Incident Stress Management (CISM) 224
Crohn's disease 93
Custody and control form (CCF) 161
Cyclizine 126

D

Dark adaptation 59
Deafness 19, 22
Deaf Pilots Association (IDPA) 189
Decompression sickness 207
Decongestant 37, 69
Deep vein thrombosis (DVT) 83, 85
Deferral 141
Degenerative disk disease 172
Dehydration 173
Deicing agent 174
Demobilization 225
Denial 23, 24, 141, 146
Dental Squadron 221
Department of Commerce 4
Depression 38, 106
Depressurization 206
Dermatitis 174
Deroche, Elise 209
Dextroamphetamine 126
Diabetes mellitus 20, 29, 55, 96
Diets 179
Dilantin 104
Diluted urine 162, 165
Diluter demand mask 205
Dimenhydrinate 126
Diphenhydramine 69, 126
Diphenoxylate 94
Diphtheria 177
Disability 148, 171
Disabled pilots 24, 149
Diuretic 88, 173
Divers Alert Network (DAN) 209
Divorce 223
Dizziness 21
Dog 182
Dominant eye 60
Doppler color blood flow 77
Dreaming 212
Driving under the influence (DUI) 131
Driving while intoxicated (DWI) 131
Drug abuse 20, 153
Drug dependence 20
Drug Free Workplace Act 154
Drug testing cutoff levels 156
Duke University Medical Center 209
Duties Not to Include Flying (DNIF) 226

E

Ear block 190
Eardrum 185, 190
Earhart, Amelia 209
Earplugs 189
Earwax 71, 185
ECG treadmill tracings 81
Echocardiogram 77, 80, 83
Economy-class syndrome 84
Effective Performance Time (EPT) 201
Electrocardiogram (ECG) 20, 76
Electroencephalogram (EEG) 52, 103
Emphysema 72
Endorphins 108
Endoscopy 92
Ephedrine 126
Epilepsy 20, 103
Equilibrium 19
Erectile dysfunction 40
Erythropoietin (EPO) 196
Esophoria 56
Estazolam 40
Ethylene glycol 174
Exercise 180, 181
Exercise stress test 76, 83, 90, 100
Exophoria 56
Explosive decompression 200
Eye surgery 63
Eyeglasses 57

F

FAA 6
Fainting 21, 51
Family doctor 11
Farnsworth lantern test (FALANT) 62

Farsightedness. *See* Hyperopia
Fatigue 215
Federal Air Surgeon 16, 22, 121, 123, 141
Fexofenadine 70
First World War 3
Flecanide 80
Flexeril 50
Flicker vertigo 129
Flight attendants 211
Flight engineer 13
Flight examiner 17
Flight path control 7
Flight Standards District Office (FSDO) 17, 62, 149
Flight surgeon 221
Fluoxetine 106
Flying Class 222
Flying Physicians Association (FPA) 28
Flying squadron 221
Food and Drug Administration (FDA) 39, 86
Form 8500-20 76, 82
Form 8500-8 28, 29, 35, 132
Frayser, Robert 192
Free Balloon Airman Certificate 13
Free balloon pilot 13

G

G Awareness Maneuvers 127
General Aviation Safety Inspector 150
German measles 177
Germany 3
Ginger root 127
Glare 58, 59
Glasses 22
  bifocal 57
  frame 57
  reading 55, 57
Glaucoma 67
  open angle 67
Glider 13
Glucometer 100
Gluteraldehyde 165
Gray out 54
Great Britain 3
Guilt 108
Guynemer 4

H

Hair testing 160
Hairpiece 31
Halcion 219
HALO 223
Handicapped 148
Hawks 56
HDL 74
Head injury 53
Headaches 21, 49, 103
  cluster 50
Headsets 189
Hearing aids 22, 190
Hearing loss 184
Heart block 80
Heart rate monitor 182
Heart transplant 20, 75
Heart valve replacement 20, 75
Height 18
Helicopter pilot 129, 192
Hemoglobin S 204
Hepatitis 178
  chronic 91
Herniated disk 172
Heroin 156
Heterophoria 56
High blood pressure. *See* Hypertension
Hilton Study 17
Histamines 69
Histotoxic hypoxia 198
HIV 140
Hives. *See* Urticaria
Holter monitor 79, 83
Hudson mask 205
Human factors 2
Humor 108
Hydraulic fluid 174
Hyperopia 54
Hyperphoria 56
Hypertension 87
Hyperventilation 199, 204
Hypoglycemia 99
Hypotension 91
Hypoxia 59, 60, 194, 198, 204
  stagnant 198

I

Ibuprofen 37
I'M SAFE 9
Imitrex 50
Immunoassay 163
Imodium. *See* Loperamide
Impairment 148
Influenza 177
Inner ear 186
Insulin 99
International Normalized Ratio (INR) 80, 83, 85
International Wheelchair Aviators 149
Intestinal disease 93
Intoxicated passengers 116
Irregular heart beat 78
Ishihara color plates 61

J

Jet A, B 174
Jet lag 217
Jet pilots 223
Jordan, Jon L. 21

K

Kaiser 4
Karvonen formula 181
Kidney disease 29, 100
Kidney stone 21, 94, 173
Kidney transplant 96
Kugel, Cole 17

L

Labyrinthitis 51
Lake Tahoe 208
Laser blindness 68
Laser thermal keratoplasty 64
LASIK 65
Law, Ruth Oliver 209
Lawrence of Arabia 123
Lazy eye 56
LDL 74
Leadville, Colorado 196
Lenses
  contact 22, 33
  corrective 22, 56, 57
Light signals 61
Lipoprotein profile 74
Lithium 40, 109
Liver cirrhosis 91
Logan, Richard 148
London Blitz 84
Loperamide 94
Loratadine 70
Lortab 50
Loss of consciousness 103
Low blood pressure. *See* Hypotension
Luke, Frank 4
Lung disease 71

M

M-Mode 82
Machado, Rod 19
Macular degeneration 63
Maintenance of wakefulness test 137
Malaria 178
Manic depression. *See* Bipolar disorder
Mannock, Edward 4
Marker beacon 188
Markham, Beryl 209
Marshall, Sheri 149
Maxillary sinus 191
Maximum Allowable Weight Table 222
Measles 177
Meclizine 126
Medical certificate
  expiration 16
  validity 16
Medical Disqualification (DQ) 226
Medical flight test 148
Medical Operations Squadron 221
Medical rejection for military service 130
Medical Review Officer (MRO) 169
Medical Support Squadron 221
Medications 42, 46
Mefloquine 178
Melanoma 138
Melatonin 219

Meniere's Syndrome 51
Mental health 223
Methamphetamine 156
Microsleep 212
Midrin 50
Migraine 49, 103
Migraine-equivalent 50
Miller, John 17
Monocular vision 63, 66, 68
Monovision contact lenses 58
Montgolfier balloons 209
Morse code 188
Motion sickness 123
Mt. Everest 195
MUGA 81
Multiple sclerosis 60
Mumps 177
Myocardial infarction 20, 75
Myopia
  empty field 54
  space 54

N

Nasal cannulas 206
Nasal polyps 191
National Driver Register (NDR) 34, 131
National Institute of Drug Abuse (NIDA) 156
National Transportation Safety Board (NTSB) 6, 8, 146, 193, 211
Navigation 8
Navigation charts 61
Nearsightedness. *See* Myopia
Needle test 4
Nephrolithiasis 94
NFL football players 173
Nichols, Ruth 209
Nicknames 31
Nicotine 172, 194
NIDA 5 156
Night flying 61, 67
Nitrox diving 208
Noise 184
Non-traffic conviction 134
Nonin FlightStat 200
Nutritional supplements 183
Nystagmus 55

O

Obesity 18, 88, 171
Occupation 32
Office of Inspector General (OIG) 131
Olestra 183
Olympic athletes 196
One-eyed pilots 63
Operational limitations 18
Ophthalmologist 62, 65
Optometrist 62
Ostomy 93
Oxymetazoline 69, 191. *See* Afrin

P

Pacemaker 20, 75, 81
Pacemaker syndrome 82
PADI Dive Manual 208
Partial Thromboplastin Time (PTT) 80, 85
Passenger airline 17
Passenger smoking 193
Passive inhalation 169
Paxil 40
Penketh, Mike 148
Peptic ulcer 92
Pericarditis 79
Peripheral neuropathy 100
Peripheral vision 199
Permanent address 31
Permanent threshold shift (PTS) 184
Personality disorder 20, 112
Pfizer Depression Self-Quiz 107
PharmChek patch 161
Phenytoin 104
Photorefractive keratoplasty 64
Physical fitness 171
Physiologic zone 195
Physiologically deficient zone 195
Pilot
  active 6
  hotline 41
Pilot-astronaut 195
Pilot-in-command 13, 24
Plague 178
Pneumococcal vaccine 177

Pneumonia 177
Pneumothorax 73
Polycarbonate 58
Polycystic ovarian syndrome 97
Polymerase chain reaction (PCR) 139
Positional Alcohol Nystagmus (PAN) 118
Post-Traumatic Stress Disorder (PTSD) 224
Practical Test Standards 150
Pre-test 26
Prednisone 39, 94
Pregnancy 211
Premature ventricular contraction (PVC) 79
Premenstrual syndrome (PMS) 173
Presbyopia 54, 64
Pressure demand mask 205
Privacy Act of 1974 36
Private pilot 14
Promethazine 126
Propranolol 41
Prothrombin time (PT) 83
Prozac 40, 106
Psychosis 20, 113
Pulling Gs 198

Q

Quimby, Harriet 209

R

Rabies 178
Radial keratotomy 64
Radionuclide angiogram 81
Radionuclide stress test 77
Raynaud's disease 85
Re-examination 16
Reactive airway disease. *See* Asthma
Receiver Autonomous Integrity Monitoring System (RAIMS) 62
Recompression chambers 209
Recreational pilot 13
Rectal examination 92
Rectal itching 174
Red Baron 4. *See* Von Richthofen, Manfred Freiherr
Red wine 74
Regional enteritis 93
Regional Flight Surgeon 22, 137, 202
Reinhart, Richard 21
Rejection for health insurance 130
Rejection for life insurance 130
Rapid eye movement (REM) 212
Report of Eye Evaluation 65, 68
Respirators 174
Rhinitis medicamentosa 69
Risk 6
Ritalin 40, 112
Rogers, Cal 189
Royal Air Force (RAF) 4
Royal Navy 225
Rubella 177
Runway lights 61

S

Saint-Exupery, Antoine de 9
Scop-dex 126
Scopolamine 125, 227
Scott Duo-Seal mask 205
Scott Executive Mark III 205
Scott Sky mask 205
Screening test 156, 163
SCUBA diving 206, 223
Second officer 13
Second-hand smoke 194
Seizure 53, 103
Selfridge, Thomas 3
Shame 108
Shell shock 224
Shingles 178
Shy bladder 162
Sickle cell anemia 198, 203
Sildenafil. *See* Viagra
Simulator sickness 123, 125
Sinus block 191
Sinus surgery 69
Skin care 174
Sleep 212
  apnea 214
  disorders 136
  hygiene 137, 218
Sleep-Eze 219
Sleeping Buddha 40

Sleeping pills 137, 219
Smith, Clyde 148, 189
Smoke 193
Smoking 73, 171, 192
  cessation 194
Snoring 213
Social Security Number (SSN) 29, 31
SODA 23, 62, 141, 147
Solo flight 13, 17
Somnoplasty 214
Space 195
Space motion sickness 123
Space-equivalent zone 195
Special issuance authorization 142
SPECT nuclear cardiology 77
Speech 19
  recognition 184
Speedboat driver 14
Spinal
  disk 172
  laminae 173
Spondylolithesis 173
Spondylolysis 173
Squamous cell carcinoma 138
SSRI 40
St. John's Wort 38, 108
Stewart, Payne 203
Strabismus 56
Stress 175
  formulas 183
Stretching 182
Stroke 104
Student pilot 14
Substance abuse 116, 225
Substance dependence 114
Suicide 8, 123
Sunglasses 58
  aviation 59
  polarized 58
  prescription 58
Super King Air 209
Suspended driver's license 132
Sweeney, Mark 131

T

Tachyarrhythmia 78
Tampered specimens 161
Tea 173
Teeth 192
Tegretol 104
Temporary threshold shift (TTS) 184
Terrorism 8
Testing Designated Position 158
Tetanus 177
Thalassemia 204
Thallium 77
Thrombin 85
Thyrotoxicosis 79
Time of Useful Consciousness (TUC) 201
Tinnitus 51, 186
Tinnitus Retraining Therapy (TRT) 186
Toothache 191
Torricelli, Evangelista 194
Tower light signals 61
Traffic conviction 131
Transient global amnesia 104
Travel compression stockings 84
Treadmill test. *See* Exercise stress test
Trial fibrillation 80
Trifocals 57
Triglycerides 74
Trimethobenzamide 126
Tuberculosis 177
Tucks 174
Typhoid 178

U

Ulcerative colitis 91, 93
Ulcers 92
Ultralight aircraft 13
United Flying Octogenarians 17
United States
  Army Signal Corps 3
  Department of Transportation 131
  Food and Drug Administration (FDA) 40
  Office of Management and Budget (OMB) 29
  Supreme Court 6
  War Department 3
Urinalysis 76
Urine sample 28
Urine testing 159

Urticaria 70
USAF Surgeon General 221
Uvula 213

V

Vaccinations 177
Valsalva maneuver 190
Varicella 177
Varicose veins 84
VASI 63
Vertigo 19, 50
Viagra 40, 60
Vibration exposure 192
Vibration white finger 192
Vigilance 7, 215
Vision
  color 60
  distant 57
  double 56
  intermediate 56
  near 56, 57
  night 59
  peripheral 57, 63
  requirements 55
  uncorrected 56
Vitamins 183
Von Richthofen, Manfred Freiherr 4

W

Western Sahara 7
White, Robert M. 195
White-coat syndrome 89
Windshield 59
Wright brothers 3
Wright Flyer 3
Wright, Orville 3

X

X-Chrom 63
Xanax 50

Y

Yoga 173, 182

Z

Zeitgebers 217
Zip code 31
Zoloft 40
Zomig 50